TABLOID MEDICINE

How the Internet Is Being Used to Hijack Medical Science for Fear and Profit

ROBERT GOLDBERG

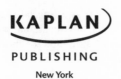

PUBLISHING

New York

© 2010 Robert Goldberg

Published by Kaplan Publishing, a division of Kaplan, Inc.
1 Liberty Plaza, 24th Floor
New York, NY 10006

Library of Congress Cataloging-in-Publication Data has been applied for.

Printed in the United States of America

10 9 8 7 6 5 4 3 2 1

ISBN-13: 978-1-60714-727-5

Kaplan Publishing books are available at special quantity discounts to use for sales promotions, employee premiums, or educational purposes. For more information or to purchase books, please call the Simon & Schuster special sales department at 866-506-1949.

CONTENTS

INTRODUCTION

I DECIDED TO WRITE THIS book because information from the Internet nearly killed my daughter. Twice.

The first time, it was material from *Worst Pills, Best Pills*, a book produced by Public Citizen, an organization that has warned America about the hidden dangers of medicines for nearly half a century. In addition to selling 2.2 million copies, generating nearly $20 million for Public Citizen, the book's dire warnings are repeated on countless websites, which is where Sara found the information.

Among the medications that *Worst Pills, Best Pills* claimed were dangerous was Abilify, the drug she had just been prescribed and which is used to treat bipolar illness and extreme panic disorders. As a result, Sara repeatedly refused to take Abilify, even though it was essential to curbing the panic she felt about eating even the slightest amount of food. Her weight and blood pressure dropping rapidly, she could have suffered heart damage or a heart attack at any time.

Meanwhile, websites and the media were attacking doctors like hers for prescribing Abilify off-label, accusing them of turning into prescribing whores for the drug companies in exchange for a few pens and some salads from Chili's for the nursing staff.

Sara's physician as well as my friend, Dr. Fred Goodwin—one of the world's leading psychopharmacologists—prevailed upon her to take the drug, and she finally agreed. Sara began to eat, and her courageous journey to recovery began.

But not without a second dangerous interruption, courtesy of another set of online experts—who actually weren't experts but only people like me, with a particular point of view, who blog about health care every day. These so-called experts began to claim that treatments for eating disorders are a perfect example of "money-driven medicine." That is, that all the girls receiving treatment were just being shaken down by insurance companies.

In turn, this belief also infected government officials and agencies seeking to slow the rising cost of health care in the United States by controlling the treatments available to patients. A federal study entitled "Management of Eating Disorders," which had been produced for the government by a for-profit consulting firm, concluded that evidence for the effectiveness of treatments for bulimia remained "weak" and that "few factors were found to be consistently related to outcomes."[1]

What neither the government technology assessment nor the Web commentary by instant experts ever mentioned was the well-known fact that the disease is still not well understood. Yet thanks to claims online and off, from private organizations and government reports, that the current treatments for eating disorders didn't work, insurance companies began to deny or limit treatments, even when their policies directly contradicted the recommendations of physicians. As a result, patients' conditions were exacerbated.

For example, insurance companies began to require a thirty-day or earlier discharge for patients admitted for eating disorders. As a consequence, Sara was discharged from the eating disorders unit the first time after she did not binge or purge in a controlled setting for a few days in a row. On two other occasions, she was discharged too early, not because she was able to get control of her illness but because her blood pressure had been stabilized.

Similarly, one of her friends at her eating disorders program had a perforated stomach from too much vomiting. Against the medical advice of her doctor, her insurance company kicked her out of the unit after a week because her heart rate was normal.

Sara made it despite the experts. But she did so because she was tough and self-possessed. If not for the medication that Public Citizen nearly scared her out of taking and that many on the Web heaped scorn on her physicians for prescribing, Sara might not have graduated magma cum laude with a degree in psychology and might not be working now with children who suffer from mental illness.

There are millions of Americans who unfortunately have not had the same happy ending. Rather, they were killed or maimed by what I call tabloid medicine.

Today we face a paradox: a society that has never been healthier or lived longer but that is more distrustful of medicines and medical technology than ever before. Are today's treatments more dangerous, or do we simply fear them more? And why are products once almost unquestionably considered safe and effective—such as vaccines, antidepressants, and painkillers—now regarded by many as unacceptably risky?

I argue that the rise of the Internet as a dominant source of information on health has been one of the key drivers behind these changes in perception. This book will describe how the Web has been used to create this new movement of tabloid medicine, driven by anecdotes and overgeneralizations, YouTube videos and flashy new websites for advocacy organizations and alternative medicine retailers. Together, they advance the belief that medical progress should be feared more than it should be trusted and that medical innovations carry hidden dangers that could strike anyone at any time.

It isn't a message entirely born of the Internet age—so long as there have been treatments for disease, there have been opponents—but the many groups and individuals that today convey this belief are able to do so with unprecedented speed, reach, and effectiveness thanks to the Web.

The purveyors of tabloid medicine do what they do for many reasons. Some seek to generate clients for lawsuits, customers for natural products, or donations for their causes and organizations. Others simply want to validate their beliefs and convert others to their point of view. As I will show, these forces share the view that the corporations producing medical advances, the scientists whom they work with, the officials who regulate them, and the physicians who prescribe today's treatments all should be viewed with skepticism.

To paraphrase risk theorist Aaron Wildavsky, whose writing on risk perception deeply influenced this book: the great struggles over the perceived dangers of medical technology and prescription drugs are essentially about trust and distrust of societal institutions—that is, cultural conflict. The Precautionary Principle reflects the cultural belief that large institutions and capitalist enterprises are corrupting influences that should demonstrate the absence of absolute harm before being allowed to market technology, whether it is nuclear power, offshore oil drilling, vaccines, or medicines to treat diabetes.

Why does this matter to the millions of Americans who look for medical information on the Web? Because we are all the targets and the potential victims of tabloid medicine, which is already shaping not only the information we receive about drugs and devices but also the treatments that are available to us, the cost of medical interventions, and the policies that govern the care we receive.

Tabloid medicine feeds us a steady diet of vivid scary stories and heartstring-tugging anecdotes, but we are seldom given the facts about the benefits or the balance between risk and benefit—facts we need to make informed and rational decisions. This is no accident; rather, it's a strategy that takes advantage of the deeply ingrained and often subconscious ways humans react to suggestions of danger in order to convince each of us that we must avoid these apparent risks at all costs, even though dangers lurk not only in what we do but also in what we do not do.

Yet the effects go far beyond individuals; after all, we ultimately decide about the adoption or risks of technology as a society. Experts in the field of behavioral economics are quick to point out how individual framing decisions about risk add up and have consequences for the community at large. Risk is a collective choice, with broad effects. Just think of how cultural or societal views about smoking or seat belts have changed laws, industry, and behavior. The framing of technological risks can therefore define what is dangerous and determine how society responds.

The Web is a spectacular tool for spreading and sharing knowledge rapidly. But it has also devalued traditional sources of expertise and allowed the rise of a class of "instant experts," who range from the dangerously uninformed to the credentialed and opportunistic. We want our information to be fast, hassle-free, and on our own terms, but because online information is unfiltered, anyone can post information about the risks of medicines (accurate or not), absent discussion of benefits. And they do. By carefully placing and repeating a handful of scary stories and articles, taken out of context, tabloid medicine has been able to influence most of the so-called facts about treatments we come across each day.

The conspiracy narrative of tabloid medicine has found its expression in manufactured controversies that consist of several elements: the emergence of an "instant expert" who bucks the establishment to courageously reveal evidence of serious danger that was previously hidden; the rapid spread and repetition of these findings on the Web; and the (mostly uncritical) validation of this new risk by the media and politicians. Finally, opposing or critical views are delegitimized and ignored, often through claims that the experts propounding these views cannot be trusted because they have consulted for or worked with pharmaceutical and device firms.

Thus, the Internet is used to deliberately manipulate the framing of risk. Tabloid medicine is not information; it is a deliberate instrument of control designed not only to shape our decisions but also to bring about changes in policies, laws, and corporate behavior. It seeks to paint medical technologies as having little benefit and many risks—none of them worth taking—and demands that we remake our institutions and our society to curb or block their use. As I will show, the individuals and groups who use tabloid medicine do so (if sometimes with the best of intentions) without regard for the public health consequences of their actions.

Today, tabloid medicine stands dominant, but it can be fought. Its proponents assume that because corporations and other institutions can't be trusted, hidden dangers will always emerge when we least expect them, but maintaining that precautionary perspective and state of fear depends on making people feel that risks are always unpredictable. This requires credulous Internet users. Skeptical, careful consumers of health care information attuned to the telltale signs of tabloid medicine are not such easy marks. Thus, Americans must learn how to be savvier Web users and recognize the ways information can be manipulated and misrepresented by those with ideologies and interests.

The Internet is being used to rapidly accumulate and share information that matches our genes, medical conditions, and lifestyles to treatments, clinical trials, and health outcomes. That information can be used to reduce uncertainty and individualize treatment based on our likely response or risk as individuals. In particular, the use of genetic biomarkers—measures of our risk of disease and our response to treatment—will lead to medical care that increases benefits and reduces adverse events.

I'm not without my own cultural biases that shape my views about the benefits and dangers of medical developments—but I have never hidden them. I don't fear technology. I know that it has saved the lives of millions of people around the world—including my daughter—and I believe that personalized medicine holds the promise of better health and fewer risks.

Nor do I believe that the social and economic institutions producing medical treatments are seeking to exploit individuals or the planet. Rather, I agree with the science writer Matt Ridley who writes,

"The world will pull out of the current crisis because of the way that markets in goods, services and ideas allow human beings to exchange and specialize honestly for the betterment of all."[2] Over the years, the organizations I have been associated with have received unrestricted grants from pharmaceutical firms to support their operations and research activities, and critics have sought to invalidate my views as a result. That is just a way to stifle debate.

Ultimately, I believe that if we organize medicine around the goal of anticipating and avoiding every risk, the result will be the production of fewer new treatments. If we eliminate the perspective of anyone who receives support from companies, we will lose the guidance of thousands of insightful clinicians and researchers. If the only people who conduct research and prescribe medicines are those approved by the tabloid medicine crowd, we will have fewer choices and less freedom.

Tabloid medicine's supporters claim we don't need many of the new treatments and that we should all be happy with the choices they give us. This book will not only show why they are wrong but will also demonstrate the damage tabloid medicine has already done, the role the Internet has played—and will continue to play—in promoting and disseminating its message, and the steps we can take to combat tabloid medicine and prevent a future devoid of innovation and rife with restrictions.

CHAPTER 1

Prospect Theory: The Risks We Choose to Live with and Why

I N 1979, IN A famous experiment, two Israeli-born psychology profes-
sors, Daniel Kahneman at Stanford University and Amos Tversky at
the University of British Columbia, conducted a survey that helped
revolutionize economic theory and thinking about risk taking. The
two scholars, who went on to win a Nobel Prize in economics, asked
their students to imagine that the United States was preparing for the
outbreak of an unusual Asian disease, which was anticipated to kill six
hundred people. They then asked the students to choose between two
programs to combat the disease: Program A, which would save two
hundred people, or Program B, where there was a one-third probability
that six hundred people would be saved but a two-thirds probability
that no people would be saved. The vast majority of students (72 percent) chose Program A.

Kahneman and Tversky then posed the same question differently. If Program C were adopted, four hundred people would die.
If Program D were adopted, there was a one-third probability that
nobody would die but a two-thirds probability that six hundred

people would die. When asked the question this way, students supported Program D by 78 percent. You might have noticed what the students apparently did not: Programs A and C are the same. So are Programs B and D.

By wording the choices differently, Kahneman and Tversky framed the same information to influence how people made a decision, and they specifically manipulated the way the question was asked to dramatize the difference between a sure gain and the possibility of a loss. From that angle, Program A was a clear winner. But when it was reframed as a sure loss in the form of Program C, Program D won hands down, because it offered the potential that no one would die. The deliberate manipulation of the question was designed to show not only how framing changes perception, but also, even more importantly, that the change is accompanied by a move from risk aversion in order to hold on to gains to risk taking to avoid loss. Prospect theory, as it is known, demonstrates that we tend to value a gain that is certain over one that is less than certain, even when the expected value of the uncertain gain is higher.

The opposite is even truer for losses: we will go to great lengths to prevent a certain loss, even if it means taking even *greater* risks. We will avoid changes that might make things worse or require us to give up something we already have and value. A concept known as the endowment effect suggests that we value something more highly when we already possess it than if we are trying to obtain it. Think of how we value our homes when we put them up for sale compared to how we price them when we are looking to buy. Similarly, my son Zach and I bought some comic books that are now worth several thousand dollars. He looks at them only once in a while, but he would never sell one or buy another comic book at their current value. We all have a bias toward the status quo and will actually incur risk to avoid losing what we have. The flip side is that, if a choice is framed in a certain way, we are unwilling to take the risk inherent in trying to gain something new.

This is clear when it comes to how people often decide whether to start taking a drug or finish the prescribed doses. Studies have shown that when people are told only about the risks of the drug or are given this information first, they are less likely to take the medication—and therefore less likely to effectively treat the disease. Similarly, when patients were presented with information about a medicine first in terms of the likely individual benefit relative to the risk incurred and then, later, in terms of the likely benefit to the population as a whole, without a description of the individual risk. They were five times more likely to chose the medicine in the second condition when no likely side effects (and thus no risks) were described than when an individual risk-benefit analysis was given.

When it comes to our health, it is clear that changes perceived as likely to make the situation worse (risks from treatments) loom larger than likely improvements. Thus, framing can be used both to push people to avoid a certain drug or treatment and to persuade them to embrace a particular remedy—in the first case by making something seem less certain and therefore posing a potential risk to be avoided, and in the second by making a benefit seem more probable. Kahneman and Tversky call this perception pseudocertainty.

In one experiment, prospect theory researchers told a group of college students about a disease that would affect 10 to 20 percent of Americans and asked the students if they would get a vaccine that protected half the people who took it. The students were then told there were two distinct strains of the virus that would each affect 10 percent of Americans and that the vaccine offered complete protection against one strain and no protection against the other. When given the second scenario, nearly 60 percent of the students said they would be vaccinated, compared with 40 percent when given the first scenario. The students valued full protection against a single identified virus more than probabilistic, or likely, protection against the disease itself, even though (as in the first experiment discussed) the level of protection was exactly the same.[1] The study showed that the way the vaccine was described and framed determined whether people accepted or avoided it and that most people will choose the option framed as a sure gain, but will risk more (even their health) if the benefit seems uncertain.

HOW DO WE CHOOSE RISKS?

As our discussion suggests, and as we can gather from our daily lives, framing transforms complex decisions and information about risks into simple choices between gains and losses. This process is guided by values and is highly intuitive. More precisely, as psychologists Valerie Reyna and Charles Brainerd have demonstrated in nearly twenty years of research, our choices reflect what we understand, not the information we are given. Reyna and Brainerd call their explanation of how we make decisions about medical risks and benefits "fuzzy trace theory":

> Judgment and decision making [rely] ... preferentially on *gist* representations of information (e.g., about risk), as opposed to verbatim representations. *Gist* and *verbatim* are defined much as they are in everyday parlance, except that *verbatim* applies to more than verbal information but also to graphs, numbers, pictures, and any other form of information. Thus, a gist representation is vague and qualitative; it captures the bottom-line *meaning* of information, and it is a subjective interpretation of information based on emotion, education, culture, experience, worldview, and level of development. A verbatim representation, in contrast, is precise and quantitative, and it captures the exact *surface form* of information (i.e., it is literal).[2]

The gist people understand is shaped by many factors. Evaluation and framing of degrees of risk or different risks are determined by experience, previous knowledge, culture, etc. In all cases, to the extent that such information appeals to what Reyna calls *gist-based intuition*, it will be used to help frame our decisions in terms of holding on to a sure thing or gambling to avoid an even greater loss.

Reyna provides the following example about how information is filtered through gist-based intuition to frame risk. She gives the scenario of a forty-nine-year-old woman curious about the chances she will develop breast cancer. She consults the Breast Cancer Risk Estimation Tool on the website of the National Cancer Institute. The questionnaire tells her that the likelihood she will get invasive breast cancer at some point in her life is approximately 22.2 percent. This 22.2 percent represents the verbatim risk. But is this high or low risk? And how worried should she be? Reyna explains that while the figure is lower than 50 percent, which is the general threshold for considering events likely, it is also nearly twice the chance that the average woman will be diagnosed with invasive breast cancer (11.3 percent), which is available from the same tool. This is the gist, the meaning of the quantitative result to the individual concerned, and it can be impacted by myriad considerations, ranging from culture, to experience, to how well the woman understands statistics to her family history.[3]

Kahneman and Tversky found that the degree of risk avoidance is cumulative over time based on experience and context. We use experience to create a benchmark for judging whether to take an action to gain something or to avoid risk. Kahneman and Tversky call this benchmark a reference point. This reference point is more important to our decisions than the actual potential outcome. For instance, one study undertaken by Angela Fagerlin, an associate professor of medicine at the University of Michigan Health System, found that asking women to estimate the average risk of breast cancer influenced their subsequent perceptions of the likelihood they would develop the disease. Fagerlin found that when the women were asked to guess the lifetime risk of breast cancer at the outset of the study their answers were much too high, averaging 46 percent. Then they were told that the real answer was 13 percent. Finally, the subjects were instructed to estimate what they thought their own risk of breast cancer was. The women who had been asked for estimates of the average risk rated their individual risk lower than women in another group who had not been asked to guess the average risk and who were more scared about their chances of getting breast cancer.[4]

Yet providing people with objective information on the risks and benefits of treatment does not translate into increased use of a medication or procedure. Fagerlin recently completed a study to determine why women with a high risk of hormone-positive breast cancer do not take the drug Tamoxifen, even though it reduces the risk of getting the disease by one-third. The study targeted women who were at high risk of developing breast cancer within the next five years, a total of 632 women with an average 2.56 percent five-year risk, and the researchers gave each one a decision aid with objective information about Tamoxifen that was tailored to each woman's health history. After reviewing the decision aid, 29 percent of women said they would seek more information from their own physician, and 6 percent said they would agree to take Tamoxifen.

But three months later, Fagerlin's research team found that less than 1 percent of participants had started taking Tamoxifen, and fewer than 6 percent had either talked to their doctors or sought more information. The researchers explained, "Participants were concerned about the risks of Tamoxifen, and many believed that the benefits of Tamoxifen did not outweigh the risks." Yet the women had been given information showing the benefits of prevention. In addition, they had also been given data on the risks of side effects, the average odds of getting cancer, and other relevant topics.[5] However, if we think of the decisions in terms of framing, we see that the numbers were used to make comparisons between a small certainty (a reduced risk of breast cancer) and uncertainty (benefit to some but not others and generalized risks). Thus, Fagerlin's study illustrates Reyna's observation that the "gist of risk is relative, that is, like any semantic interpretation, meaning that it depends on the context."[6]

WHY WE OVERREACT TO RARE DANGERS AND UNDERREACT TO COMMON ONES

Over time, as we choose risks and establish reference points, most of us tend to overweigh or overestimate the occurrence of rare events and underweigh the risks associated with everyday activities. Security expert Scott Plous explains in his book *The Psychology of Judgment and Decision Making* that, "[i]n very general terms: (1) The more *available* an event is, the more frequent or probable it will seem; (2) the more *vivid* a piece of information is, the more easily recalled and convincing it will be; and (3) the more *salient* something is, the more likely it will be to appear causal."[7] Images that engage our emotions and our imaginations are more likely to stick in our minds and become part of the shortcuts, rules of thumb, and stereotypes we use when we judge the risk of an event or situation.

The more often we hear about a new peril—and in the more places—the more dire and immediate it feels and the more we think that it really poses a threat to us personally. This plays into what is called the availability heuristic. The easier it is for us to conjure up examples of something, the more common and likely it seems as a result. Says Dr. Craig Fox, a colleague of Kahneman's and co-director of the UCLA Interdisciplinary Research Group in Behavioral Decision Making, "Typically, people assess the likelihood of an extreme event by the ease with which they can recall instances of that event."[8] The Internet has only amplified this effect by making claims of nascent risks nearly ubiquitous, present not only on news sites but also on blogs, website sidebars, Twitter, Facebook, and email. Further, it has provided a soapbox for people to trumpet a wide variety of supposed risks, leading Internet users to feel constantly beset by danger. The Internet also does not differentiate between legitimate and illegitimate, scientifically supported and not, minor and major.

Our mental methods for gauging and acting on danger, and their tendency to fail us when it comes to making accurate analyses, are deeply hardwired. International security expert Bruce Schneier explains:

> Assessing and reacting to risk is one of the most important things a living creature has to deal with, and there's a very primitive part of the brain that has that job. It's the amygdala, and it sits right above the brainstem, in what's called the medial temporal lobe. The amygdala is responsible for processing base emotions that come from sensory inputs, like anger, avoidance, defensiveness and fear. It's an old part of the brain, and seems to have originated in early fishes.

He notes, "Humans have a completely different pathway to cope with *analyzing risk*. It's the neocortex, a more advanced part of the brain that developed very recently, evolutionarily speaking, and only appears in mammals. It's intelligent and analytic. It can reason. It can make more nuanced trade-offs. It's also much slower."

Much like the difference between the gist and verbatim approaches to dealing with uncertainty, humans have two systems for framing risk: a primitive intuitive system and a more advanced analytic system. The two are supposed to work as a team, but more often than not, our amygdala runs the show and the neocortex is the understudy. Here lies the biological explanation for our instinct to process the most vivid potential risk—no matter how rare—as the most serious threat. In the modern world, this often makes us fearful without doing much to keep us safe.

In his book *Mind Wide Open*, journalist Steven Johnson describes how once, during a storm, the glass in a large window in his apartment was hurled inward by strong winds. He was standing near the window and came within inches of being killed. Just before the window came hurtling out of its frame, Johnson heard the wind whistling. Now, despite knowing that the new window is safe, "when the wind kicks up, and I hear that whistling sound, I can feel my adrenaline levels rise ...

Part of my brain—the part that feels most me-like, the part that has opinions about the world and decides how to act on those opinions in a rational way—knows that the windows are safe ... But another part of my brain wants to barricade myself in the bathroom all over again.[9]

The amygdala is designed to process and respond to risks quickly. But that speed is not always paired with efficiency or accuracy. Steven Johnson's reaction to the whistling of the wind causes him to fear death whether or not it is a real risk, and it takes very little effort emotionally to react to an immediate image of risk no matter how illusory. The cognitive process required to analyze and evaluate actual risk and plan for it is another matter. Daniel Gilbert, the author of *Stumbling on Happiness*, puts it this way:

> The brain is a beautifully engineered get-out-of-the-way machine that constantly scans the environment for things out of whose way it should right now get. That's what brains did for several hundred million years—and then, just a few million years ago, the mammalian brain learned a new trick: to predict the timing and location of dangers before they actually happened.
>
> Our ability to duck that which is not yet coming is one of the brain's most stunning innovations, and we wouldn't have dental floss or 401(k) plans without it. But this innovation is in the early stages of development. The application that allows us to respond to visible baseballs is ancient and reliable, but the add-on utility that allows us to respond to threats that loom in an unseen future is still in beta testing.[10]

It is the "unseen future" that contributes greatly to uncertainty and disturbs our status quo. When an event disrupts our reference point, it essentially wipes out the narrative, or prior understanding, that made life certain. The norms, shortcuts, and rules of thumb become useless when the unforeseen danger lands on our doorstep. Our lack of knowledge of what the event means or what the future will bring is a risk unto itself because our sense of control has been stripped from us. Indeed, as Kahneman observed, "What actually happens with fear is that probability doesn't matter very much. That is, once I have raised the possibility that something terrible can happen to your child, even though the possibility is remote, you may find it very difficult to think of anything else. People do not fear the unknown *per se*; they fear what they *know* they do not know."[11]

How we perceive risks is partially determined by whether they are under our control. People underestimate dangers they believe they have control over and overestimate those they feel helpless against. That's why people are more afraid of SARS than cardiovascular disease, of being killed by strangers than by someone they know, of terrorist attacks than accidents at home, even though the latter risks are all larger. Indeed, many activities we choose to undertake without a second thought, from riding a bicycle to doing household repairs, are much more dangerous than those we worry about. All of the following have an equal mortality risk: "[f]lying 1,000 miles by jet; [t]raveling 10 miles per bicycle ... [h]aving one chest X-ray taken in a good hospital; [s]moking 1.4 cigarettes," yet how we view these risks varies considerably.[12]

Dr. Craig Fox has pointed out that people try to buffer fear of many extreme events with the illusion of control. Our response is often one of an overresponse, which can consist of focusing time and attention on rare events to the exclusion of more common risks or seeking to control the superficial reasons for a rare event. In trying to control the future, we ignore other, more fundamental problems. As Fox notes, driving a car is more dangerous than flying, and yet we continue to fear plane crashes far more than car accidents because we have more control over the car than over the plane. (Another contributor is that the majority of Americans believe that they are above-average drivers, so they overestimate their ability to avoid danger.)[13]

In fact, Michael L. Rothschild, a professor at the University of Wisconsin, argued that if a plane were seized and crashed each week by terrorists, then someone who flies once a month would have a 1 in 135,000 chance of being aboard one of those planes in the course of a year. In contrast, the chances of being killed in a year by an auto accident are 1 in 7,000.[14] Consider that, after 9/11, Americans suddenly began to drive more and fly less, and as a result, according to German scientist Gerd Gigerenzer, an additional 1,595 died in car crashes.[15] People may also take certain risks as a way of asserting control. Since there is seldom an option that carries no danger, people may choose the one that makes them feel autonomous or that reinforces their desired image of themselves in order to counter their feelings of uncertainty or powerlessness, even if their choice is riskier than other available options.

This helps explain why some patients turn to alternative medicine or other unproven therapies. Alternative practitioners can often provide attention that is lacking from busy physicians and give patients the sense of empowerment and agency that they crave. This provides a way to escape the sense of helplessness that may come from the diagnosis of a serious illness and makes patients believe they can do something to make themselves healthy again. A recent study shows that we are more likely to choose alternative medicine over Western medicine when we are uncertain about the cause of an illness because alternative medicine better tolerates uncertainty. We believe that an alternative can or might provide an underlying cure (versus symptom alleviation by Western medicine) without any of the risks.[16] Likewise, believers in toxins in the environment or conspiracies to conceal dangerous health risks find a sense of control and power as activists and have a ready scapegoat for the bad things that befall them or others.

Furthermore, new or unfamiliar risks receive more emphasis both online and in the media (and therefore in many patients' minds) than ones we have already experienced or we constantly live with. This can create in people a tendency to overreact to immediate, sudden risks and pay less attention to long-term or gradually developing ones. A recent example is the outbreak of H1N1, or swine flu, in April 2009. Quickly, news coverage of new cases consumed television networks, websites popped up to track the disease's spread, face masks began to sell out in stores, and schools began to be closed. Each death from swine flu was given extensive coverage, at least in the early stages of the outbreak.

But deaths from seasonal flu, which every year far, far outnumber deaths from swine flu, seldom receive any notice in the news at all. In fact, regular influenza kills around thirty-six thousand Americans every year.[17] Even the panic surrounding swine flu died down by the time scattered cases began popping up again in the fall of 2009, just a few months after the initial outbreak of the virus. As people got used to swine flu, their fears began to abate. To observers, it was a familiar picture. This phenomenon had occurred just a few years before, over avian flu—which killed exactly no one in the United States—over SARS a few years before that, and over many supposed crises before that.

While we panic over SARS, or over the presence of the chemical BPA in water bottles, or over whatever today's terrifying threat is, we are ignoring the everyday causes of diseases that actually kill millions, ranging from heart disease to diabetes. Indeed, the small activities of our daily lives—driving to work, taking a walk, sitting in front of the television—are all more likely to kill us than the foreign disease du jour or the phthalates in our vinyl flooring.

NEW AND OUT OF CONTROL: MAKING THE FUTURE UNCERTAIN

The effect of novelty or exoticism is especially pronounced when new dangers are also highly publicized and this constitutes a second determinant of what we fear and how much we fear it. These days the media is quick to seize on every new danger, natural disaster, Amber Alert, or impending outbreak, to fill the twenty-four-hour news cycle and attract viewers. Whether it is the day, now long past, when big cities each had several newspapers running three daily editions or our current Internet-driven age, news is often not good news. Not only are there claims of new health risks and hidden dangers all around us, but such stories now spread far beyond conventional media outlets in a flash, multiplying on blogs and personal websites, through social media tools such as Twitter and Facebook, and via email. Every time they are repeated, these stories gain in apparent authority until they are popularly held to be the truth.

In the case of medical myths, researchers and scientific authorities struggle to contain their spread and convince the public the risk isn't real or is much smaller than portrayed. Just one example is an email hoax about the spread of H1N1 circulated in the summer of 2009, which caused the Centers for Disease Control and Prevention to issue repeated denials:

Subject: Fw: Latest on H1N1 Straight from the CDC and Johns Hopkins

I'm not a bearer of "fear," but think we all should pay attention to THIS one ... Evelyn.

Wise council [sic] from Julie, who also sells Enzacta, and she agrees, HFI and PXP from Enzacta will keep your immune system strong and help fight off H1N1 ... these are more practical steps we can take ... Kevin.

From Julie: I have an ex-husband who is a research physician at an Ivy League University. I decided to contact him to get the real and full scoop on H1N1. Since he does government research, he was able to access everything we want to know about H1N1, and he also contacted top docs in infectious disease at Johns Hopkins. Here is the dirt:

The CDC says H1N1 is currently wiping out entire villages in Asia. They expect it to hit the U.S. in Jan/Feb where it will kill six out of ten people. It HAS mutated. (Throw out the conspiracy theory.) They will attempt a program of mandatory vaccinations but probably will not have enough time to enforce it. I will not be vaccinated. The last time they did mandatory vaccinations at least one person died and many others developed Guillain-Barré syndrome, which is a devastating illness.[18]

Websites, emails, or videos describing the dangers of medical technologies are in many ways an offshoot of urban legends: stories told through word of mouth that have a grain of truth so that we think they might be worth believing. (Think of the $250 cookie recipe or the "free Microsoft computer" emails. In my time, it was the fried rat in the bucket of Kentucky Fried Chicken.) But there is meaning in the method by which such stories are constructed and spread. Mikel J. Koven, a folklorist at the University of Wales, observed, "By looking at what's implied in a story, we get an insight into the fears of a group in society," and these tales "need to make cultural sense." The status of these stories as a reflection of our environment also explains why some of them persist for years, popping up again and again in different forms, while others are short-lived. Koven points out that "it's a lack of information coupled with these fears that tends to give rise to new legends. When demand exceeds supply, people will fill in the gaps with their own information ... they'll just make it up."[19]

What's more, the vivid, immediate nature of medical urban legends tends to make them stick more than factual discussion or debunking. As urban legend expert Jan Harold Brunvand says, "The Internet has increased the speed at which some of these stories are circulated. Just like 'that' they are all over. They are transmitted very quickly. I think the media plays a big role ... Even if the context of a newspaper article is to debunk the story, *some people tend to remember the story rather than the discussion of it* [emphasis mine]."[20]

With the growing immediacy of what is broadcast, published, and uploaded, the coverage of new risks is almost never in proportion to the danger those risks actually pose. Broad strokes, bold headlines, and instant analysis that follows a simple narrative (with a bit of hyperbole and alarmism thrown in) are much better at drawing audiences and selling publications than sober, conservative analysis. Web pages and news programs alike often present the likelihood of the danger in a way specially designed to make readers and watchers worry (if they include such information at all) and ignore research that finds no risk.

Moreover, journalists for traditional media outlets are increasingly relying upon the Web as a source for stories and information. This compounds the failings of both news coverage and online information and creates a vicious circle in which journalists draw from the Internet and their stories in turn end up back on the Internet, reinforcing misinformation and impeding coverage of other points of view. A recent study of 166 professional journalists found that while 67 percent of them use websites for work purposes, only 22 percent said they verify Web information with another source before using it. Further, 36 percent of reporters said they conduct interviews via email, and 68 percent said they use email press releases for story ideas.[21] The reliance on the Web, with its wealth of events that are immediate, vivid, and usually rare, shifts the perception of more traditional media outlets, as it does that of individuals. The rare event becomes more salient and the circumstances or information surrounding it are used to fill out a narrative that does little to allow people to determine the real nature of the risk or its source.

Years ago the syndicated columnist Art Buchwald observed that "television has a real problem. They have no page two. Consequently every big story gets the same play and comes across to the viewer as a really big, scary one." The Internet has only amplified this effect. Not only is it akin to a giant page one, where every story is out of proportion and scary, but the fact that the media is increasingly relying on material it obtains from Web-based sources to fill pages and television segments leads to extended and inflated coverage that goes far beyond page two. Online information is now everywhere: in our morning paper, on daytime talk shows and the evening news, in our email, on Twitter, and on the blogs we read. But there is little confirmation of its accuracy and lots of overstatement and scaremongering.

The Web is the ultimate platform for trumpeting a wide variety of alleged risks, cataclysms, and conspiracies. Dr. Tammy Boyce, deputy director of the Risk, Science and Health Group at the Cardiff School of Journalism's Media and Cultural Studies Unit, looked at the effects of journalists using the Web as a source for their coverage of the allegation (and the research supposedly supporting it) that there was a link between the measles vaccine and increased risk of autism. What she found was a case study of how uncertainty about the future had not only framed risks about medical technologies, but had also been used to promote an agenda of fear.

Boyce looked at news stories, both on television and in print, during seven months in 2002 and spoke with both the writers who produced these articles and their sources. She found that the media overwhelmingly had come down on the side of those against the vaccine and distorted the information it gathered to fit the predetermined conclusion that immunization was unsafe or, at least, that its safety was in doubt. The result was a fundamental disconnect between the science and the message being disseminated to society:

> In reality, there was very limited evidence to show that MMR [measles, mumps, and rubella vaccine] was unsafe. Almost all scientists agreed that MMR was safe. But still the media tried to create a balance between pro-MMR and anti-MMR. Journalists deliberately selected sources that made for easier story making and quoted comments made not by scientists and health professionals but by politicians, parents and pressure groups. This media attitude led their reports to become *political stories* [my emphasis] which were not necessarily fact-based, and gave the misleading impression to the public of an equivalence of evidence.[22]

Boyce also emphasized that rather than speak with physicians, the journalists whose work she surveyed turned to the Internet. She believes that when it comes to medical questions, nonspecialists try to sensationalize the issue, rather than getting involved in the scientific nuances and statistical details. This is exactly what makes a lot of media coverage of health issues so damaging; it fails to inform readers because it shies away from the difficult task of understanding and analyzing the science in favor of presenting a conventional narrative of conspiracy and risk. The impact of sensational media coverage associating MMR with autism was huge, as Dr. Boyce points out.[23] The vaccination rate in the United Kingdom dropped thanks to these stories, and the incidence of the diseases it was designed to prevent, especially measles, shot up.

On the Internet, anything goes and the truth is less important than getting the biggest audience. Organizations and individuals use histrionic rhetoric about supposed dangers to promote their agendas, without any check on their claims, and can drown out contrary information since search results are ranked by hits, not accuracy. There is good information and valuable analysis buried beneath the morass of personal opinion, prejudice, and half-truths, but finding them requires patience and skill. When it comes to health information, the task is especially difficult because differentiating fact from fiction requires a level of scientific and medical literacy and knowledge that few Internet users possess. That's why self-interested groups often successfully fool readers, even those who start out unconvinced, with lists of studies that supposedly support their contentions but that actually have nothing to do with the topic or do not in fact show what the site is claiming.

When it comes to understanding statistics or science or the realities of research, journalists are seldom more knowledgeable than the rest of the population, so they, too, get caught in the web of the Internet, even when they begin with the intention of bringing the readers the facts. But if we want to end up with accurate information, journalists—indeed all of us—have an obligation to verify the "facts" we find on the Web. That's more work than most of us are willing to do; we want immediate answers, the truth in two pages of hits. And that is why Internet users, whatever their profession, whatever their goal, are all too often easy prey for those who have learned to use the Web to advance their agenda and attack their opponents.

I KNOW SOMEONE THAT HAPPENED TO . . .

One of the most effective tactics of fearmongers, Internet charlatans, and nightly news shows alike has been the use of anecdotes. Not only are these stories vivid, but they also put a face on today's danger, one with which we can identify. Research has repeatedly shown that we see risks as more likely if they are personified than if they are anonymous, because this makes the risk more immediate and, in our minds, more real. If a family member is hurt by a product with an otherwise excellent safety record, suddenly we want to spread the word that that product is dangerous. If a colleague develops an unusual side effect from a drug, we become reluctant to take it or to allow others we know to do so.

Yet there are a thousand diseases, equally rare and equally serious; a thousand cases of products that may, on a few occasions, cause harm; a thousand drugs that have worrying complications in a very small percentage of patients. Yet we never think about them because we don't have a person to associate them with. Risks don't become real or salient to us until we can put a face on them. Once a risk becomes personalized, our frame around it has shifted. No longer is it abstract. Now it is something that happened to "John at work" or "my friend Sue" or "my neighbor's mother." We worry about the dangers even if the chances of their happening to us are extremely small or if the risk of our not taking the medication or using the product is higher.

The media, and subsequently the Internet, plays an important role in allowing us to stay connected in real time, and seemingly in person, with events as they happen. My son Zach was in the Israeli Defense Forces during Operation Cast Lead, a campaign to eliminate rocket attacks from Gaza. I was able to keep myself informed round the clock through Facebook, blogs, YouTube postings of the military operation, and Internet radio feeds from Israel. These didn't make me any less (or more) apprehensive about his safety, but, as for thousands of other parents, these sources allowed me to share the experience with others and have some sense of control over the events. Firsthand experiences and accounts, real-life examples (including those used in this book!), or statements from experts provide more convincing evidence of a position than dry statistics. This is also the case for claims made about the risks and benefits of medical treatments.

The Internet has also extended the ability of the media to take personalization of risk far beyond the circle of people we encounter in our daily lives. Suddenly we "know" the people we meet online or see on television, whether on news programs, talk shows, medical programs, or even on sitcoms and soap operas. There's a reason why news stories, whether they appear in print or pixels or on television, love to fill medical segments with the stories and faces of the victims. We often do not register that the medical facts have been twisted to fit an exciting narrative or that only the oddest and most exciting cases are being used, even if a case is one in a million or the chances that the scenario will occur in real life are vanishingly small. (Indeed, it is precisely because these situations are made especially dramatic that we are more likely to remember and therefore worry about them.) Now add in blogs chronicling the lives of people with various diseases or advocating medical causes and websites and forums that cater to people who have a specific condition or have someone close to them who does, filled with photos and emotional accounts. Web users landing on these sites suddenly worry about risks that were never previously on their radar or dramatically revise their estimation of whether such risks are worth being concerned about.

It is easy to see how "instant experts" on medicine can rapidly multiply. The many information sources constantly at our fingertips put a face to experts of all sorts, be they doctors interviewed for an article, or guests on talk shows such as *Oprah*, or authors of Internet articles who may or may not be what they claim. Because people feel they "know" them, they trust them more than they should. Even those who are legitimately credentialed may mold their stories to fit the demands of the media, which favors catchy sound bites and dramatic narrative. They give no time for scientific detail or nuance (or, often, competing opinion) and may have agendas of their own lurking off-screen, unacknowledged. More dangerous yet are the so-called experts who do not have a scientific or medical background but whose words are nonetheless taken as gospel.

Two egregious examples are Jenny McCarthy, who along with her former boyfriend, actor Jim Carrey, was regarded as an "expert" on immunizations because of her leading role in the anti-vaccine movement, and Suzanne Somers, who masquerades as an authority on both cancer cures and hormone replacement therapy. To a considerable extent, their legitimacy is the result of their previous celebrity and the willingness of major talk show hosts, such as Oprah Winfrey, to allow guests lacking medical credentials to use their shows as an infomercial for various brands of quackery and anti-science and anti-medical rhetoric. Other instant experts, reveling in their very ordinariness, may nonetheless be considered authorities on the Internet, selling a poignant personal story that convinces readers they're for real. The objective risk of the dangers being trumpeted by instant experts may be minimal and the scientific support for the alternative they are peddling even smaller, but those in the audience, on the couch at home, and in front of the computer feel they know the risk is real because someone with a face and a name has told them so.

The online world has taken our problem of sifting truth from fiction and expanded it a thousandfold, giving new exposure to stories of people with just about any illness or injury and victims of any possible (or impossible) complication. Some of these stories are true, some are not, but there is no way to tell one from another. Often, the tellers, consciously or not, frame an issue in a personalized way so that it will stick in people's minds and help convince them. The common refrain is that they are an "every person" who has been hurt or wronged, with the not-so-hidden message being: it happened to me, so it could happen to you. And because faces or names are put to these risks, our estimation of how common and serious those risks are rises. This misinformation is not always malicious. For every person who is deliberately deceptive, there are many others who are simply misguided. Still, it is misinformation and made no less dangerous by good intentions.

IS NATURE REALLY BENIGN?

The flip side of fears about the safety of drugs and conventional treatments is often a faith in alternative medicine, however unproven or scientifically implausible. The emphasis on herbs, New Age treatments, and homeopathy as safe alternatives for treating serious illnesses because they are "natural" is based not in science but in a conscious effort to frame medical technology and its commercialization as a source of hidden dangers.

The natural-versus-artificial frame is one that instinctively resonates with many people. Yet nature is not inherently benign. In many ways, our lives are much safer now than when we lived in a "natural" world. Life expectancy and well-being are both much greater as a result of technological advances. No longer are we beset by an endless array of potentially fatal illnesses, from smallpox to polio to tuberculosis, and many conditions that were once fatal, including diabetes, heart disease, and even many kinds of cancer, are now survivable chronic conditions. Injuries that killed our forbears are now treatable. Advanced sanitation saves us from cholera and other diseases transmitted from dirty water, heating keeps us from freezing in the winter, and modern cooking and cooling appliances make our food safe and longer lasting.

Furthermore, the natural can be just as dangerous as the man-made. Think of all the poisons that are derived from plants (e.g., oleander, nightshade). Many other supposed natural treatments have little or no actual effect, a risk that might be small when it comes to treating the common cold but that looms large if you are trying to treat cancer. In cases where the alternative preparation is actually pharmaceutically active, it is no different and no less risky than a conventional drug. Natural substances also have dangers when combined, just as artificial ones do, so alternative treatments may interact badly when taken at the same time as conventional medication or other alternative treatments. St. John's Wort reduces the efficacy of many drugs, including anti-virals, some antihistamines, calcium channel blockers, antidepressants, and some lipid-lowering medications. Feverfew increases the risk of bleeding, especially if taken along with anticoagulants such as warfarin or aspirin, and may react badly with non-steroidal anti-inflammatories (NSAIDs). Ginseng inhibits anti-psychotics, MAOI inhibitors, steroidal hormones, drugs for hypoglycemia, and many more. The list of these interactions is long, and due to lack of testing, the potential of many alternative preparations to react with one another or with conventional medications is unknown.[24]

Further, investigations of many alternative remedies have found that they are not always as advertised. They may contain little or none of the supposed active ingredient or have additional undisclosed components. Alternative remedies may also be contaminated with toxic metals, such as lead and mercury. But perhaps most important, there is little scientific data to back their use for whatever condition (or, often, for a wide range of conditions) they are purported to treat. Rather, their efficacy claims are founded on anecdotal evidence and poorly designed and biased small studies. For instance, advocates of bio-identical hormones promote them as safer than synthetically produced hormones for treating conditions associated with menopause. Yet there is scant scientific evidence to support these claims. On the contrary, such products have never undergone any study in women to determine the safest and most effective dose or combination of hormones.[25] The number of alternative medicines that have been shown to be effective in well-designed large, randomized, controlled trials is very small, and the same is true for other types of alternative treatments, such as acupuncture and Reiki.

This is true, and particularly worrisome because, while medications made by drug companies have to undergo extensive testing before they are allowed on the market, and are closely monitored by the FDA, alternative drugs are regulated very differently. Considered "dietary supplements," they are subject to little scrutiny, either of their ingredients or their claims of efficacy. So long as they bear a disclaimer that reads, "These statements have not been evaluated by the Food and Drug Administration. This product is not intended to diagnose, treat, cure, or prevent any disease"—known to opponents as the "quack Miranda warning"—the makers and advocates of these treatments can claim just about anything they want and sell pretty much whatever combination of ingredient they please.

Yet the narrative of unspoiled nature or pure bodies corrupted or damaged by big corporations only to be redeemed by the destruction of those organizations and a return to natural order is, as Wildavsky and Douglas argue, even more powerful today than it was in explaining the unexpected in less advanced societies. And the supposed ability to identify the source of hidden dangers from conventional medicine is a powerful tool for framing risk and influencing the public, far more so than the verbatim information or data any one agency or scientist can offer. Framing, like all social or economic tactics, is a group exercise. It is not a product of cost benefit analysis, but the result of an interplay of emotions, values, experience, and information that influences the risks we choose.

The Internet, because of the role it plays in delivering the kind of vivid information that is critical to framing risk decisions immediately and to millions of people, can and has become a powerful tool for influencing what risks we focus on. Increasingly, the Web is being used to make people fearful and uncertain about medical technologies, creating a duality between corporate medicine's corrupting essence and lurking danger and the natural order's healing power.

RISK AND CULTURE: UNCERTAINTY AND FEAR AS A POLITICAL WEAPON

Despite the myriad risks, actual and imaginary, that surround us, most of us are not constantly consumed with fear. Nor do communities, societies, or families live in reaction or overreaction to unforeseen events. Rather, we choose the risks we want to face and those we want to avoid. This goes beyond our human tendency to fear the foreign, and overlook the everyday. As I have argued, the introduction of certain types of information changes our frame to increase uncertainty and fear, and the common feature of this framing process is determining what level of uncertainty individuals can accept and how it contributes to a shared perception of the risks of medical technology. Kahneman and Tversky were thinking of the way anxiety can be manipulated by the labeling of outcomes when they concluded their most famous article by saying, "The framing of acts and outcomes can also reflect the acceptance or rejection of responsibility for particular consequences, and the deliberate manipulation of framing is commonly used as an instrument of control. When framing influences the experience of consequences, the adoption of a decision frame is an ethically significant act."[26] Because of the manipulation of these frames, what Americans fear most in the twenty-first century (apart from terrorism) is the impact of science and technology on the physical world.

As Aaron Wildavsky and Mary Douglas wrote in *Risk and Culture*, "What are Americans afraid of? Nothing much, really, except the food they eat, the water they drink, the air they breathe, the land they live on and the energy they use ... Once the source of safety, science and technology have become the source of risk."[27] How is it that the safety and reliability of medicines—and the scientific processes that produce medical technologies—have come to be regarded by many Americans as some of the most significant dangers? More precisely, at a time when we are living longer than ever before, with greater well-being than ever before, in large part because of advances in science and medicine, why have the risks of medical technologies become one of the main dangers the public seems to worry about?

These risks follow a pattern or narrative: they are unforeseen, rare, disastrous events that poison or pollute our bodies. The source is always technological contamination hidden by companies seeking profit, and the consequences are always the result of corporate callousness. I argue that the Internet has become an important and powerful tool for people and groups who seek to frame risk to increase public uncertainty about the dangers of medical technologies. They do this by increasing the sense that unforeseen tragedies are immediate and intentional and that individuals and organizations act without considering the public health consequences of their actions.

CHAPTER 2

The Precautionary Principle:
The Politics of Pseudocertainty

S INCE WHAT WE FEAR most of all is what we know we do not know, it is not surprising that increasingly our approach to an uncertain and risky future is to reject new technologies and overreact to their risks. Bisphenol-A, or BPA, an industrial chemical found in hundreds of plastic products, including plastic baby bottles and food packaging, has become one of the latest battlegrounds for those who believe that industrial chemicals in our food, household goods, and construction products are polluting the globe into extinction. There is also concern that BPA "might have subtle but deleterious effects on the neurological and reproductive development of kids." And it has been linked to a wide range of problems, including declining sperm counts, shorter penises, obesity, and diabetes.[1] Frederick vom Saal, a scientist at the University of Missouri who has led the charge against BPA for over a decade, told *Discover* magazine that the chemical is the biological equivalent of global warming.[2]

But not so fast. In 2008, after reviewing the available evidence, the Food and Drug Administration issued a draft report that concluded that BPA was safe, that "there is reasonable certainty in the minds of competent scientists that the substance is not harmful under the intended conditions of use." This included evaluating studies sponsored by the National Toxicology Program, which does research on the effects of chemical and environmental factors on human health for the federal government. Although most data on the effects of BPA came from studies on rats, the media's reporting focused on its use in baby bottles and sippy cups. Yet in simulations of typical use to determine how much BPA leached out of baby bottles, the bottles produced *no* detectable BPA. The estimated maximum total infant exposure to BPA from bottles was 1.7 parts per billion (yes, per billion). Total maximum BPA exposure from infant formula containers was 6.6 parts per billion. The FDA also found that the "no adverse effect level" of BPA was more than 2,000 times the predicted exposure of infants to the chemical, and more than 27,000 times in the case of adults.[3]

But the finding did nothing to convince environmental activists, who claimed there was a cover-up or whitewash of the real dangers of BPA, which they identified ominously as an "endocrine disruptor," making the substance sound like the advanced weaponry from a video game or science-fiction movie. The media was quick to jump on the story, hyping the danger until many parents were terrified that they had inadvertently been damaging their babies and furious that the government had allowed the danger to go unexposed for so long. Parenting blogs and communities buzzed with their anger and fear, and the debate spilled over into many other sites and blogs. Environmental and safety websites took advantage of the opportunity to wax hyperbolic about BPA's risks, citing scary-seeming scientific results that were almost always mischaracterized or taken out of context.

Meanwhile, the Endocrine Society issued a "scientific statement" on endocrine-disrupting chemicals that listed BPA among many substances that could act as endocrine disrupters. The statement invoked what is known as the Precautionary Principle, the idea that where the risks are unknown or uncertain, continued use or development of the source of the risk should be curtailed or stopped. In other words, better safe than sorry. This approach seems sensible. After all, we use it every day, and it works well for dealing with things such as busy streets and hot stoves. When it comes to science and medicine, though, the principle acts as a mechanism to control and constrain the development of new technologies, which does not make us much safer and makes us a lot more afraid. In asserting the Precautionary Principle, the Endocrine Society moved away from the FDA definition of "safe" and embraced the notion that because it was impossible to establish no risk for endocrine disruptors, society should eliminate them from the planet.[4]

Despite the fact that its initial findings had indicated that the available evidence showed little reason to worry about BPA, the FDA soon partially bowed to the fears of parents and the howls of environmental and safety groups that BPA's dangers were being hidden or ignored. The agency eventually issued a lukewarm statement that reaffirmed the National Toxicology Program position that it had "some concern about the potential effects of BPA on the brain, behavior and prostate gland of fetuses, infants and children."[5] Did the FDA think BPA was unsafe? No, not really. According to Dr. Joshua Sharfstein, the FDA's deputy commissioner, "If we thought it was unsafe, we would be taking strong regulatory action."[6] Yet the FDA also suggested ways people could limit their exposure to BPA, including disposing of old bottles or cups made with the chemical and checking the labels on containers to make sure they were microwave safe. The agency also recommended that mothers breastfeed their infants for at least twelve months, since liquid formula can contain traces of BPA due to the containers it is sold and stored in. Finally, the FDA assured the public it was working with companies to produce BPA-free baby bottles and baby food cans, and would support further research into the issue.

But for those who were convinced that BPA was endangering America's children, this was not enough. If we need to eliminate BPA because of its effect on the endocrine system, they asked, why not eliminate all endocrine disruptors? Indeed, if we follow the Precautionary Principle, as the Endocrine Society advocates and the FDA recommends, we have no choice but to do so. And there are many endocrine disruptors to choose from. For instance, the Environmental Working Group, an advocacy group seeking to eliminate BPA from all products, also urges parents to give up beef because it, too, impacts estrogen production, reduces sperm counts, and could adversely affect fetal development. Instead, the EWG encourages soy for infants and pregnant women instead of beef.[7]

But wait a minute. Soy—along with whole grains, pumpkin, zucchini, carrots, garlic, and cabbage—contains endocrine disruptors called phytoestrogens. At low levels and with prolonged exposure, phytoestrogens have been associated with reduced fertility, smaller penis size, lower sexual activity, and reduced brain formation. Even writing about endocrine disruptors can lead to endocrine disruption. "Laptops are becoming increasingly common among young men wired into the latest technology," said Dr. Suzanne Kavic, director of the Division of Reproductive Endocrinology at Loyola University Health System. "However, the heat generated from laptops can impact sperm production and development making it difficult to conceive down the road."[8]

No plastics. No beef. No soy. No pumpkins. No grains. No laptops. When you believe that anything that could possibly pose a danger must be regulated, the effects are endless, and they strike at the heart of our daily lives. The decision to redefine risk as the absence of proof of absolute safety and to limit action or access to technologies until that proof is established is the core of the Precautionary Principle, and it has extensive implications for how we understand the potential dangers that come with progress, especially in medicine and science.

THE RISE OF THE PRECAUTIONARY PRINCIPLE

The Precautionary Principle first took hold in the public debate in Europe in the 1970s and '80s, primarily in the context of environmentalist concerns, and has its roots in the German *Vorsorgungsprinzip*. It is simply a political process for establishing that any industrial activity or technological advancement carries hidden and uncertain risks that must be determined before introducing or allowing it into the environment. The principle emerged, not surprisingly, as the benchmark for framing environmental risks and establishing standards for what is safe from the perspective that technology corrupts nature. It wasn't really new—there have always been those who prefer safety to progress—but it was a renaming and repackaging of the age-old attitude that has proved both influential and detrimental. Perhaps the earliest important use of this idea was in the United Nations World Charter for Nature in 1982, which advised that where "potential adverse effects are not fully understood, the activities should not proceed," but it has also been used in many other national and international environmental documents.[9] By the 1990s, the principle had extended its influence into a broader range of issues and countries.

It was only a matter of time before the Precautionary Principle took hold in the United States, where it became codified in 1998 in the Wingspread Statement, which said, "Where an activity raises threats of harm to the environment or human health, precautionary measures should be taken even if some cause and effect relationships are not fully established scientifically. In this context, the proponent of the activity, rather than the public, should bear the burden of proof."[10] It is a neat reversal of the principle of the justice system; if we applied the Precautionary Principle to crimes, it would be up to the defense to prove that the defendant was innocent, rather than the prosecutor to show that he was guilty. So long as there is "reasonable ground for concern," in the words of the European Commission, the development in question should be stopped or stringently regulated.[11] The danger does not even have to outweigh the benefit. Indeed, no cost-benefit analysis need be done. Merely raising the potential for risk or demanding proof of safety is enough.

Not surprisingly, given the intertwined nature of environmental and health concerns, the Precautionary Principle quickly became part of the debate in health care as well. Indeed, it has perhaps been most successful when it grounds its concerns in public health rather than in pure environmentalism, since doing so strongly engages the media and the population by making the threat feel more direct and personal. The Precautionary Principle, whether or not it goes by that name, resonates with the lay public in the context of medical decisions because people instinctively recoil from placing their own health and that of their families in potential danger. This is especially true when children are involved: parents simply refuse to do anything that might harm their child, and they insist on absolute safety, however unfeasible. What they fail to grasp is that there is a risk in doing everything, including regulating against risk and doing nothing.

DEMANDING 100 PERCENT

Proponents of the Precautionary Principle believe that absolute safety is possible, but when it comes to scientific and medical developments, they are asking the impossible. Science can never provide 100 percent certainty about whether a technology does or does not pose a danger. It can only give a probability. Even where the evidence is strongest, it will never be absolute. Furthermore, where it is possible to establish a high degree of certainty that there is no risk, doing so takes a long time and extensive study; such a finding cannot be produced immediately and it often evolves over time. Therefore, all science runs afoul of the Precautionary Principle, since nothing is ever "fully established," as the Wingspread Statement demands, but rather is always subject to revision or rejection if new data contradict or challenge the current consensus.[12]

Science certainly cannot anticipate adverse events that have not happened yet or that cannot be predicted by what we know now, yet this is what the Precautionary Principle demands: total safety for all time. Science journalist Ronald Bailey uses a striking analogy to illustrate the absurdity of the situation: "It's like demanding that a newborn baby prove that it will never grow up to be a serial killer, or even just a schoolyard bully, before the baby is allowed to leave the hospital."[13] The proponents of the Precautionary Principle allow—indeed, encourage—the public to believe that scientists have perfect information about the risks of new technologies or medications at the time they are developed and that any downsides later discovered are the result of negligence or malice. This is why newly revealed risks of drugs or medical devices are greeted with anger and accusation and fuel distrust of doctors, researchers, and companies. But just because science doesn't have all the answers or fails to produce a verdict immediately doesn't mean that it is useless or corrupt.

Unfortunately, too many people agree that all danger is too much danger. Prospect theorist Paul Slovic asked subjects whether it was true or false that a one-in-ten-million lifetime chance of developing cancer due to a particular chemical was an insignificant danger that was not worth fearing. But more than 30 percent replied that they would indeed be concerned and held that this minuscule probability of harm constituted a serious threat.[14] This shows profound risk avoidance and a lack of understanding of statistics and of the scientific method. But it also reflects a human tendency to catastrophize that is very apparent in those invoking the Precautionary Principle. They envision the worst possible outcome and even conjure various fantastic scenarios of what could go wrong, even when there is nothing to suggest that these results are likely or even possible. The ultimate image of disaster can seem so clear that the complex chain of events, each highly improbable, required for it to occur is lost. Suddenly, the end result seems inevitable when in fact it is a one-in-a-billion outcome.

Journalist Daniel Gardner quotes a scenario given by John Weingart, once a member of a panel charged with identifying locations for radioactive waste storage sites. Weingart recounted the following about public meetings:

> People would invent scenarios and dare Board members and staff to say they were impossible. A person would ask, "What would happen if a plane crashed into a concrete bunker filled with radioactive waste and exploded?" We would explain that while the plane and its contents might explode, nothing in the disposal facility could. And they would say, "But what if explosives had been mistakenly disposed of, and the monitoring devices at the facility had malfunctioned so they weren't noticed?" We would head down the road of saying this was an extremely unlikely set of events. And they would say, "Well, it could happen, couldn't it?"[15]

Further, we remember the cases where technology went wrong, and take for granted the myriad advances that we and those around us use—indeed, depend on—every day. Because people tend to forget the predictions that came true rather than those that did not or that proved less dire than anticipated, there is a confirmation bias that makes it seem that worst-case scenarios are more common and likely than they actually are. This renders us more willing to accept the Precautionary Principle.

Even technologies that have shown success and safety are maligned because of the scary possibilities imagined by their opponents. Take genetically modified foods, another poster child for Precautionary Principle supporters of what is wrong with the current regulatory approach. Over the course of the development of GM foods during the last several decades, there have been many scary scenarios proposed for both the environment and human health—and none has actually materialized. Moreover, genetically modified foods have benefits, including reduced reliance on pesticides, increased yields from

33

less land, and the ability to thrive in climates where growing crops is ordinarily extremely difficult.

But you wouldn't know this from listening to opponents of the technology. In the vacuum of the media coverage or the Internet, where the dangers of GM crops are taken for granted and dissenters are shouted down, it seems there isn't even a debate. And it isn't just one issue; it's dozens, hundreds, thousands, each with its hyperbolic story. So, in the end, Americans can be forgiven for believing that eliminating genetically modified foods, endocrine disruptors, or whatever the threat will ensure absolute safety, carry no risks, and entail no trade-offs.

WHEN GOOD AND EVIL MEET RISK AND BENEFIT

In another experiment, Slovic and two colleagues were curious about why assessments of dangers diverged so significantly between experts and the public at large. They discovered that the experts based their estimation of each of the risks presented by the experimenters on the potential mortality of the threat. Not so for the laypeople they asked. Even when this group of subjects knew how many people were likely to die as a result of each of the dangers discussed, there was no clear relationship between this knowledge and how dangerous they believed the activity to be. Rather, their perception was swayed by the emotional elements discussed in chapter 1: novelty, control, personalization, natural versus man-made, immediacy, etc. The laypeople were also very confident in their estimates of risk, even when these guesses bore no relation to the actual probabilities. When Slovic had them give the chance that they were incorrect, 25 percent said that the probability they were wrong was below 1 percent.[16]

But that wasn't the whole story. Slovic and his colleagues also found that laypeople judged things they perceived as having little redeeming value to be dangerous and things that seemed useful and positive to be negligible threats, whatever the true risks were.[17] In

Beyond Fear, Bruce Schneier explains, "When someone says that the risks of nuclear power (for example) are unacceptable, what he's really saying is that the effects of a nuclear disaster, no matter how remote, are so unacceptable to him as to make the trade-off intolerable. This is why arguments like 'but the odds of a core meltdown are a zillion to one' ... have no effect. It doesn't matter how unlikely the threat is; the risk is unacceptable because the consequences are unacceptable."[18]

To Slovic's subjects, that *both* the value and the risk of something could be low or high seemed impossible, but it happens all the time in the real world. A medical procedure may offer the chance of substantial improvement in a patient's condition but also carry significant potential for something to go wrong. Another treatment may be risky but not do much to help the patient. Slovic's subsequent experiments indicated that providing the subjects with information on the benefits of new developments made them rate the upside of those technologies more highly and reduced their estimates of the dangers.[19] On one hand, that means good information can help bring perceived risk closer to real risk. On the other, the spread of false information about the potential benefits of a procedure or technology reinforces or creates inflated fear.

Our perceptions of risk are caught up in emotional value judgments, words like *BPA* or *nuclear power* or *vaccines* are themselves invested with *good* and *bad* and therefore *safe* and *dangerous*. At one time, scientific and medical technologies symbolized hope and progress, from drugs to pesticides, from water treatment to preservatives. No longer. Perhaps one indication of this is that, these days, there is hardly a word that carries a more sinister association than *chemical*. We are beset by articles and websites about how our water supplies, our soil, even our bodies are contaminated with dangerous chemicals and toxins. No surprise, then, that whether you ask people in the United States, Canada, or France (or, undoubtedly, most other developed countries), all but a quarter of respondents say they "try hard to avoid contact with chemicals and chemical products in daily life" and "if even a tiny amount of a cancer-producing substance were found in my tap water, I wouldn't drink it." In fact, 60 percent opined, "It can never be too expensive to reduce the risk from chemicals."[20] That's a strong statement. And an unrealistic one. Budgets are finite and threats innumerable when you include anything with even a minute potential for harm.

But, of course, chemicals can be natural—water, for example—as well as artificial, and we couldn't live without them. The next time you hear a scare story about yet another researcher who has found a dizzying array of chemicals in the bodies of subjects or you read an article on chemicals detected in city water, ask yourself an easy and fundamental question: What is the *concentration* of these chemicals? Chances are very, very good that the answer is given in parts per billion or indeed parts per trillion. We're constantly creating better and more sensitive tests that can identify the presence of substances in the tiniest of tiny amounts, but surely only the most paranoid of us believe there is a risk in a concentration, even of a dangerous substance, that amounts to "a grain of sugar in an Olympic-size swimming pool."[21] Similarly, studies that find that chemicals cause cancer in rodents (and it's usually rodents, even if the news story glosses over that) use much, much higher concentrations of those chemicals to conduct the experiment than those to which any human is likely ever to be exposed.

Perhaps you remember Alar and apples. Alar was a chemical used to make apples ripen more quickly and evenly, improve their appearance, and allow them to remain fresh for longer. In the 1980s, reports that Alar caused cancer launched public fear and devastated apple growers—even those who had never used Alar. The genesis was a 1973 article that suggested that Alar was connected to cancer in mice, which was followed by two government studies that found a weaker but still present link. All these studies used very high levels of Alar, far, far above those found on the apples sold in the supermarket, and tested the chemical in rodents rather than humans. Indeed, in the late 1970s, the EPA asked Uniroyal, the maker of Alar, to test one of the chemical's byproducts, 1,1- (unsymmetrical) dimethylhydrazine (UDMH), at concentrations so high the researchers believed it would kill the mice before evidence of cancer-causing effects could be seen. And even then, the results showed that the risk of developing cancer due to Alar was 1 in 5×10^5 over seventy years of exposure.

In the mid-1980s, the EPA opened a special review, asking the manufacturer for more data rebutting the original study, and in the fall of 1985, it indicated that it planned to have the chemical pulled from the market. However, the agency's Scientific Advisory Panel held that proof that Alar was carcinogenic was not strong enough to remove the chemical. As a result, Alar was simply restricted and more research by the company required. Nonetheless, Massachusetts and New York prohibited the use of Alar and several foreign countries refused to allow the chemical or apples treated with it to be imported.

But for those who grew apples, the real pressure to abandon Alar came from companies making apple juices and sauces, which said they would not buy apples from growers using Alar. Their decision came in part from the efforts of "safety advocates," such as Ralph Nader, who had pushed the producers to take action against Alar, even though much of the scientific evidence didn't back up their accusations, especially at the levels of the chemical consumed by humans. An executive at the parent company of Mott's told the public that the firm's decision "has nothing to do with the safety of Alar or the position that the EPA has taken ... The reason is simple. There has been so much negative publicity that continued use of apples treated with Alar could hurt consumer confidence in the Mott's brand name." A scientist at the Natural Resources Defense Council opined, "It's a scandal that EPA allows a suspected carcinogen to remain in our food supply ... The processors' stand is laudable."[22] So growers dropped Alar, and sales, once around $20 million a year, plummeted. The chemical's manufacturer, Uniroyal, sold its entire chemical division to another company but claimed that the fears about Alar were not the cause.

But the controversy was just beginning. In 1989, the EPA reversed its earlier decision and prohibited the use of Alar after a public panic created by a piece on the news program *60 Minutes*. The show was sparked by a publication entitled "Intolerable Risk: Pesticides in Our Children's Food," disseminated by an environmental lobbying group called the Natural Resources Defense Council and based on an analysis the NRDC had carried out using a computer model and some dubious assumptions. In fact, the EPA had already rebuffed its conclusion several weeks earlier. But the study's shortfalls were something neither the group nor the news media were interested in discussing. That would have ruined the compelling narrative of hidden harm, endangered children, and thousands of invisible deaths. The *60 Minutes* show led with an image of an apple covered by a skull and crossbones and alleged that Alar was "the most potent cancer-causing agent in the food supply today."[23]

Via a PR firm, the NRDC also coordinated dozens of press conferences trumpeting its findings and persuaded actress Meryl Streep to serve as a spokesperson for the dangers of Alar. Predictably, the population went crazy, and so did the press. Parents were convinced their children were being poisoned. Schools forbade children to bring apples for lunch. Stores threw out their stocks. Apple sales plummeted. The EPA, FDA, and Department of Agriculture said that Alar was not dangerous in the levels in which it was found in food. No one listened. The manufacturer soon had no choice but to stop selling Alar.

The furor over Alar fell hard on apple growers, endangering yield and quality and disrupting their picking and the jobs it created. Some had to pull back the percentage of orchards that could be harvested. Others eventually went out of business. Because apple sales fell overall due to public fears of Alar, even growers who had never used the chemical were impacted. In fact, fewer than 15 percent of growers treated their orchards with Alar. The EPA put the cost for growers, in 1986, at $31 million, but later data by the Department of Agriculture raised the figure to a minimum of $125 million. The growers launched a suit against the NRDC, Fenton Communications (which had been retained by the NRDC to promote its findings), and CBS News's *60 Minutes* over the damage the media coverage had done to the apple business. However, they lost several times in court.

In the end, the scientific data failed to confirm the supposed risks of Alar. Not only had most of the early research, including the 1970s study that set the whole thing off, used doses tens of thousands of times those found in normal consumption of apples, but later reviews of the evidence by the British government, the United Nations, and even the EPA itself all confirmed that Alar posed no real danger. Dr. Joseph D. Rosen of Rutgers University explained, "There was never any legitimate scientific study to justify the Alar scare."[24]

THE END OF SCIENCE?

Even if 100 percent safety were possible, would we really be willing to pay the price? If your answer is "of course!" think about it carefully. Look around you. Now imagine that anything that could potentially carry a risk to people, animals, or the environment were banned. That means no electricity or anything that runs off of electricity, no micro-wave, no refrigerator (coolants are dangerous), no oven, no car in the driveway, no cellular phones. And forget about trains and planes. It also means that probably none of the pills you have in your medicine cabinet would exist, not even aspirin (which, after all, has a toxic-ity risk if you take too much of it), cough syrup (likewise), or birth control pills (increased risk of blood clots). You certainly would not be allowed to have antibiotics, undergo any kind of surgical procedure, get a vaccine, or receive a scan, whether an X-ray or an MRI. We might as well remove any food that has sugar or fat in it, since that can cause obesity, type-2 diabetes, and many other health problems.

This scenario isn't crazy. It is simply taking the Precautionary Principle literally: if any item or action could at *any* point cause harm of *any* kind and magnitude to *anything*, living or otherwise, then it should not be developed. And I didn't make up this list; these are just a few of the answers given when a British news site asked doctors and scientists what technological developments would not exist if we had stuck throughout history to the Precautionary Principle.[25] Still, at a session on the Precautionary Principle in 1999, Jeff Howard, a one-time member of Greenpeace International's Toxics Campaign, advocated for making the principle yet more stringent. *More* stringent? Why, yes! He proposed five further requirements be added, one of which was: "Even the most fundamental of past decisions must be subject to re-examination and precautionary reform."[26]

Think about this. At its most extreme, the Precautionary Principle threatens not only the technologies of the future but every technology ever developed: our gadgets and conveniences but also the drugs, devices, and procedures that keep us alive and improve our quality of life and the initiatives to save millions in developing countries through vaccination, safe water, anti-HIV medications, and more.

The Precautionary Principle's defenders have countered accusations that the principle paralyzes science by saying that it actually calls for *more* science. The editorial chair of a European Environment Agency report published in 2002 argued, "The use of the Precautionary Principle can bring benefits beyond the reduction of health and environmental impacts, stimulating both more innovation, via technological diversity and flexibility, and better science."[27] Yet an article in the British online news magazine *Spiked* put well why this is not so: "The Precautionary Principle does not merely ask us to hypothesize about and try to predict outcomes of particular actions, whether these outcomes are positive or negative. Rather, it demands that we take regulatory action on the basis of possible 'unmanageable' risks, even after tests have been conducted that find no evidence of harm. We are asked to make decisions to curb actions, not on the basis of what we know, but on the basis of what we do not know."[28]

Furthermore, since science cannot produce 100 percent certainty, and, indeed, it often offers results that differ and even contradict one another, opponents of a technology can always argue that we don't know enough and need more study, holding developments perpetually hostage or killing them outright. This is exactly what we have seen from vaccine opponents who continue to tell the public we don't know whether immunizations cause autism or brain damage, despite dozens of large studies that show that they do not. Even when the Precautionary Principle can be applied judiciously and carefully, the risk of bypassing or halting important scientific research and discoveries is large. The potential of some developments is not immediately apparent, and risks tend both to emerge and to be mitigated over the course of time and further research. Think about aspirin, a versatile medication with myriad uses and more being found all the time. Many believe that it would be considered to have unacceptable risks if it were being developed today.

INVISIBLE VICTIMS

Those who invoke the Precautionary Principle often publicize the small dangers of scientific developments while ignoring the larger risks inherent in the status quo. They also fail to acknowledge that human health and environmental protection sometimes are goals in opposition to each other. Or, rather, many of them choose environmental protection without ever acknowledging that they have done so. One of the hallmarks of the use of the Precautionary Principle in environmental discussions is the assumption that man-made developments are ipso facto malevolent and dangerous and things that are natural are fundamentally safe. As the previous chapter suggests, the principle has easily been carried over into health, particularly in the case of alternative medicine, yet natural remedies can be just as dangerous as ones developed in a lab.

The principle's backers frequently presume that every chemical, every technology, every change, is a threat to nature and that none of them offers benefits that outweigh their environmental impact. But a lot of dangers from our environment have been reduced significantly because of technology. Award-winning science journalist Ronald Bailey describes how, at a symposium on the Precautionary Principle, one of the panelists asserted that in the last two hundred years the quality of drinking water has decreased.

Clearly, the panelist had deffcient knowledge of history; as Bailey writes, "Two hundred years ago, drinking from any stream, well, or spring could expose one to typhoid, typhus, cholera, and other diseases. In fact, chlorination has so improved drinking water quality with regard to health that people in the West no longer even think twice about drinking tap water. Unfortunately, more than a billion people in the developing world can't say the same; millions still die of water-borne diseases each year."[29] For some in the developing world, life is the same as it was a hundred years ago, in a purer, more natural time. But I doubt even the most hardened environmentalist really wants to live their life.

What about the case of the pesticide DDT, which is regularly invoked in support of the Precautionary Principle? The story of how Rachel Carson exposed the danger of DDT in her book *Silent Spring* is a famous one. But what made Carson's narrative popularly compelling wasn't her account of the damage done by the chemical to bird eggs—after all, most of us are not inspired to act in response to such abstract risks—but her contention that DDT was driving an epidemic of cancer in humans, especially children. Yet the reason the percentage of children killed by cancer, although still tiny, was rising was that they were no longer dying of measles and polio and diphtheria. This was true not only of children but of people in all age groups.

In fact, rather than endangering our lives, DDT could be credited with saving millions. During and after the Second World War, it was a critical part of preventing the spread of typhus, marking the first time that the disease had been controlled effectively. DDT also prevented millions of deaths by reducing and, in Europe and North America, eliminating malaria. It's easy for those of us in rich nations to trivialize that benefit, but today millions in developing countries, particularly in Africa, continue to be killed by malaria. In some countries, the disease has been resurgent since the use of DDT was stopped, and the death toll has again risen. These are victims, too. The environmental and health consequences of DDT are serious—but so are the millions of lives it saved and the millions lost in its absence.

The same mechanism is present when the Precautionary Principle is applied to medicine: for example, when critics want to ban a cholesterol drug that has severe side effects in a few patients but pay no mind to the number of people who do not suffer heart attacks, strokes, or other complications because they are on the drug. As Australian researcher Ronald Brunton writes in an article in *Australasian Biotechnology*, "Approving a new medicinal drug which turns out to have harmful side effects—such as thalidomide—can produce highly visible victims, heart-rending news stories, and very damaging political fallout. But incorrectly delaying a drug produces victims who are essentially invisible."[30] We can see the victims of drugs; we may even know their names and faces, thanks to the media and the Internet. But we don't see those hurt by lost opportunities. No one ever puts them on *Oprah* or creates a Web page memorializing them. So the trade-off between risk and benefit, between those who were helped by a new technology and those who were hurt, is hidden.

OUT OF TRAGEDY, HOPE

Even the case of thalidomide, a favorite example of those who support increased use of the Precautionary Principle, is not a case of unmitigated harm. Rather it is an extreme example of the difficult decisions and the complex balance between risk and benefit that exist in the development of drugs. The important cases—the ones that tell us something about the risks we are and are not willing to take, about the nature of progress and regulation and science—are not simple or straightforward; they are hard, agonizing, and without satisfying answers. And yet we also should not let them dominate everything so that it seems preferable to do and allow nothing than to confront tough issues or take a chance of something going wrong.

Developed in Germany in 1954 and marketed as a sedative, thalidomide was sold in forty-six countries under dozens of brand names by Chemie Grünenthal and by various other firms that had purchased the license. At one time, thalidomide was the third leading drug in Europe, and in some nations it could be purchased without a prescription. Contrary to the common contention, the ability of thalidomide to reach the market wasn't the result of negligent testing. Because the deformities it causes appear only in primates, they were not visible in the animal studies done. Testing in humans did not show the risk either because, although pregnant women were included in the tests, none were in their first trimester, when the damage is caused. Many people turned to thalidomide because it was portrayed as safer than barbiturates, and even large doses of it did no apparent harm, so it could not be used to commit suicide and it wouldn't hurt children who got into their parents' medicine bottles. One ad, which would eventually prove terribly ironic, showed a child holding a pill vial from the bathroom cabinet that bore the legend, "This child's life depends on the safety of Distaval [one of thalidomide's brand names]."[31]

One of the uses for which the drug was prescribed was morning sickness in pregnant women. Over time, thalidomide produced certain characteristic birth defects in a significant percentage of babies born to these women. Two doctors, one German, Widukind Lenz, and one Australian, William McBride, were the first to begin noticing the proliferation of cases of phocomelia, a rare defect producing very short, flipper-like limbs, and to connect them to thalidomide. By 1961, reports were coming in from many different countries of the risk associated with the drug. Grünenthal and the other companies distributing the drug were slow to take action, but eventually thalidomide was pulled from the market. Around eight thousand surviving children worldwide were affected by thalidomide. What allowed the teratogenic effects to slip through for so long was that they appeared only when the drug was taken between the twentieth and thirty-sixth day of pregnancy. Not only was this a very narrow window, and so many pregnant women who took the drug delivered healthy babies, but many women did not yet know they were pregnant at the time they were given thalidomide.

Thalidomide was never approved by the United States because its 1960 FDA application was famously delayed by a medical officer named Frances Kelsey, who noticed that the drug failed to act as a sedative in rats, as it did in humans, and wondered whether its mechanism was different in rats and humans. If it was, she believed, then it wasn't certain that animal testing was sufficient to show that thalidomide was safe in humans. However, the fact that the drug was never approved there didn't mean there was no thalidomide use in the United States. Samples were given out by the drug's U.S. manufacturer to thousands of patients, including some pregnant women, as part of what was billed as a clinical trial but which was aimed mostly at promoting the drug, and for which there were only spotty records. Thalidomide was tremendously symbolic for the FDA, the policy community, and the American public, and it remains so today. In the wake of the revelations about the birth defect risks of the drug, the United States strengthened laws governing the approval of new medications.

For most people the story ends there. It's an open-and-shut case, they say: thalidomide was a horribly dangerous and deforming drug allowed to get and stay on the market due to grossly inadequate safety testing and monitoring and the callous actions of companies interested in profits over patients. *This*, they believe, is why we cannot be too careful about any drug that might be risky. But the tale of thalidomide doesn't end with its withdrawal—and millions have lived better, longer lives because of it.

In the mid-1960s, thalidomide came back to life. As many discoveries in medicine are, its reemergence was due to chance. One day, Dr. Jacob Sheskin, the head of the Jerusalem Hospital for Hansen's Disease (or what most people call leprosy), was sent a patient with extremely advanced erythema nodosum leprosum, or ENL, a very painful and debilitating side effect of leprosy that causes boils, joint pain, inflammation, and intense pain. Patients waste away, unable to eat or sleep and dependent on morphine and sedatives to control their agony. About 60 percent of people with advanced leprosy get ENL.

The patient who arrived at the Jerusalem Hospital in 1964 was close to death and had received almost no benefit from any sedative available. While trying to figure out if there was anything that could be done for him, Dr. Sheskin stumbled upon a small stash of thalidomide, now no longer being sold. Remembering the use of the drug in mental patients who similarly responded to no other sedative, the doctor decided it was worth a try. It worked. Spectacularly. Not only was the patient finally able to sleep, but his ENL began quickly to improve radically. The same thing happened in other patients with ENL. Sheskin then embarked on a series of controlled clinical trials in Venezuela, where thalidomide could still be purchased, and confirmed his findings. Soon the drug was promoted by the World Health Organization for use in ENL patients, and even the United States allowed highly controlled use of thalidomide for ENL beginning in 1975. Thanks to Dr. Sheskin's discovery, the vast majority of facilities that treated leprosy have been able to be closed.

In the 1980s, thalidomide found another use: in AIDS patients. Like those with ENL (and tuberculosis patients, who had also been helped by thalidomide), people with AIDS suffered from severe wasting. They also got sores in the mouth and esophagus called aphthous ulcers, caused, like the wasting, by a chemical called TNF-α (tumor necrosis factor alpha) and a rare cancer called Kaposi's sarcoma. All of these conditions responded well to thalidomide. But the drug was hard to get a hold of, and many AIDS patients had to obtain it from abroad, mostly via Mexico, through buyers' clubs. However, these channels were dubious, and the quality and purity of the drug uncertain. Researchers into the uses of thalidomide had likewise found that it was difficult to obtain and so one, Dr. Gilla Kaplan, finally managed to persuade a small pharmaceutical firm called Celgene to apply to the FDA for approval to produce thalidomide.

While the process to get the drug approved by the FDA was ongoing, research into its potential use as an anti-cancer drug was being conducted by leading cancer researchers Dr. Robert D'Amato and Dr. Judah Folkman. They were working on angiogenesis, the growth of blood vessels, and hoped that finding a way to inhibit such growth would allow the development of drugs to fight cancer and several other diseases. It was thalidomide's anti-angiogenic effect that had caused the birth defects, but that also made it a perfect candidate from the perspective of D'Amato and Folkman's research. Subsequent study found that the drug is also very effective at fighting multiple myeloma, a difficult-to-treat cancer that attacks the plasma cells in the blood.

In July 1998, after a long and spirited debate and heartfelt stories from both victims of thalidomide and those helped by it, the drug was approved by the FDA under the condition that patients be carefully monitored and that extensive safeguards be put in place to prevent pregnant women from taking thalidomide. New uses, especially for rare autoimmune conditions, are still being discovered, even as old ones are sometimes superseded. If the Precautionary Principle had been in force, thalidomide would not have been allowed on the market in the 1990s, when Celgene was seeking to have it approved to treat cancer, even without its history.[32] Yet, in its new uses, the drug has benefited millions of patients around the world.

SLEEPING DANGERS

In other cases, science has been so successful at eliminating or severely reducing risks that people forget how common and how serious those risks can be and how easily they can return. But since all treatments carry risks, the ebbing of the diseases they prevent can lead to evocations of the Precautionary Principle and calls for investigations into these dangers. This is especially evident in discussions of immunization, since parents today do not remember a time before vaccines for diseases such as measles, pertussis (whooping cough), and polio. Furthermore, the prevalence of vaccines has made these illnesses very uncommon in rich nations—and given parents a false sense of security that no harm will come to their children if they are not vaccinated. But as the uptake of immunizations drops, diseases begin to come back, especially in our globalized and interconnected world, and they bring with them their dangerous complications.

The first chapter in the history of the contemporary anti-vaccine movement was written in the 1970s and '80s with the controversy over the pertussis vaccines. It began with a 1974 article by a British scientist that was picked up by the press. The article claimed to show that the immunization against pertussis was responsible for irreversible brain damage and/or seizures in twenty-two children. The media grabbed the results and ran with them, setting off a panic. Seemingly reasonable voices argued that as long as there was even a possibility that the vaccine led to brain damage, it should not be used.

Before the article, there was 80 percent uptake of the pertussis vaccine in the United Kingdom. Soon that figure was 30 percent. Between 1974 and 1976, 100,000 British children landed in the hospital with the disease and 40 died. But the damage was not confined to the United Kingdom. Halfway around the world, in Japan, the government took the pertussis immunization off the vaccine schedule in 1975, and in the next three years, 113 children lost their lives to pertussis.

Then the controversy hit the United States. The drop in vaccination rates was less dramatic than overseas, but fear spread fast and manifested itself in other ways beyond declining immunizations. Lawyers reacted by suing companies that produced pertussis immunizations, alleging that the vaccine was responsible for "epilepsy, mental retardation, learning disorders, unexplained coma, Reye's syndrome (a sudden onset of coma, later found to be associated with aspirin), and sudden infant death syndrome."[33] Over the next thirteen years, eight hundred lawsuits were brought, demanding over $21 million in damages. The cost of the vaccine skyrocketed to $11.00 from a mere $0.17. Three of the four manufacturers stopped production.

The furor was ratcheted up further by a 1982 NBCTV program called *DPT: Vaccine Roulette*, which showed harrowing images of children supposedly hurt by the pertussis portion of what is correctly called the DTP (diphtheria, tetanus, and pertussis) vaccine and offered interviews with government officials, doctors, and parents designed to reinforce this premise. Scientists interviewed for the show later said they were interrogated until they made comments that could be edited to make it seem they believed DTP was dangerous. As is typical, the risks of pertussis were downplayed. The conspiracy narrative was taken up by parents who believed that they had found a reason for their children's illness and by anti-vaccine organizations such as the National Vaccine Information Center, founded as Dissatisfied Parents Together in 1982 and still headed today by Barbara Loe Fisher, who believes her son was one of DTP's victims.

The vaccine did have some risks, including an elevated chance of side effects compared to other immunizations, but by the late 1980s, science had studied the question of whether the pertussis vaccine increased the risk of mental retardation or epilepsy and produced extensive evidence against this theory. The incidence of these conditions, the data showed, was the same in children immunized with the vaccine as in those who did not receive it. DTP could cause harm—all vaccines, all medications, all treatments can—but science suggested it was nonetheless innocent in the vast majority of cases. Yet the courts gave the "victims" compensation anyway, blatantly ignoring the medical evidence. One received $1.13 million, more than half of the $2 million brought in by the pertussis vaccine that year for all the companies making the vaccine.

To bring an end to this, the government stepped in and set up the National Vaccine Injury Compensation Program, under which special judges review the scientific data and, where it speaks in favor of a vaccine-caused injury, dispense compensation from a fund created with a tax levied on each vaccine given. The system has not always hewed to the science, nor has it stopped companies from getting out of the vaccine business, but it is a dramatic improvement.[34]

But the work of DTP's opponents has proved lasting and has been far from benign: in children who have not received an immunization against pertussis, the risk of contracting the illness is raised twenty-three-fold. Babies, many of them too young to be fully vaccinated and therefore in need of protection by immunizing older children and adults, are at special risk of death from pertussis. In 1976, a thousand people were struck by pertussis in the United States. In 2005, that figure was more than twenty-five thousand. The death rate from pertussis is small, approximately 1 percent, but the mortality from the vaccine, even before the new and safer DTaP replaced the DTP, is a tiny fraction of that. The story of DTP is an example of the worst potential consequences of the Precautionary Principle: legal and cultural opposition, willfully ignoring the science, left hundreds of thousands of children around the world unimmunized, sickened or killed thousands more, and almost drove the pertussis vaccine off the market. In trying to vanquish an illusory risk, the movement against the pertussis vaccine created a real risk.

FACING THE FUTURE

Helen Keller famously observed, "Life is either a daring adventure or nothing. Security does not exist in nature, nor do the children of men as a whole experience it. Avoiding danger is no safer in the long run than exposure."[35] Yet if we live in a world of risks and if all of choices have trade-offs, then why has the Precautionary Principle become the predominant approach to viewing and avoiding risks? Because the principle, in all its flavors and variations, plays upon the human tendency to equate uncertainty with risk or danger. But it is not an objective method for determining the impact of technology or for ranking risks. Indeed, the threshold for applying the principle is minimal and varies from issue to issue, and "once it is met, there is something like a presumption in favor of stringent regulatory controls."[36]

In these cases, what kind of guidance is provided by the Precautionary Principle? If the burden of proof is on the proponent of the activity or process in question, the Precautionary Principle would seem to impose a burden of proof that cannot be met. And indeed, the point of the principle is not to establish a standard for safety. It is to create uncertainty about safety; provide groups with a sense that they can protect themselves or the environment against the hidden dangers of technology by simply rejecting all new developments; and delay or halt scientific, medical, and technological progress by making sure there is never enough proof of safety.

The Precautionary Principle is a means for choosing what to fear. It focuses on those risks and avoiding them even at the expense of ignoring possible benefits. Those who invoke the Precautionary Principle to seek regulation of cloning of embryonic stem cells neglect the possibility that without therapeutic cloning, we will have to wait longer for real cures to fatal diseases. Want to eliminate salt consumption in the United States to reduce heart attacks from hypertension? Then be prepared to accept a likely risk that a reduction in the use of salt—the primary source of iodine—will lead to an increase in birth defects and impaired cognitive development in children.

As we discussed in chapter 1, people are more likely to avoid or fear the most immediate and vivid dangers, especially rare ones. And even more so when that danger is a technological or industrial action or product that might corrupt "benign nature." The Precautionary Principle weaves these two beliefs into a powerful tool for blinding us to the probabilities of the risks identified, to other risks triggered by our choice of fears, and to the possible loss of benefits. The Precautionary Principle is powerful in part because it speaks to the belief that if we only do the right things and avoid things that undermine nature, we can provide ourselves and our children harbors for ultimate safety.

Even more, it promotes the view that we are in charge of our fate and that all dangers can be eliminated or mitigated by making the right decisions. The feeling of control is a critical element in determining which threats people fear and how likely they judge each hazard. Ultimately, we must relearn to accept that we live in a world full of risks. Past generations had no choice but to acknowledge that they were surrounded by dangers. But all our advances have given us the illusion today that we have a choice, that we can reject the risks of life and, in so doing, keep ourselves safe from everything. We cannot and we never will be able to do so.

As we will see in the next chapters, the Internet has become a source of pseudocertainty for those of us seeking protection from risks and a return to a time and place where technology did not undermine our bodies or our planet. The Precautionary Principle has found a new force and a new reach in the Internet age. The websites, blogs, forums, and search engines that occupy our days didn't exist when the principle first became codified, but they have been some of its most valuable tools. The Web has stretched its tendrils into every aspect of our lives, transforming them from what they were only twenty years ago.

Medicine has not been spared. A slower convert perhaps than other areas of society, it is now forced to confront head-on the challenge of the Internet and the power that it has wrested from the hands of doctors and researchers. The Internet has its good points: greater and easier access to information and research, the growth of communities where patients can find people who understand what they are experiencing, and the means for patients to engage more deeply with their own health. But it also has the potential to become an echo chamber for ideologies and a repository of misinformation. Also, Americans have approached medical information on the Web with less skepticism than it warrants. It is to these trends that I now turn.

CHAPTER 3

Insta-Americans: The Rise of Online Self-Diagnosis

THERE WAS A TIME when doing your own research on health information meant a trip to the library and a slog through thick, technical, jargon-heavy medical books and hard-to-understand articles unearthed from piles of journals or rolls of microfilm. So most people just asked their doctors, and the vast majority trusted what they were told. But today the picture is very different, thanks to the Internet and the wealth of information it has put at our fingertips. The Web has made possible near-instant answers to questions on even the most obscure treatments and diseases, has fostered community among patients dealing with the same condition, and has given people the tools to have informed discussions with their doctors about their care and to participate in their own health.

But it has also given charlatans—as well as the well-intentioned but ill-informed—the power to influence millions. Sites that seem authoritative but that lack transparency and fail to reveal their sources entrap unwary would-be health care consumers and empower not patients but lawyers, alternative medicine advocates, industry opponents, and those with ideological axes to grind. In addition, it has led some patients to disregard the advice of their doctors in favor of Internet answers, destroying the potential for a true patient-physician partnership and endangering their health. Doctors now find that some patients are scared of safe treatments because of information found online, while others are combative and demanding, insisting that they know better than their physician which medication or procedure is best.

These developments are indicative of the evolving *insta-American*: the fast-growing segment of the population that doesn't want to be slowed down by writing and mailing checks to pay bills, reading an entire newspaper to be informed, or plodding through the phonebook to find a number. Such trends are also one facet of the democratization of knowledge throughout contemporary society and the devaluation of traditional sources of expertise. Insta-Americans want their information fast, hassle-free, and on their own terms. Scheduling a doctor's appointment weeks in advance and reading medical literature to investigate prescription drugs are tedious and time-consuming processes. For the insta-American, seeking out medical information is most likely to begin with Google. These realities hold potential for both good and ill, but if we are to harness the benefits of Internet health information and avoid the risks, we must examine how we use the Web to make medical decisions.

INSTA-AMERICANS BY THE NUMBERS

For nearly a decade, the Pew Research Center's Internet and American Life Project has examined Internet use and habits among Americans looking for medical advice and information. Their results indicate that Americans are overwhelmingly turning to online medical advice despite serious shortcomings in the quality of Internet information and problematic questions about the appropriateness of self-diagnosis and treatment. In 2008, 74 percent of American adults had Internet access and more than 82 percent of them (61 percent of total adults) looked online for health information at some point.[1] More than eight million do so every day. Medical searching is "at about the same level of popularity ... as paying bills online, reading blogs, or using the Internet to look up phone numbers or addresses."[2] These numbers continue to grow as Internet access becomes more ubiquitous and as those raised with computers and the online world become adults. In 2002, a total of 63 million Americans over age 18 consulted the Web for health facts; six years later, that number was 146 million.[3] In December 2008, data collected by Microsoft indicated that health or medical questions make up about 2 percent of all Internet searches.[4]

According to the Pew Research Center, women are slightly more likely than men to use the Internet to look for health information: 64 percent versus 57 percent.[5] On some health websites, however, women predominate; for instance, 78 percent of visitors on WebMD are female. Women are also overrepresented on interactive components of these sites, such as message boards. This is true in part because women often search for information concerning their children or spouses, not only for themselves. WebMD said in 2007 that the site's "fastest-growing segment ... is the woman over 50 managing her health and that of her family."[6]

Age also affects Internet use, but less than you might think. While those over sixty-five are less likely to use the Internet to find health information than younger adults, only about 27 percent of the population in this age range have done so; 59 percent of those age fifty to sixty-four have. In the eighteen to twenty-nine and thirty to forty-nine groups, usage was almost identical, at 71 and 72 percent. Not only will the percentage in the lowest age group continue to go up in the years to come, as today's Web-addicted kids become adults, but the aging of Baby Boomers also promises to further raise traffic in the over-sixty-five segment. This will increase searches not only on medical problems but also regarding more general health topics such as diet and exercise as this generation works to remain healthy as they grow older.

Another factor impacting the use of the Internet for medical information is education. In general, the more degrees someone has, the more likely it is that he or she will go online for health answers. Part of this trend comes from that fact that those with less education are more likely to be poor and therefore to lack easy access to the Internet. The same is true of the data showing that 51 percent of African Americans and only 44 percent of Latinos (compared to 65 percent of whites) have looked to the Web for health information. Finally, not surprisingly, Pew found that computer literacy and connection speed have a significant effect: the faster the Internet connection and the more tech-savvy a user is, the more likely it is that he or she will search for health topics. Again, these indicators may be partly a proxy for income and other socioeconomic factors.[7]

Patterns have also emerged regarding which Web resources people use to gather information. In 2006, a search engine was the first stop for about 66 percent looking for answers to medical questions online, while 27 percent of Web users went straight to a particular health-related site. Those eighteen to twenty-nine years old tended to start with a search engine, with 74 percent saying they made this their first stop, while those over sixty-five were most likely to start with a certain site they knew and trusted (34 percent). Nearly three-quarters (72 percent) of users went to multiple sites, but few visited more than five, which means that the first sites they saw had a disproportionate influence on the impression they took away. In nearly half of searches conducted in 2006, the information sought was for another person (a figure that went up to 52 percent by 2008), while 36 percent of inquiries were solely for the Internet user. Parents of children under eighteen were 10 percent more likely to seek health facts for someone else (54 versus 44 percent) than those with no children or whose kids were grown.[8]

New uses of the Internet for learning about health issues and making medical decisions are also emerging. Blogs, personal sites, and forums catering to medical information or to a specific condition have become important for people turning to the Web for health answers, with 41 percent of users saying they have visited such sites. Furthermore, rating sites for doctors and hospitals have been gaining in traffic, although only about a quarter of e-patients have used them so far. The numbers for other types of online interactions are lower: 13 percent have listened to a health-related podcast, 6 percent have contributed to an online health site, 5 percent have commented on a blog, 5 percent have left a review of a doctor, while only 4 percent have reviewed a hospital.[9]

The Pew Research Center indicates that the information these users seek spans a wide range of health topics. Whether it is a specific medical problem, such as arteriosclerosis, or general diet tips, evidence suggests that Americans see the Internet as an encyclopedia of medical advice and expertise. In 2008, topping the list of search topics were "specific disease or medical problem" and "certain medical treatment or procedure," at 66 and 55 percent, respectively, a little higher than in previous surveys. Questions having to do with diet and exercise came in third, at 49 percent, and questions about doctors and other health professionals came in fourth, at 47 percent. Drugs were fifth, at 45 percent.[10] A study the same year by Manhattan Research put the number of people who use the Internet for information on prescription drugs at ninety-four million, up from twenty-six million six years earlier.[11]

For better or worse, not only are Americans consumers of online health and medical information, but they also use what they find on the Internet to determine the choices they make about their care. In general, 57 percent of those who searched the Web for answers to health questions in 2008 indicated that doing so had an effect on their medical decisions, with 44 percent saying the impact was minor and 13 percent saying that it was major. A majority said that online research affected their treatment decisions (60 percent), "changed their overall approach to maintaining their health or the health of someone they help take care of" (56 percent), or led them to seek another medical opinion or more information from their doctor (53 percent). Also affected were health habits, chronic disease management, and the choice of whether to visit a medical professional.[12] According to a 2007 survey by the online advertising firm Prospective, 75 percent of users believe that the Web is "their most trusted and reliable resource for researching ailment and drug information."[13]

CONFIDENCE, CONVENIENCE, AND COMMUNITY

Americans turn to the Internet because it is easy and accessible, but they also do so because the health information they find online makes them feel empowered and in control. Many patients use the Internet because they want to learn about symptoms, understand a recent diagnosis, or explore treatments in order to interact knowledgeably with their doctors and be partners in their own health care. Doing so, they believe, will improve their care by ensuring that they receive the correct treatment, both medically and in terms of their goals, and avoid or mitigate side effects. In other cases, Americans seek to use knowledge gained online to be advocates for family members or friends or to help loved ones through a health problem.

In many cases, this is a good thing and can legitimately arm patients and health care consumers with valuable information. When Pew asked in 2006 how people felt during their Internet research, large percentages said they felt "reassured that they could make appropriate health care decisions" (74 percent), confident in talking to their doctors about health worries (56 percent), and "relieved or comforted by the information they found online" (56 percent). A quarter or fewer reported being "confused," "frustrated," "overwhelmed," or "frightened."[14] In 2008, Pew found that 41 percent of the Americans surveyed believed that what they'd discovered online benefited them and improved their treatment, while only 3 percent perceived themselves or those around them as having been injured by Internet information, a number that had not changed from earlier polls.[15]

People with life-threatening or long-term illnesses, a constituency called e-patients, are particularly frequent users of the Internet, to understand and further their care. An article in the *Journal of Health Communication* in March 2006 found that among people who had recently received the news that they had cancer, "Patients who used the Internet to gather health information were more likely than nonusers to be confident about participating in treatment decisions, asking questions, and sharing feelings of concern with their doctors."[16] Research has indicated that among patients with chronic problems, only around half access medical information online, but those who do both spend more time doing health research on the Web and are much more likely to change their behavior in response to what they find.[17] Recent medical emergencies or new diagnoses have an effect similar to chronic health problems, raising the percentage of patients who ask for a second opinion or seek more information from doctors as a consequence of Internet research from 48 percent to 59 percent. People in this group were also found to be 12 percent more likely to communicate the information they found online to others: 57 versus 45 percent.[18]

These trends are important because the chronically ill are not just a small minority of Internet users. In fact, an estimated 133 million adults, or about half the adult population of the United States, are afflicted with long-term conditions of varying degrees of severity, and many have more than one.[19] Furthermore, this number is rising for several reasons. First, due to advances in medicine, many diseases that once killed quickly, including cancer and HIV/AIDS, or that prevented children from living to adulthood have been turned into illnesses with which patients live for many years. Once-fatal injuries are also now survivable but may have lasting effects. Second, as life expectancy is extended, the elderly may spend decades dealing with multiple conditions that can be mitigated but not cured. Third, negative consequences of modern life, such as the rising prevalence of obesity, create long-term health issues and increase the likelihood of people developing secondary problems such as type-2 diabetes.

One result of this new medical landscape is that patient blogs, personal websites, and even Twitter streams now provide intimate coverage of daily life for patients with just about any condition you can name. Sites such as the Association of Cancer Online Resources (ACOR) and PatientsLikeMe host or link to dozens of patient communities and keep up on research and news. Online sites where users can talk with one another and ask questions have proved a boon for patients with serious or chronic ailments, since they provide firsthand experience and may be more up-to-date on the latest research and potential therapies than some doctors. Even specialist physicians find themselves overwhelmed by the thousands of articles in thousands of journals that come out every week, and the lag time between research and publication can be long. But new treatments are developed constantly, and the use of existing ones is always evolving; the one-time last-resort treatment may have become more common, the intolerable initial side effects may now have been mitigated, or a limited efficacy profile may have been expanded.

Participants also have far more time than busy doctors to help those facing bad news, to research new leads, or just to talk, so users of these sites get the personal touch that is often missing in the maze of clinical facilities and medical terminology confronting them in the real world. Personal expertise from fellow patients can also help when it comes to recognizing dangerous problems or early signs, or that an error in treatment has occurred. Certainly, few physicians, no matter how expert, can duplicate the insight of those who have lived with a disease and gone through treatments for it. Just feeling connected can improve patients' well-being and confidence, and the encouragement and advice they get online may make them more likely to stick to their treatment regimen, even if it is difficult, or voice concerns to their doctors that they might otherwise keep quiet about. Furthermore, these online communities are beginning to provide the basis of new "experimental interactive modules for managing chronic diseases" that bring together patients and medical professionals.[20] However, none of these benefits come without risks, as we will see.

Some physicians have jumped on the Internet bandwagon, too. Practices that use email, instant messaging, and other online resources to reach patients more efficiently are starting to spring up. Online consultations hold promise for making care more efficient for both parties by allowing patients to ask a quick question, find out whether a visit is indicated, or request a prescription refill without the time and hassle involved in coming in to the office. Furthermore, electronic communication may help patients voice their concerns, since it is less intimidating and gets them faster answers. The result may be better compliance with prescription dosage and administration and a way to catch problems at the first sign. In addition, new ways to communicate can help doctors and patients feel more connected to one another, and can aid patients in forging the partnership they crave. Increased use of electronic medical records, driven by federal incentives for their adoption, will further facilitate and support this trend.

Many of the offices most advanced in reaching out to patients through the Internet, however, are concierge practices that do not accept insurance and are therefore less tied into the existing paradigm of how medicine is practiced. A lot more doctors would move into these new communications methods (and many already participate in online health discussions on blogs, forums, and websites on their own time) but are impeded by a system in which they are not reimbursed by public or private payers for time spent dealing with patients outside the office setting. Web-based consultations also raise questions of privacy and confidentiality and concerns that doctors will miss important information by not having the patient physically present.

THE RISE OF CYBERCHONDRIA

The promise of Internet medicine is bright, but it also presents substantial risks. One concern is the accuracy of the information posted on websites or conveyed through online communities or blogs.

Online information can be alarmist or can overrepresent the potential for serious illness or side effects, and many websites represent an agenda that can be at odds with the existing scientific data or that distorts contemporary information in a way that is misleading and disingenuous. Furthermore, the online world is unfiltered and not moderated, providing no check on misinformation or even fraud, and it lets the ill-intentioned or merely ill-informed reach thousands of potentially vulnerable users. These elements are made worse by a lack of transparency about where Internet content comes from and by a lack of sufficient skepticism by those who turn to the Web for health facts.

Although Web users often say they are reassured by what they find online, Googling the symptoms of an illness has a dark side that many of us are deeply familiar with: cyberchondria. In November 2008, research by Microsoft showed that, as many have long believed, simple symptoms typed into search engines often point users to highly unlikely serious illnesses rather than to milder, more common causes. In one section of the study, the authors inputted "muscle twitches" into three types of Web searches: a Web crawl, a general search engine (Live Search), and a specialized search engine (MSN Health and Fitness). The results linked the symptom to amyotrophic lateral sclerosis (Lou Gehrig's disease) in 7 percent of cases for the Web crawl and a whopping 50 percent for the general search engine, but not at all for the specialized search engine.

In fact, the real probability that ALS was the cause of the muscle twitching was tiny, way below even the 7 percent returned by the Web crawl. A milder explanation, benign fasciculation, was mentioned by 53, 12, and 34 percent of returned sites for the Web crawl, general search engine, and specialized search site, respectively, and another likely cause, muscle strain, by 40, 38, and 66 percent, respectively.[21] Microsoft obtained similar results with a search for "headache," with many sites indicating that the symptom could be the result of a brain tumor. As one of the authors of the study remarked, "People tend to look at just the first couple results ... If they find 'brain tumor' or 'ALS,' that's their launching point."[22]

Not only are these results misleading, but many people are too quick to perceive them as indicative of the actual probability of a given illness. When Microsoft polled around five hundred of its own employees, 50.9 percent said they regularly or occasionally "consider the ranking of Web search results as indicating the likelihood of the illnesses, with more likely diseases appearing higher up on the result page(s)." In addition, 24.5 percent said yes to the question "Have you ever used Web search as a medical expert system where you input symptoms and expect to review possible diseases ranked by likelihood?" Even when users did not see the Internet as a medical opinion, they were likely to overestimate the likelihood of the worst possible explanations.[23]

While arguably cyberchondria merely sends patients running to their doctor's office, it can produce unhealthy worry and stress and make some patients wary of their own physicians, convinced that their doctor is not being honest with them. Cyberchondria also forces patients to spend money on a doctor's visit that might be unnecessary and makes doctors devote scarce time to deflating patients' Internet-fueled fears when the real cause may go away on its own.

But perhaps more immediately dangerous is information on the risks of drugs and treatments that has proliferated online in a similar way. Just as Internet searches tend to overstate the likelihood of the more serious cause for simple symptoms, they also overemphasize the dangers of side effects and harm from medications and procedures. Like ALS and brain tumors, the serious side effects of FDA-approved drugs are rare—sometimes very, very rare—yet many patients attribute all symptoms they experience while on a drug to the medication. This is especially true because side effects listed on the label may also have many other causes, unrelated to the drug. In other cases, cyberchondria uses the power of suggestion to make patients believe they have developed a feared side effect.

Consequently, physicians have repeatedly reported that they are seeing a rising number of patients who are worried about drugs or other treatments based on information uncovered on the Web. In some cases, doctors are facing enormous patient pressure due to incomplete or incorrect understanding of the data on benefits and risks. Dr. Randy Fink, an obstetrician/gynecologist in Miami, Florida, told the media in 2007:

> Every day, I spend time undoing damage done by patients reading faulty or misleading information from the Internet. I am fond of telling patients that the Internet is the world's biggest bathroom wall. It is a natural tendency to either over-interpret or under-interpret information about one's health, so there is no substitution for an objective opinion from a clinician who knows your personal history.[24]

The emergence of fears about drugs such as Vioxx has increased fear about medications in general and led to an expansion of sites stoking such fears. In a poll sponsored by Pfizer in March 2008, 89 percent of the doctors questioned said they worried that if concerns about drugs were publicized prematurely then patients would quit taking prescribed medications.[25] Patients do not always speak to their physicians before discontinuing drugs and may refuse to resume the treatment or switch to a similar one.

Too much Googling can also increase nonadherence to medication regimens or reduce office visits if patients are scared of following their physician's advice due to online information. Furthermore, Internet-induced fear can lead to frantic visits to other doctors or "diagnosis shopping."

HIDDEN MOTIVES ON THE INTERNET

Not only can patients be scared needlessly by Internet research but an untrained user who is making health care decisions based on Google results will find a plethora of material of questionable worth. And in much the way that our email boxes are filled with spam urging us to collect millions by helping Nigerian princes or asking us to confirm our banking information from phony eBay or Bank of America security sites, much of the medical information on the Web is designed to sell, deceive, or frighten, rather than inform. Those who promote these biased answers are many and varied: "Well-intentioned individuals may provide information based on personal experience; quacks promote unproved remedies giving false hope and inaccurate information about outcomes; cranks have some scientific background but are disenchanted with traditional science; most alarming are charlatans who 'engage' in fraudulent practices with the intent to deceive."[26] Americans seeking online health information must be aware that the motives and intentions of those on the Internet are not always pure. Medical advice and research websites may be operating under the influence of special interests and politics that may not be immediately visible to the average online health information seeker. Unfortunately, "science and snake oil may not always look all that different on the Net."[27]

Even more troubling, the majority of individuals researching health information on the Internet are not appropriately scrutinizing the sites they find. "Fully three-quarters of health seekers say they check the source and date 'only sometimes,' 'hardly ever,' or 'never,' which translates to about 85 million Americans gathering health advice online without consistently examining the quality indicators of the information they find." Half of the people polled fall into the "hardly ever" and "never" categories, with greater education making people more likely to check the site's source. This is compounded by the fact that many sites make details about who writes the content, when it was updated, and who sponsors the website difficult to find or fail to include such information at all.[28]

Much of the medical misinformation online comes from three types of sites: alternative medicine pages, litigator-run or -affiliated sites, and anti-industry groups. Many operate largely through fearmongering, attributing every possible negative side effect to a given treatment, and exaggerating real risks. Industry critics may produce highly credible-seeming websites, often casting themselves as consumer advocates or safety activists in order to conceal the fact that their agenda is political rather than scientific. Similarly, lawyers may present themselves as interested solely in obtaining justice for wronged patients or may create sites that seem objective—except for the links to litigators seeking patients for class action suits. Alternative medicine sites mix scare stories about conventional drugs and procedures with hyperbolic claims about the efficacy of various herbs and diets. They are in the business of miracle cures and usually have dozens of glowing testimonials that prey on the hopes of patients.

To determine what patients typically see when searching for information on prescriptions drugs that are in the headlines, in 2007 the Center for Medicine in the Public Interest took a snapshot of the first three pages of Google search results on two controversial drugs, Crestor and Avandia. Since a 2005 Pew study places the average depth of a search at 1.9 pages, the sample threshold of 3 pages (30 individual sites) used by CMPI thus allowed for a wide range of results without surpassing the limits of content that an average user would view.[29] CMPI used Google because it accounted for 65 percent of all online searches in the United States in 2007 (and would make up 71 percent of queries in 2008).[30] This places the search engine in an enormous position of power. Companies can be made or broken based on where their sites fall on a Google search results page. Similarly, the sites a Google search returns for a patient looking for information on medications can greatly influence prescription patterns and patient decisions. It is no wonder then that many companies and organizations pay extra or manipulate Google results to make sure their site appears at the top of the page. Three other commonly used search engines, Yahoo!, MSN Search, and AOL, make up 42 percent, 20 percent, and 15 percent of medical searches, respectively.[31]

The results of CMPI's search produced unequivocal results. The think tank found that the information displayed in search engine results was not only misleading and confusing, but potentially dangerous for patients. An analysis of search results revealed that online real estate was dominated by websites paid for and sponsored by either class action law firms or legal marketing sites searching for plaintiff referrals. Other sites belonged to groups or individuals selling alternative medicines. With few exceptions, the information online was presented in a way that made the sites appear legitimate although they had no medical authority whatsoever.

For this analysis, CMPI divided the sites into seven groups, reflecting the results of a typical online search of a high-profile prescription-related medical topic.

1. **Official government or pharmaceutical sites**—These sites are among the best sources for online information on medical topics. Although it may seem counterintuitive to some people to look to pharmaceutical companies' official sites for sound information, both types of sites are carefully scrutinized for accuracy, and companies who give misleading or even confusing information can get hit with stiff fines.

2. **Reputable medical and professional organizations**—Websites such as those of the American Heart Association or the American Cancer Society represent another good source for health information. They have earned a reputation of trust and credibility and often feature links to peer-reviewed medical journals or the recommendations and conclusions of medical professionals.

3. **Impartial news/database sites**—Information pulled from news sites should be carefully evaluated. While the information found there may be valuable, it may not necessarily reflect the conclusions and points of view of the medical community as a whole. The articles may be chosen based on their ability to attract readers, as opposed to their containing sound research, or may lead to misunderstandings due to the lack of science backgrounds on the part of their authors.

4. **Forums or blogs**—Blogs represent the personal point(s) of view of one or more people. They are not objective sources of information. Forums contain the opinions of any number of individuals, and those participating in these discussions may be patients, physicians, and even attorneys or activists. Any information found on such sites should be verified using credible sources, and users should be wary of supposedly scientific content presented without citations that would allow it to be confirmed.

5. **Anti-pharmaceutical activist sites**—There are a number of groups online that for various reasons pursue an anti-pharmaceutical agenda. Individuals searching for health information should pay extra attention when evaluating inflammatory statements about medications. These attacks may be rooted in an ideological view rather than in sound science.

6. **Alternative treatment sites**—Another class of sites which users should be wary of are those that offer information on alternative treatments. Such sites often have financial interests in selling herbal remedies or other products. Opting for such treatments without consulting a trained physician may result in medical complications or allow serious problems to go unchecked.

7. **Class action/litigation sites**—A new technique for gathering parties for class action lawsuits is to create websites that patients will find when searching for medical advice. Such sites

cannot be relied upon for balanced and accurate information, and any site that provides links to class action firms should not be trusted.

CRESTOR

The first drug for which CMPI examined Google results was Crestor, one of a class of drugs called statins. It was approved by the FDA in 2003 to treat high cholesterol and to slow the progression of athero-sclerosis (hardening of the arteries), both of which can lead to heart disease. Dozens of clinical trials have concluded that Crestor is safe and effective. Nearly 2,400 Americans die of cardiovascular disease each day, an average of one death every 36 seconds, and the disease claims more lives each year than cancer, chronic lower respiratory diseases, accidents, and diabetes mellitus combined.[32]

Statins are especially important because just a 10 percent decrease in total cholesterol levels (population-wide) may result in an estimated 30 percent reduction in the incidence of coronary heart disease, and it is estimated that, in 2007, the direct and indirect costs of cardiovascular disease in the United States added up to $431.8 billion.[33] Heart disease, cholesterol, and atherosclerosis are, in many cases, preventable diseases, but fewer than half of the people who qualify for any kind of lipid-modifying treatment for coronary heart disease are actually receiving it.[34]

However, a fretful patient Googling the drug may not readily find information on Crestor's benefits or the extensive positive safety data on the drug. On the first three pages of results for a search for "Crestor side effects," a full 47 percent (nearly half) of the results were from class action/litigation sources and another 14 percent were from anti-pharma activists or alternative medicine practitioners (7 percent each). In contrast, 17 percent came from official government or pharmaceutical pages. Another 17 percent were drawn from news or database sites, which are good preliminary sources but are written for, and usually

Online Environment for Crestor*

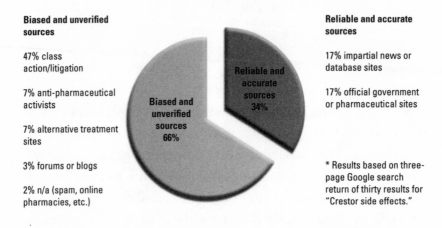

Biased and unverified sources

47% class action/litigation

7% anti-pharmaceutical activists

7% alternative treatment sites

3% forums or blogs

2% n/a (spam, online pharmacies, etc.)

Reliable and accurate sources

17% impartial news or database sites

17% official government or pharmaceutical sites

* Results based on three-page Google search return of thirty results for "Crestor side effects."

by, nonmedical personnel and can be inaccurate, misleading, or sensationalistic. Overall, 66 percent of the resulting sites were biased and unverified sources, and only 34 percent were reasonably reliable and accurate sites—and even then, most of them would require caution and careful checking on the part of the user. A search of the Crestor online environment thus clearly indicates that Americans who go online are finding mostly information which is intentionally biased, tainted, or misleading.

Much of the available information found online regarding Crestor can be characterized as the replication and repetition of a single complaint submitted to the FDA by Public Citizen, an anti-pharmaceutical industry group. Dr. Sidney Wolfe, director of Public Citizen's Health Research Group, has insisted that Crestor is unacceptably dangerous because it carries a rare and reversible risk of muscle damage and kidney problems.[35] The FDA and data in clinical trials flatly contradict Public Citizen's contention.[36] In fact, an FDA reevaluation of Crestor data (following a petition by Public Citizen to restrict or remove the drug from the market) reconfirmed that the medication is safe.[37]

In addition, a 2008 study suggests that the benefits of the drug are broader than initially thought and that it may help even those who do not have high "bad" cholesterol but who have another risk factor: high C-reactive protein.[38] In response to these results, which showed a 44 percent drop in cardiovascular issues in this group of patients, in December 2009 an FDA panel backed wider use of Crestor to reduce stroke and heart attack, even in patients whose cholesterol was still in the healthy range.[39] Two months later, the FDA followed suit and gave formal approval for increased use of the medication.[40] The lack of availability of complete information on Crestor on the Internet may make patients who would benefit from the drug reluctant to accept a prescription for a statin from their doctors or could lead to non-adherence to a recommended cholesterol drug regime.

AVANDIA

The same picture emerged when the test was repeated for another drug, called Avandia, which was approved by the FDA in 1999 for treatment of type-2 diabetes, a serious and life-threatening disease that affects about eighteen to twenty million Americans,[41] a number that is on the rise in the United States and in other countries. Having type-2 diabetes increases the risk of many serious complications, including heart disease, blindness, nerve damage, kidney problems, and limb amputation.[42] The total annual economic cost of diabetes in 2007 was estimated to be $174 billion, and the per capita annual health care costs incurred for people with diabetes were $11,744. That is 2.3 times the cost for those without diabetes. One out of every ten health care dollars spent in the United States is spent on diabetes and its complications.[43]

But a search for "Avandia side effects" in 2007 resulted in 65 percent of sites from biased sources, with 40 percent of those sites created by personal injury lawyers and another 12 percent representing forums or blogs where anyone can say anything. On the other side, news sites represented 28 percent of the search results, and official government and pharmaceutical sites, 7 percent.

Online Environment for Avandia*

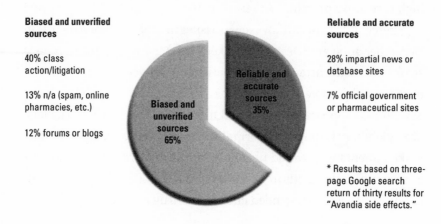

Biased and unverified sources

40% class action/litigation

13% n/a (spam, online pharmacies, etc.)

12% forums or blogs

Reliable and accurate sources

28% impartial news or database sites

7% official government or pharmaceutical sites

* Results based on three-page Google search return of thirty results for "Avandia side effects."

Again, the information our search found online regarding Avandia centered on a single unfavorable source. In May 2007, Dr. Steven Nissen submitted an article based on a six-day meta-analysis of publicly available studies on Avandia to the *New England Journal of Medicine*. Nissen's article was given special, expedited peer review and was published that same month. The piece was accompanied by an editorial commissioned from two long-standing critics of the FDA's post-approval regulation of drugs, Drs. Bruce M. Psaty and Curt D. Furberg, who believed that the agency was lax in reacting to information suggesting new risks. The respect afforded to the *New England Journal of Medicine* resulted in instant credibility for the article. Relatively few questions were raised about the expedited peer review process or the fact that the study was compiled in only six days. That single article elicited a flurry of congressional action and exploded onto the radar of the media, both traditional and online, and quickly dominated Internet sites discussing Avandia.

The accusations leveled at the drug and the inflammatory language used by Dr. Nissen had dramatic results. By September 2007, Avandia prescriptions had declined by about 60 percent, but there was no corresponding increase in the use of other drugs for diabetes, indicating that some patients who had stopped taking Avandia had not replaced it in their drug regimens.[44] In a statement to the House Committee on Oversight and Government Reform, FDA commissioner Andrew C. von Eschenbach, MD, advised, "It would be counterproductive indeed if patients stopped taking rosiglitazone [Avandia] to avoid a small and potential increased heart risk, only to incur a much greater risk from their underlying diabetes."[45]

Yet, that is exactly what happened. Doctors reported, "Patients have already formed their own opinions based on press reports of this study. In many cases, I have a tough time pushing a patient toward something they're already afraid of based on lay press awareness."[46] According to the Centers for Disease Control, the percentage of people on oral diabetes medications declined 5 percent between 2007 and 2009, and the percentage of diabetics on any medications also dropped in 2007 after rising steadily for the previous decade. Meanwhile, the proportion of Americans diagnosed with diabetes has steadily increased.[47]

Nissen's attacks on Avandia have not abated in the ensuing years. Two large trials of Avandia, ACCORD and RECORD, had both found no link between Avandia and more heart attacks or deaths, but critics of the drug were far from satisfied. In 2010, a few months before an FDA advisory committee panel was to review additional clinical trial information about Avandia's risks and benefits, Nissen leaked to the *New York Times* a set of tapes he had secretly recorded of conversations he had with Glaxo executives in 2007 prior to the release of his *NEJM* article. Although the tapes contained nothing new or explosive, despite Nissen's allegations otherwise, the newspaper ran a story alleging that Glaxo executives had tried to pressure Nissen into not publishing his study.

The article was timed to run just after the release of a U.S. Senate Finance Committee investigation charging that Glaxo "threatened scientists who tried to point out Avandia's risks, and internal memorandums from the Food and Drug Administration show that some government health officials want Avandia withdrawn."[48] The message emerging from the Senate Finance Committee report was that Glaxo-SmithKline had hidden the fact that Avandia carried a cardiovascular risk. However, these claims were part of the conspiracy narrative advanced by Nissen and another safety zealot, David Graham, that alleged that Avandia killed people.

As the FDA advisory committee meeting came closer, the campaign against Avandia increased further. A second *New York Times* article, which ran one day before the committee convened, alleged that Glaxo "hid" data on tests showing that "not only was Avandia no better than Actos, but ... also ... that it was riskier to the heart."[49] Both Nissen and Graham published new studies maligning the drug, both of which became available online just days before the meeting.[50] In fact, neither article revealed anything new about Avandia or was able to demonstrate more than a small additional risk. Nissen's update of his 2007 meta-analysis had all the same problems as the original, while Graham's comparison of Avandia with Actos use post-hoc analyses to try to produce the results he wanted and failed to sufficiently account for changes in Avandia prescriptions after 2007. Most concerningly, both Nissen and Graham neglected to look at changes in patients' blood sugar, making it impossible to judge how successful the drug was in achieving its purpose and therefore preventing real discussion of Avandia's balance of risk and benefit.

Ultimately, the FDA advisory committee voted 20-12 to keep Avandia on the market, while also asking for additional warnings and restrictions on the drug's use. Its decision was an acknowledgment that the clinical data on the drug continue to show that, although Avandia may carry a slightly higher risk of a heart attack in a small group of patients, this danger is outweighed by benefits for most patients. Nissen and Graham have not succeeded this time in forcing a useful drug off the market, but the latest controversy over Avandia continues to highlight a troubling trend in medical science: the legitimization of campaigns—using medical journals as a platform—that are designed to generate headlines or advance a political agenda.

Ultimately, such attacks scare off both potential patients and doctors who might prescribe the drug, not because of the medication's safety but because of its reputation.[51]

Crestor and Avandia are but two examples of drugs unfairly vilified on the Internet, often because of a single report or study that may have been poorly done or poorly understood. While the exact percentages may change and certain biased groups are more active in some areas than in others, the general pictures is clear: Internet searches turn up far more inaccurate information than they do facts you can trust. For charlatans and critics, websites are a cost-effective means of reaching more people than was ever possible in the pre-Web age. This is made worse by the fact that many websites may look credible, and most Internet searchers do not know how to look for concealed bias or are not willing to take the time to do so.

Biased and misleading sources are dangerous not only because of the incorrect information they disseminate but because, as we will see in the next chapter, they dominate the online environment and, in doing so, create an echo chamber in which their other views cannot be heard. The influence of such actors works like a series of gears: each turns the other and amplifies the dubious material found online. A striking feature is that no consistent catalyst drives the process; different groups can be found at the center depending on the issue. The result is a widespread dispersal of biased or inaccurate information throughout the online community.

THE DANGERS OF GOOD INTENTIONS

People with hidden agendas are not the only risk involved in trusting online information. In addition, the Internet gives a soapbox to people who may mean well but who lack medical training or scientific knowledge and who give advice based on nothing but their own experience. In general, the Internet tends to elevate anecdotes above sound medical studies, especially in the context of communities and boards in which people ask questions and exchange ideas. As I discussed in chapter 1, human beings are programmed to give extra weight to events that they have personally experienced, that happened to people they know, or even that they have recently heard about. This phenomenon is called *availability bias* because such risks are more available in the forefront of our minds, and it leads people to inflate the likelihood of an event they fear and underestimate the probability of alternative scenarios. The result may be that a patient is terrified she is developing breast cancer because her friend was just diagnosed, while ignoring the fact that she has strong risk factors for lung cancer.

This can mean that patients refuse to take a new drug because a fellow e-patient had a bad reaction to it or they believe they will be cured by an unproven treatment because someone they met online claimed miraculous improvement. This is especially dangerous when unverifiable personal stories found online persuade patients to discount the recommendations of a doctor or the statistical results of scientific studies. Humans also naturally tend to blur correlation and causation, attributing one event to another because they occurred in sequence or around the same time. So patients may believe that a treatment worked because symptoms improved after they started on that treatment, even if the condition would have gotten better anyway, or if other therapies were being used simultaneously. And they may then spread this belief to others through the Web.

Online communities do offer valuable support to people struggling with a serious illness or looking for answers from others who have been there themselves, but the frequent anonymity and the unfiltered nature of the information, two attributes that draw some to these online message boards, also mean that there is no check on misrepresentation and inaccuracy. The vast majority of participants are also not medical professionals, and the best or worst outcomes may be overrepresented, offering a distorted view of the prognosis for people with a given condition. The flip side of exhaustive attention to new treatments and emerging information on existing ones is that benefits may be overstated and risks minimized—or vice versa. Patients may also be encouraged or inspired to demand access to treatments that are not appropriate for them or try to circumvent scientific procedures governing access to experimental drugs.

The ultimate danger of Internet searching—particularly for information about risks and benefits—is that there is no arbiter of truth to let users know whether what they are being told is accurate.[52] Rather, "the Web has become the world's largest vanity press, allowing anyone with Internet access to act as an author and publisher of material on any subject."[53] If research is gathered in a vacuum, without the benefit of input from a credible physician or certification of the information from an official medical organization, such as the FDA or the American College of Cardiology, the results can be dangerous. This is especially true of chronic or life-threatening conditions, where fear can be high and treatments may be limited. For instance, *The Oncologist* expressed concern in a July 2006 article that cancer patients made a vulnerable audience for untested and inefficacious alternative treatments promoted through the Internet.[54] Some patients are aware of these pitfalls but are willing to "just take a leap of faith," as one woman with ovarian cancer said of her interaction with other patients via the Internet. While this is understandable, it can also be damaging to their health.[55]

Finally, even when the information found online is sound, the ability of patients to understand the science involved may be limited, especially in a case of papers and presentations directed at a medically trained audience. Internet users tend to bridle when their health literacy is questioned, but such concerns are not reflective of a belief that consumers of online content are stupid or inferior. Rather, they are an acknowledgment of the reality that doctors and scientists undergo years of training to do their jobs, and that process cannot be duplicated by a few clicks of the mouse. Most of us do not expect to understand the inner workings of the electronics that fill our homes, including the computer on which we access the Web, without any instruction, so why should we expect to comprehend medical studies, replete with statistics and specialized language, without a single lesson?

Even when Web users turn to journal articles, studies about the risks and benefits of treatments can and do diverge in terms of quality and accuracy. Increasingly, the scientific articles that make it to the top of an Internet search or that end up widely cited on websites, blogs, and news sites, are not carefully designed studies of people receiving care. Rather, they often consist of meta-analyses (studies that reanalyze data from previous studies with a particular question or goal in mind), surveys, or epidemiological exercises that fail to control for all the relevant variables. They may, therefore, reflect a bias toward the Precautionary Principle and fail to take into account the range of benefits and risks.

Furthermore, a significant percentage of Internet users have only a high school education—or less. Others are not native English speakers. As a consequence, since even sites directed at the public may require high levels of literacy, they are especially difficult to understand for exactly those who are most in need of sound medical advice and who are the least able to access a doctor about concerns.[56] One study evaluating information on health care sites in both English and Spanish concluded that high school or greater reading comprehension was needed to understand all or the vast majority of sites in both languages.[57] Poor literacy also reduces users' ability to tell accurate information from inaccurate and to unearth concealed biases within the material.

EMPOWERMENT?

The proliferation of "empowered" patients is also not without its shadows. The presence of Google has made some patients believe that they are experts, even in areas in which they have no training, and has led them to dismiss the knowledge of doctors and scientists. For some, empowerment doesn't mean forging a cooperative relationship with doctors and other health care providers, but dictating terms and making decisions—whatever the medical recommendation—based upon information that confirms existing beliefs or concerns. Despite the many problems and pitfalls of Internet health information, too many Americans have come to see online sources as more authoritative than the clinical judgment of their own physicians. And when they choose to follow the advice of websites instead of that of their own doctors, they achieve just the opposite of empowerment and imperil their health.

Kelton Research found in July 2008 that 85.6 million Americans, or 38 percent of adults, had "doubted the opinion of their doctors or other medical professionals when it conflict[ed] with information found online." And that figure rose to 43 percent in the eighteen to thirty-four age group.[58] Those with chronic conditions were especially likely to act on the results of Internet searches, even without discussing them with a medical professional: 75 percent of this group said they did so versus 55 percent of the general Internet population.[59] Many physicians report that patients come to appointments with dozens of printed out Web pages. Others say that Internet information leads some patients to reject diagnoses and prescriptions because they are convinced they have a different illness or that the drug they were given is dangerous. Refusing to comply with the demands of such patients may prompt anger and the departure of the patient to another physician. Patients who refuse to listen to their doctors are undermining the very foundation of the partnership they claim they want and making themselves not empowered but vulnerable to anyone who tells them what they want to hear.

In 2002, Carina von Koop and her colleagues classified patients into four types: In Control, Involved, Informed, and Accepting. At that time, they estimated that the In Control, who "believe in making their own medical choices and will often insist on managing their own medical tests and treatments in the ways they think best, even if their clinicians disagree," were about 4 percent of the population, but this number has probably increased precipitously over the years. Also probably more prevalent today are those who fall into the Involved and Informed categories, who are knowledgeable about their disease and the treatment options and who participate in their care but leave the ultimate decisions, to varying degrees, to the doctor. In 2002, it was estimated that around 24 percent of the patient population were Involved and about 55 percent were Informed.[60] The benefit of the Internet is in increasing the ranks of the Involved and Informed categories, allowing more patients to understand their treatment and work with their doctors, but Web searching often changes from a positive to a problem when Googling patients enter the In Control group.

Doctors are not altogether innocent in the way the relationship between physicians and patients is evolving. They have, in some cases, been dismissive of the information patients have found on their own and possessive of their own authority. Doctors today must be prepared to have a dialogue with patients, not just to hand down pronouncements, and should realize that, when used properly, the Internet can produce informed, knowledgeable patients. They must also be willing to engage the information found online and explain why it is or is not valid, despite the constraints placed upon them by increasingly short office visits. But the patients, in turn, must be ready to listen to their doctors and recognize that partnerships are not inherently equal. Dr. Rahul K. Parikh summarized the situation well when he wrote in his blog, "We all agree that patients don't like to be treated like children, talked down to, or told to just 'take two of these and call me later.' But doctors don't like to be treated like waiters—taking orders from a menu prepared by the patient."[61]

USER BEWARE

Charlatans selling spurious cures and false panaceas are hardly an innovation of the twenty-first century, and medical misinformation has been passed from person to person for eons. After all, our culture is replete with old wives' tales and bizarre home remedies, ranging from swallowing a teaspoon of kerosene to cure a cold to sleeping with a bar of soap to prevent leg cramps to eating raisins soaked in gin to treat arthritis. But what makes today's trends especially worrying is their reach; the snake oil salesman of a century past did not connect with millions of people every day. As a result of its potential for harm, concerns about Internet health information have existed almost as long as the Web itself and have been the subject of scholarly debate in the medical community since at least the mid- to late-1990s, when the number of Web users was much lower and turning to Google for answers to medical questions was still a nascent trend. As the use of online sources for health information has become more and more prevalent, so have the worries about the content that users are finding and how it is being used. Among teenagers today, 95 percent are online, and there are already indications of cyberchondria in children, for whom Googling is a natural reaction to uncertainty or worry.[62] Nor is the rest of the world exempt. Rather, patterns in Europe and Japan resemble those in the United States.[63]

The rise of the Internet as an all-purpose and highly trusted source for medical knowledge reflects an environment where traditional sources of medical authority have been eroded, not only doctors but also government agencies.[64] These patterns are part of a larger societal shift in which old bastions of knowledge are being devalued and the advice of the amateur, the man on the street, is being increasingly emphasized and esteemed. As one commentator put it, "In the age of Web 2.0, authoritative expertise is slowly waning. The layman reasserts herself as a fount of collective mob 'wisdom.' Information—unsorted, raw, sometimes wrong—substitutes for structured, meaningful knowledge. Gatekeepers—intellectuals, academics, scientists, and editors ... are summarily and rudely dispensed with."[65]

The Internet has democratized knowledge through not only Google and Wikipedia but also the multiplicity of blogs and individual websites. Perhaps the most worrying aspect of this evolution is that the cult of the amateur places little weight on accuracy, and online commentators authoritatively proclaim information that is untrue or half-true—some out of ignorance or confusion; some, deliberately. The very concept of truth is alternately deified by people in search of absolute answers (and those who claim to provide them) and diminished by those who try to cast all perspectives as equally valid. Knowledge has all too often become relative and mutable, determined by majority vote rather objective evidence. In chapter 5, we will show how groups use these online realities to create instant experts to promote their viewpoints, often drawing on those who have little or no formal expertise but who possess marketing savvy, celebrity, or simply an intractable belief.

As a culture, we are increasingly prone to want answers instantaneously. But when it comes to obtaining advice on medical decisions, going online may not be the wisest course of action. In most cases, there is no better resource than a trained physician who knows an individual's health history. Online information can add tremendous value for patients when used as a research tool for discussions with a doctor, but users should be aware of the sources of the information they find online and the possible ulterior motives of site owners. In particular, they should beware of sites or links that seek to compel a choice based on the immediate and rare risks of a treatment, even if seemingly supported by scientific study.

Internet medicine is a reality that requires all of us to learn to navigate its benefits and its risks, not only patients and doctors but also companies and government agencies. We no longer have the choice to ignore it and hope it will go away, we must instead become increasingly aware of how we make choices about risks and benefits and what type of information will allow us to think about all the implications of a treatment decision, not just the first or most prominent site or YouTube video we come across. Much information on the Web is there for a purpose: to encourage decisions based on the Precautionary Principle and to promote the view that technological and new medical products are harming nature and our health. And decisions based on this perception have a direct impact on our own health and that of society.

CHAPTER 4

A Damaging Precedent:
The Side Effects of the Vioxx Panic

IKE THOUSANDS OF PEOPLE with multiple sclerosis, Lissa Gifford, aged forty-five, had to struggle against her body and brain to feel what she touched, to walk from one room to another, to taste food. And since the disease would recede and then roar back without warning, worse than before, the intervening days or weeks would be filled with fear and anxiety about a future onset or episode. When she was first diagnosed, Lissa's neurologist put her on a series of drugs, none of which alleviated her symptoms. Lissa even pursued alternative therapies, such as bee stings, to no avail. Ultimately, she had to abandon her doctoral work at Brandeis University as a result of her worsening illness.

So when a new drug called Tysabri was immediately approved by the Food and Drug Administration after a clinical trial showed significant improvement in MS patients who had failed to respond to other drugs, Lissa sought out treatment. She recalls, "Within three days of my first infusion, I could feel my fingers and toes again. My toes went off in 1986. Within the week, I swam for half a mile. Now, I go up and down the stairs, I go grocery shopping whenever I want to, I can put on mascara, I can stand on one foot."

Yet almost as soon as the drug was approved, it was suddenly pulled off the market. Three people on Tysabri had died after contracting PML, an extremely rare virus that is more likely to affect people with severely weakened immune systems, such as those with HIV or Crohn's disease. The FDA and Biogen, the company that developed the drug, decided less than six months after Tysabri was available to withdraw it, leaving thousands of patients, including Lissa, without the medicine that had given them back their lives. Lissa's condition quickly deteriorated. She again lost feeling in her feet and toes. She could no longer swim or put on mascara. And the doctoral studies she wanted to resume were put on hold once more.[1]

Tysabri's withdrawal had little to do with the safety of the drug. Rather, the medication—and the people with MS who were using it— had the bad luck that the rare deaths took place on the eve of congressional hearings about the risks of Vioxx, the painkiller pulled from the market two months earlier, on September 30, 2004, based on data that showed it raised the risk of cardiovascular complications. The inquiry, led by Senator Charles Grassley, claimed that the problems with Vioxx were the result of the FDA's willingness to be misled and manipulated by industry-generated studies that hid the true dangers from an unsuspecting public for the sake of profit. As one former FDA drug safety reviewer who was closely involved in the Tysabri approval told me, "The decision to take the drug off the market was purely a reaction to the politics and fear surrounding Vioxx. Meanwhile, thousands of people who had no other effective MS treatment suffered, and thousands more are now avoiding a medication that is highly safe and using others that could have more side effects."

Tysabri was eventually returned to the market, but it took a year and a half, and it was reintroduced only after patients packed an FDA meeting on the issue demanding its return and the company agreed to implement a strict monitoring and tracking program. Meanwhile, many other drugs for MS that had a higher incidence of side effects, including leukemia, were kept on the market. Tysabri was one of the first drugs to fall victim to the Vioxx panic, but it was far from the last, that the controversy would claim. Vioxx changed the very landscape of medicine and health policy—becoming a symbol for those that thought any risk was too much and a template for future fights over drug safety.

THE BEGINNING OF THE VIOXX SCANDAL

Prior to the late 1990s, for some arthritis patients, relief came at a price: traditional anti-inflammatory and pain drugs, called non-steroidal anti-inflammatory drugs, or NSAIDs, improved their pain but, in susceptible persons, also caused irritation and damage to the lining of the stomach and small bowel, which in turn could lead to ulcers and bleeding. In some cases, these complications were severe enough to require major surgery and could even be fatal. About 4.5 million people who have arthritis are in danger of developing gastrointestinal bleeding or other complications.

Commonly used over-the-counter drugs such as aspirin, ibuprofen (Advil), and naproxen (Aleve) all fall into the NSAID category, as do many stronger prescription drugs for arthritis. Gastrointestinal-adverse events are not a negligible risk; 2 to 4 percent of people who take NSAIDs for the long term may develop such complications, well above the percentage that had cardiovascular problems on Vioxx. As many as 16,500 Americans, or 1 in 1,200 people taking NSAIDs for two months or more, may die from gastrointestinal events every year. More than 100,000 end up in the hospital.[2] In addition, several large studies found that the ulcers and bleeding caused by NSAIDs, even when it did not lead to hospitalization, caused persistent pain and a reduced quality of life.

However, in the early 1990s, scientists began making new discoveries about the COX enzyme, a protein linked to both pain reduction and protection of the stomach lining. They found that there were two types of COX, both of which were blocked by NSAIDs. While COX-1 helps to prevent damage to the gastrointestinal system, COX-2 is involved in inflammation, giving the drugs their ability to help arthritis patients.[3] The research culminated in the introduction of COX-2 inhibition drugs, commonly referred to as coxibs. They were believed to provide all the benefits of pain reduction without the ill effects of ulcers or other gastrointestinal complications because they blocked only COX-2 and left COX-1 alone.

Indeed, after COX-2 inhibitor drugs entered the market, the number of people in the hospital for NSAID-caused stomach bleeding went down 8 percent.[4] The first coxib to receive FDA approval was Pfizer's Celebrex, on December 31, 1998, followed closely by Vioxx on May 20, 1999. From its introduction, Vioxx was a huge success. By 2003, despite heavy competition with Celebrex and other lesser known coxibs, it reached sales of $2.5 billion, accounting for 11 percent of Merck's total revenue.[5] It was also, at the time of the recall, one of the world's top twenty best selling and most prescribed medicines.[6]

The "narrative" about Vioxx is that Merck kept the risks of its product carefully hidden. But even before the first coxib was placed on the market, the scientific literature suggested the possibility of increased heart problems for those on the drugs. In the mid-1980s, before scientists understood about the existence of two types of COX, pharmacologist Garret FitzGerald demonstrated that COX potentially served to inhibit clotting in the blood. He theorized that blocking the enzyme might raise the likelihood of complications such as stroke and heart attack.

More than a decade later, FitzGerald told Merck, during the pre-approval studies on Vioxx, that the COX-2 inhibitor could increase clotting in patients, and the company initiated a new evaluation of its information on the drug's safety, taking into account FitzGerald's concerns.[7] Nonetheless, at the time of Vioxx's introduction, FitzGerald's theory was still just that. During the early 2000s, he continued to study the effect of COX-2 on clotting and whether this actually increased cardiovascular complications.[8] Even today, exactly why coxibs seem to have cardiovascular side effects is a subject of some scientific dispute.

Moreover, as Vioxx began to be prescribed by doctors, research about the risks and benefits of the drug in real-world settings appeared in medical journals. The patients placed on a new COX-2-specific inhibitor were those who had a greater lifetime history of adverse reactions of all kinds, but particularly gastrointestinal complications. They also had higher pain scores, greater "functional disability, fatigue, helplessness, and global severity," and were higher consumers of inpatient and outpatient care when compared to patients who did not switch to COX-2-specific inhibitors.[9] Furthermore, COX-2 inhibitors were prescribed particularly to patients who were at an increased baseline risk of cardiovascular events compared with patients prescribed nonspecific NSAIDs, and physicians were aware that all COX-2 drugs, like other NSAIDs, carried a small risk of pulmonary edema.[10]

VIGOR

When Vioxx was approved by the FDA in the spring of 1999, the agency did not have any concerns about the drug, and clinical trials did not show an elevated risk of cardiovascular problems—rather, the opposite. For instance, for myocardial infarction (heart attack), of nine early trials, seven in fact showed benefit from Vioxx (another showed even odds; and a second, only a slight increase in risk).[11] These trials constituted more than five thousand patients.[12] However, the results of the Vioxx GI Outcomes Research (VIGOR) trial, begun in 1999 and completed the following year, raised questions about Vioxx's potential risks. VIGOR compared Vioxx with naproxen (Aleve) and found higher rates of cardiovascular complications, including a significantly higher risk of myocardial infarction, in the Vioxx group. This was largely due to a big rise of such complications among those patients in the trial who had the greatest existing danger of a cardiovascular adverse event, and the "difference in the rates of myocardial infarction between the rofecoxib (Vioxx) and naproxen groups was not significant" in other patients.[13]

VIGOR also showed, as intended, that Vioxx was less dangerous for the gastrointestinal tract. There were only 2.1 gastrointestinal adverse events per 100 patient years in people in the Vioxx group versus 4.5 for those taking naproxen. Furthermore, the Vioxx group had only 0.6 cases per 100 patient years of "complicated confirmed [GI] events (perforation, obstruction, and severe upper gastrointestinal bleeding)," compared with 1.4 for the naproxen group.[14] Given the millions of arthritis sufferers at risk for GI complications, this was an important benefit.

While the cardiovascular results of VIGOR were worrying, they were hardly the smoking gun they were portrayed as in subsequent years. In fact, they were fairly equivocal. There was no difference in the overall risk of death from cardiovascular problems between the two groups and little or no difference in many types of cardio- or cerebrovascular events.[15] Dose was important as well; VIGOR used 50-milligram doses, twice what was recommended for long-term use and a dosage intended to be given only for acute short-term pain relief.[16] The majority of the earlier studies had used 12.5- and 25-milligram doses.[17]

Merck also suggested that naproxen might have a cardio-protective effect that was affecting the data. This explanation, although subsequently much dismissed as a dodge, was based on the fact that other drugs of the same type as naproxen *have* been demonstrated to have such effects.[18] Furthermore, the Vioxx studies themselves show a similar pattern. Early studies generally did not use naproxen as a comparator, instead choosing other NSAIDs, and they tended to be positive or neutral about Vioxx's cardiovascular safety. It was later studies, most of them using naproxen, that started to show that the drug carried a danger of heart attack.[19]

Furthermore, a 2001 analysis of trials on Vioxx, published in *Circulation*, found that while Vioxx had higher risks of cardiovascular problems than naproxen, it had lower risks than a placebo or than NSAIDs other than naproxen, even in high-risk patients. The authors attributed this difference, at least partly, to the fact that naproxen had strong anti-platelet properties.[20] Finally, experts such as Garrett FitzGerald considered the naproxen question to be a relevant and plausible one, even if it did not necessarily account for all of the variation between the two groups in VIGOR. Whatever the truth about naproxen's ability to protect the heart, it was clearly a theory worthy of being engaged.[21]

Contrary to later assertions, Merck did not hide the VIGOR data, nor did the FDA ignore it. However, some critics have suggested that the company soft-pedaled the dangers, and internal documents show that Merck employees were debating the safety of the drug for years before the recall. Certainly the company was less forthcoming than it might have been, and the impression of secrecy, whether real or not, was damaging both at the time and later. It is unclear whether greater transparency would have changed the situation significantly, especially with regard to the press and public opinion, but it probably would have mitigated some of the criticism from within the scientific and medical establishment and thereby, perhaps, somewhat deflated the later scandal.

After the VIGOR data were revealed, the FDA brought in a cardiologist to look at the evidence and asked a group of independent experts to analyze the existing information on Vioxx. The conclusion of these evaluations was that there was not sufficient evidence to take further action to restrict or ban the drug. While members of the panel disagreed on the risk-versus-benefit ratio, none of them expressed a belief that action needed to be taken to remove Vioxx from the market. The FDA panel also called for more trials to get more data, and as part of this effort, the agency set up a study using data from the insurance company Kaiser Permanente to track whether Vioxx was correlated with cardiovascular events and to gain more information from which to make a decision about the drug. The man chosen to run this study was a longtime FDA employee in the Office of Drug Safety named David Graham, a man who was later to play a central role in the Vioxx scandal. The FDA also subsequently changed the Vioxx label to reflect the new risk information. These are hardly the actions of an agency involved in a cover-up.

But some believe that the FDA should have taken stronger action. Dr. Eric Topol of the Cleveland Clinic has argued that the FDA could have, and should have, demanded that Merck conduct trials focused on cardiovascular complications. A 2004 Swiss study by Jüni et al. concluded retrospectively that the drug "should have been withdrawn several years earlier."[22] But given the complexity of the VIGOR results and the heterogeneous nature of the data on Vioxx at that point—with some studies showing benefit; others, no significant difference; and others, a risk—it seems that it would have been quite premature to pull Vioxx from the market in 2000 or 2001. In addition, contrary to popular belief, the FDA cannot compel recalls of drugs (although drugmakers do comply with requests for voluntary withdrawals).

THE *JAMA* ANALYSIS OF VIOXX

In August 2001, Steve Nissen and Eric Topol, both cardiologists at the Cleveland Clinic, catalyzed these concerns over Vioxx when, along with another colleague, they published an article noting the dangers of COX-2 inhibitors in the *Journal of the American Medical Association,* which highlighted the disquieting data from the VIGOR trial. The article was based on data from a statistical technique called meta-analysis, in which trials meeting certain criteria, in this case all available trials that tallied cardiovascular endpoints and were of adequate sample size, are combined and analyzed. Doing so gives a much larger sample than any one study, which can help to identify which patterns are real and how strong they actually are in a larger population. While concerns regarding Celebrex were raised, Nissen and Topol held that the signal for heart attack was worse with Vioxx, which they said significantly raised the risk of heart attack and other cardiovascular problems.

Meta-analyses are fraught with potential problems. First, they are only as good as the trials they incorporate; problems within the trials can taint the larger analysis. Second, the studies that a researcher chooses to include or exclude will shape the outcome. Topol and Nissen included only four trials: VIGOR, a large Celebrex trial called CLASS, and two smaller Vioxx trials, as well as adverse events data from the FDA. Among the trials excluded were most of the pre-approval studies on Vioxx.[23] Consequently, Merck complained that the meta-analysis "is based on only three studies of thirty available, and we think very relevant data was excluded." Third, the explanatory power of a meta-analysis can be compromised by variations within trials that make the trials difficult to compare. This is relevant because the *JAMA* article included data on two different drugs and incorporated trials with divergent methodologies.[24]

It is as a result of these limitations that scientists frequently distrust meta-analyses as evidence for establishing both the relative and the absolute risks of a medicine. Indeed, Topol and Nissen also compared the rate of heart attacks in the Celebrex and Vioxx data to a general rate obtained from a very different population. Consequently, the authors were aware that it was unlikely that the frequency of cardiovascular problems would be the same, whether or not COX-2 inhibitors affected the danger of heart attack and stroke. The authors noted, however, that their research was designed to encourage further research and raise concerns that there was a safety signal that should be examined. Indeed, Topol shared his concerns and data with Merck, where he had previously worked.

Topol and Nissen ultimately came to the same conclusion that studies of Vioxx patients in the real world had: "Rheumatoid arthritis increases risk of [heart attack], making intertrial comparisons difficult." Finally, they acknowledged that "[b]ecause of the evidence for an antiplatelet effect of naproxen, it is difficult to assess whether the difference in cardiovascular event rates in VIGOR was due to a benefit from naproxen" or a danger from Vioxx.[25]

Nissen admitted later, "Even in August, 2001, when we published our first report on the risks, it was highly speculative. We didn't have hard data. We had some soft data and some suspicions about the mechanism of action. We could just as easily have been wrong."[26]

APPROVe AND THE WITHDRAWAL OF VIOXX

Over the next several years, controversy over Vioxx simmered and spread. Stories about the "controversial" drug trickled through the press, and online sites belonging to industry opponents, risk-intolerant "safety" advocacy groups, and FDA critics warned Internet users of the dangers of Vioxx. Beginning in 2002, the drug's label included a warning about the possible cardiovascular risks and a recommendation not to use the highest dose for the long term. The package insert offered extensive information on the cardiovascular risks, and the same warnings were added to the next edition of the *Physicians' Desk Reference.*[27]

Then, in 2004, things came to a head with the release of the results of a second large post-approval study called the Adenomatous Polyp Prevention on Vioxx (APPROVe) trial, which was designed to see if Vioxx reduced the growth of colon cancer cells compared to a sugar pill. (It did.) Merck had designed the study about a year after Vioxx was approved to address the issue of cardiovascular risk in a relatively healthy patient population and had carefully watched the number of cardiovascular incidents in APPROVe in hopes of answering some of the questions posed by VIGOR and other studies.[28] The results of the new trial found that after eighteen months of use, patients on the drug were twice as likely to have a heart attack or heart failure as those who took the placebo, providing what many regarded as the final proof that Vioxx did increase the relative risk of cardiovascular disease in otherwise healthy patients.

Belying their effect, the APPROVe data were again not totally unambiguous. Neither the overall number of deaths (ten in both groups) nor the number of deaths from cardiovascular causes differed significantly. There were actually three deaths from heart attack in the placebo group compared to two in the Vioxx group, although the number of heart attacks was higher among Vioxx users. Those on Vioxx also had under half the number of "peripheral vascular events." Unsurprisingly, the relative risks were especially high in people who had "a history of symptomatic atherosclerotic cardiovascular disease" and were also elevated among people with a history of diabetes.[29] However, the press distorted the data to exaggerate the risks, as did critics such as Nissen.

The APPROVe data could have been framed to answer some of the questions posed by Topol. Yet Merck did not seem interested in identifying which patients would benefit from Vioxx. As Topol told me, if Merck "wanted to do it right, it would have been likely to be able to find the patients (through genetic testing) who were at risk of thrombotic events and improve the safety profile of their drug. But Merck did not want to publicly discuss such a possibility." Instead, in September 2004, the company, acting on the Precautionary Principle, made the unexpected decision to take Vioxx off the market altogether. The FDA had not mandated the drug's removal, and it is unlikely that the agency would have asked for a withdrawal, but would probably have opted for a black box warning, in which the risk information is surrounded by a black border to make it stand out. The company's decision did not come from a belief that the drug was fundamentally unsafe; after all, Merck's CEO allowed his wife to stay on the medication right up to the time it was pulled from the market. Certainly Merck did not foresee the public reaction that ensued. Rather, it was focusing on the fact that it had a new—and, it believed, safer—coxib, called Arcoxia, in development.

By pulling Vioxx voluntarily, Merck felt it would be demonstrating it was acting proactively and responsibly. It believed that removing Vioxx would calm the conflict, and it could then get approval for Arcoxia, which Merck believed had fewer cardiovascular risks even if taken in high doses for long periods of time. Potential liability if Vioxx continued to be sold may also have played a role in the decision. But while Merck executives may have hoped to persuade people that they were acting responsibly, plaintiffs' attorneys took the withdrawal as an admission of guilt. The company's decision to pull the drug—against the advice of the FDA—in hopes of calming the public backfired. The Internet, which was already becoming filled with information about the danger of Vioxx and other COX-2 medicines, became the rallying point for lawyers, alternative medicine practitioners, critics of the pharmaceutical industry, and safety crusaders, who turned the debate over the drug into a cause célèbre and the watchword for those promoting the Precautionary Principle. They cast Merck not as a responsible corporate citizen going the extra mile on behalf of patient safety, but as a company who hid danger and death as long as possible to protect profits. Terrified patients who'd been prescribed coxibs frantically contacted their doctors, and many stopped taking any medication at all for their arthritis.[30]

The tone of the scientists who raised questions about the appropriate use of coxibs changed, too. Eric Topol, who had until now confined criticisms to private exchanges with Merck and the FDA, wrote on the website of the prestigious *New England Journal of Medicine* that Vioxx represented a "catastrophe" for which "[t]he senior executives at Merck and the leadership at the FDA share responsibility for not having taken appropriate action and not recognizing that they are accountable for the public health." Others held that the company and the FDA were outright negligent.[31] One was *Lancet* editor Dr. Richard Horton, who opined in the *British Medical Journal* that "[w]ith Vioxx, Merck and the FDA acted out of ruthless, short-sighted, and irresponsible self-interest." Another doctor held that "the FDA was either extraordinarily lax or frankly complicit."[32] In the United Kingdom, *The Times* accused the FDA of collaborating with Merck to hide the dangers of Vioxx and reduce the fallout from the data once it became public.[33]

Meanwhile, the trial lawyers saw the potential to make huge profits, and the withdrawal of Vioxx, coupled with subsequent revelations about the risks of other similar drugs, sent them into a feeding frenzy that targeted not only Merck and other companies that made COX-2 inhibitors but also drug companies in general.[34] Finally, stories put out by reporters interested in sensationalism stoked the panic, and ultimately, "[s]ome pundits have done the trial lawyers' heavy lifting for them by portraying Merck as an evil corporation concerned only with making money and not at all worried about killing innocent customers in the process."[35]

Nissen, who originally was circumspect about his *JAMA* findings, now reserved particular vitriol for Vioxx. Although the study he completed with Topol actually showed a higher risk of heart attack on Celebrex than on Vioxx, he now focused only on Vioxx. He also ignored the fact that Celebrex, unlike Vioxx, had not been proven to have a reduced rate of gastrointestinal complications. And he immediately proposed a study to demonstrate Celebrex's relative safety—with himself as the lead researcher. Meanwhile, as lead author of the *JAMA* article, Topol was subpoenaed to testify about Vioxx. Days after his testimony, he was asked to step aside as chief academic officer of the Cleveland Clinic.

The news accounts of the Vioxx withdrawal led many patients on arthritis medication to phone their doctors. However, some former Vioxx users reacted with a different kind of alarm to the news because they faced a return to continual pain. These patients had never received relief from any drug except Vioxx and were more than willing to take the chance of having a heart attack, especially if they were at low risk anyway, in order to get the benefits they derived from the drug. Some lived in terror of the day when their existing prescription ran out and there would be no more pills.[36]

Many patients and physicians had turned to Vioxx after several previous medications failed to work or were not strong enough. "If you live with intractable pain every day of your life, would you take a [small] chance that you would have a heart attack? A lot of my patients would," explained one doctor. One such patient was Dave Ellis, a sixty-six-year-old retired pharmacist from Edmond, Oklahoma, whose spine had been afflicted with degenerative arthritis for three decades. Speaking to the *Wall Street Journal* in the aftermath of the Vioxx withdrawal, he explained that he would be out of the drug by mid-February of 2005, an eventuality he "dread[ed]."[37]

The FDA reminded the public that "No drug is fully safe ... Our job is to appropriately balance our decisions, based on the risk-benefit profile for a drug and the societal need and desire for new drugs." The agency also explained that it experienced "pressure from all sides— allegations that we're too fast, too slow. We make decisions on the basis of the science. We weigh the benefits against the risk ... and we make the tough calls." And that's the way it should be. Medicine can never remove all doubt, innovation is inherently uncertain, and the FDA must balance safety with the need to get new drugs onto the market so they can help patients. It is this need for balance that critics often fail to grasp. As one doctor succinctly summed it up, "The FDA is not going to hold up a medication for a generation to make sure it's safe. And similarly, they're not going to require you to study half a million people."[38] The original *JAMA* article on Vioxx was intended to encourage proactive steps on the part of Merck, including limited postmarket evaluation of groups of patients likely to be at higher risk for heart problems. But that approach would soon be tossed aside. Few would focus on the science or listen to what the FDA had to say. Instead, many considered no testing requirement too onerous in the pursuit of the mythical 100 percent safe drug.

SHOW TRIAL

Then, in November and December 2004, just a couple of months after Vioxx had been withdrawn, Senator Charles Grassley of Iowa used his position as chairman of the Senate Committee on Finance to create a hearing at which Vioxx had been convicted and sentenced before the opening words were ever spoken. It would be hard to imagine a more biased proceeding or one more designed to cause shock and fear. His star witness was whistle-blower Dr. David Graham, a longtime employee in the FDA's drug safety arm with a vendetta against a number of different drugs, of which Vioxx was only one. Graham's rhetoric was consistently and wildly inflammatory, full of conspiracy theories and inflated estimates of Vioxx's dangers. He called Vioxx "the single greatest drug safety catastrophe in the history of this country or the history of the world."[39] He also alleged that 88,000 to 139,000 strokes or heart attacks had been caused by Vioxx and that 30 to 40 percent, or 30,000 people, had died. He compared the number of dead to 500 to 900 commercial airplane crashes, or 67 percent of the population of Des Moines.[40]

To back up his assertions that Vioxx was responsible for tens of thousands of deaths, Graham cited the study the FDA had commissioned him to conduct after the concern occasioned by VIGOR. Yet, like Topol and Nissen's meta-analysis, it was dogged by problems and politics. Graham had used information on 1.4 million Americans enrolled by Kaiser Permanente to conclude that Vioxx users had a higher risk for heart attack or cardiovascular-related fatality than those on Celebrex.[41] But using this kind of data is tricky because you cannot control for variations among patients, as you can in a controlled trial, leaving significant potential for factors other than the one you are studying to be causing or contributing to what you observe. This can include other drugs that patients are taking, co-morbid health conditions, and preexisting risks. Observational studies also obscure differences in dosage and cases in which the drug is being taken or prescribed incorrectly. Since the cardiovascular dangers of Vioxx appear dependent on dose and length of usage, such omissions may have serious consequences for the accuracy of the conclusions drawn.

Another issue was that, as Vanderbilt University pharmacology chair Alastair Wood explained, heart attacks have many causes other than drugs, and "there was no possibility that you could discern a heart attack due to Vioxx from a heart attack not due to Vioxx."[42] Finally, Graham's observational study was an anomaly. Between 2000 and 2004, eleven analyses were done comparing Vioxx and naproxen using observational data, but only Graham's found that Vioxx was more dangerous. Several found that it was considerably less risky. The overall combined odds ratio from all these studies was 0.86—that is, people on Vioxx had only 86 percent of the chance of having a heart attack that naproxen users had.[43] Later observational studies agreed; for instance, a study in the *Archives of Internal Medicine* in January 2005 showed that Vioxx was no more dangerous than non-naproxen NSAIDs, even in a high-risk Medicaid population.[44] Given Graham's strident statements that he had always believed Vioxx was dangerous, it is clear that he created data that said what he wanted them to say rather than letting the data tell their own story.

Graham was also not content simply to promote panic and malign Vioxx. He went on to tell the Senate Committee that without changes at the FDA, he could "guarantee that unsafe and deadly drugs will remain on the U.S. market," and he called the agency "incapable of protecting Americans from another Vioxx." He proceeded to attack five other drugs by name.[45] The problem, according to Graham, was that the FDA had some scientists charged with approving new drugs and others who monitored the ones already on the market for safety, and the work of the latter were impeded by the former, who did not want to admit problems with products to which they had given the okay.

While there is probably some truth to this, it is clear that Graham's threshold for risk is a low one. A co-worker at the FDA opined of Graham that "[h]e virtually always believes that a drug is dangerous, but he rarely takes into account the business of the benefit of the drug."[46] Others have echoed the sentiment: FDA official Dr. Sandra Kweder testified that Graham did not take into account Vioxx's potential benefits, especially in light of the fact that trials of other COX-2 drugs had not demonstrated the same reduction of GI problems as Vioxx.[47]

Graham explained that he went to work for the FDA because he "thought, 'Well, I can be honest. I can follow my conscience. I can do what's good for people.'" Conscience was also the explanation he gave for his fearmongering congressional testimony.[48] But there is a problem when conscience becomes an impediment to science, when it becomes an ideological crusade instead of a dispassionate analysis of data. There is something telling about the fact that Graham went into research because he became too emotionally involved with patients to work with them directly; being a doctor means being able to make judgments based on scientific and medical facts, not on personal beliefs or feelings.

Graham also claimed that the FDA had sought to conceal his findings. Senator Grassley told the committee that "Dr. Graham described an environment where he was 'ostracized,' 'subjected to veiled threats' and 'intimidation,'" allegations that were false or distorted. Graham also claimed that his employer tried to prevent him from revealing his damning results at a conference in France. This is simply not true. Prior to that August 2004 conference, he duly submitted to his boss the poster presentation he planned to give, as is standard procedure at the agency, and it was looked at by a variety of FDA experts. According to FDA official Sandra Kweder, they then "provided comments and raised questions." Graham willingly took some of these suggestions into account and noted on the poster that it represented his own views.[49] Yet when asked about the criticism of his conclusions about Vioxx by other scientists and by his employer, Graham replied, "I know that FDA is responsible for 100,000 people being injured. And FDA wants to keep that swept under the rug nice and quiet."[50]

What apparently upset Graham was that the other FDA scientists tasked to review his Kaiser Permanente study were less enamored of it—and of his grandiose conclusions—than he was.[51] But that's the way peer-reviewed science sometimes works. While the emails offered by Graham as "proof" indicate that the FDA felt that he should pull back on his claims, urging responsible and cautious science is a far cry from the threats and cover-up portrayed by Graham and Grassley.[52] Given the inflammatory nature of Graham's comments and his tendency to hype the dangers of Vioxx beyond what the data warranted, the FDA was quite justified in being concerned that Graham was indulging a personal vendetta against the drug and the FDA rather than engaging in science.

Following the Vioxx hearings, a journalist asked Graham why instead of simply stating his case he chose to "take a baseball bat and hit the FDA upside the head." Graham replied, "Oh, I don't view it as taking a baseball bat ... I know what I said. But the fact is that I didn't imagine that my testimony would attract the attention that it did. I honestly didn't."[53] Yet this seems hard to believe, considering his exaggerated and provocative testimony. He did everything possible to scare the public and further his personal grudges, at the expense of the scientific truth.

ACT TWO?

The Vioxx saga subsequently had another chapter when, in 2005, the FDA agreed that Vioxx could return to the market with prescription restrictions and with a new label bearing a black box around the outside of the warning to reflect the increased potential for adverse events. Looking at the same data that had precipitated Merck's withdrawal decision, an expert FDA panel held that, for certain types of people, the advantages of the medication were greater than the possible dangers.[54] Later the same year, a panel in Canada, where Vioxx had been pulled as well, likewise opened the door for it to be reintroduced.

Dr. Raymond Gaeta, director of Stanford's pain management clinic, called the decision "good news for patients overall. Clearly, there are side effects with every medication, but it's really important to weigh the potential side effects versus the benefits for an individual patient." Other doctors said that they were still worried about the dangers and advised patients to take a different drug if possible. Nonetheless, physicians recognized that Vioxx could help some patients who did not respond to other drugs or who had risk factors that affected their use of alternative medications, such as susceptibility to ulcers or gastrointestinal bleeding. Many echoed Dr. James F. Fries, who said, "As a physician, I like to have a choice of treatments, because people are different and some respond well to them."[55]

Situations in which a withdrawn drug is returned to the market are uncommon, but they do happen and have become more frequent in recent years. This trend may come from a post-Vioxx tendency to react too precipitously to safety concerns, only to see the error later. Tysabri, the drug discussed at the beginning of this chapter, was such a case. Often, the decision to let a drug reenter the market is triggered by demands from patients who were benefiting from it. Reintroduced drugs come with heavy warnings, patient restrictions, and sometimes monitoring programs. As a result, they are prescribed to only a small group of patients.

In the end, Vioxx was never returned to market, although Merck had originally said that it would consider bringing it back if the FDA panel opened the door for it to do so. Throughout 2005, the company was besieged by lawsuits over the drug, and the company initially fought each one individually, winning more than it lost. Merck eventually decided to settle. There were troubles for other coxibs; despite positive votes by the same FDA panel that had okayed the reintroduction of Vioxx, Bextra was withdrawn, and Celebrex received a black box warning. The end of the year saw renewed debate over three additional heart attacks in VIGOR that were not included in the article publishing the results in the *New England Journal of Medicine* because they had occurred after the predetermined study end point. Although the three disputed heart attacks in the full data had been sent to the FDA and posted on its website, which Nissen and Topol then had used for their *JAMA* article in 2001, there were now new accusations of a cover-up.[56] Merck also continued to hope that Arcoxia, its successor to Vioxx, would be approved by the FDA, but it ultimately was rejected in 2007. It seemed better to just move on rather than re-ignite the fight over Vioxx. Again, political and legal considerations had unfortunately trumped scientific ones.

VIOXX'S SHADOW

Science is full of surprise and uncertainty in both results and measurement. Reaping its benefits requires accepting that there will always be things we do not know and understanding that with benefits also come risks. But in an era of tabloid medicine, when a drug doesn't work as planned or a side effect is discovered, it is quickly portrayed on the Internet and in the media as a concealed danger of untold proportions. When doctors do not accurately weigh risks and benefits or fail to predict dangers, it is regarded as an exercise in scientific conspiracy, and the effects go far beyond the immediate use of a particular product. The resulting fear and controversy reverberate throughout medicine as a whole, shaping what the FDA does, scaring people into avoiding drugs for years, and leading the population to look at every medicine with suspicion.

In this regard, what has become known as "the Vioxx crisis" marks the triumphant emergence of tabloid medicine as a legitimate and objective source of scientific information. In the wake of the withdrawal and the furor of the Grassley/Graham hearings, Vioxx was transformed from a troubled drug into a symbol of corporate malfeasance and regulatory weakness. Merck had thought when it pulled Vioxx that it would soon be replaced by a safer successor product. But it failed to consider that in yanking the drug, it would give the proponents and beneficiaries of tabloid medicine both a platform and the resources to sustain and expand their enterprise.

The controversy mobilized pharmaceutical industry opponents, critics of the FDA, "safety" crusaders for whom all risk was too much, and others who believed that the scandal provided proof positive that companies were corrupt and government agencies helpless. Industry critics seized on it as a way to undermine popular confidence in government scientific institutions such as the FDA, spread fear about drugs in general, and advance their own position and agenda. The press had a field day. Those who had long warned about Vioxx basked in the glow of media attention, apparently vindicated. Lawsuits mounted against Merck and other companies making coxibs, and litigators gleefully anticipated huge fees. The Internet was flooded with stories about Vioxx's dangers, conspiracy theories ran rampant online, and sites popped up warning of evil drug companies and corrupt or clueless FDA officials. Those who disputed this view were effectively silenced, drowned out by more vociferous voices.

Amidst the fear and blame set off by the Vioxx scandal, some of the drug's detractors reaped big benefits from the panic they created. David Graham has proven unwilling to abandon his position in the public eye. He lobbied vigorously against approval of Arcoxia, attacked other coxibs, and assailed other drugs ranging from diabetes treatment Avandia, to new asthma drugs, to the cholesterol medication Crestor. In the process, he has become a hero to those who believe that the FDA is lying down on the job and that the drug companies are irretrievably corrupt. His accusations against various drugs are taken as fact by journalists, who often report them uncritically.

Steve Nissen has profited as well. Two months after Merck withdrew the drug, he heavily lobbied his friends at Pfizer to allow him to head a twenty-thousand-person trial of Celebrex sponsored by Pfizer, an endeavor that was believed to cost over $100 million.[57] He has made a career of attacking drugs and demanding more study—and then convincing the companies to let him carry out the trials himself.[58] Nissen has relished his role as a self-appointed drug regulator, often using threats about the safety of drugs to block new products, hurt those already on the market, and intimidate the FDA.[59] The *New York Times* has described him as "among a new cadre of activist scientists demanding greater vigilance on drug safety." But Dr. Michael A. Weber of SUNY Downstate Medical Center has called his statements "inflammatory" and has said, "In some of his comments to the media, Dr. Nissen has gone beyond discussing the scientific findings of his study to language that frightens patients."[60]

Nissen is also willing to promote drugs with serious risks when it suits him. In 2004, he was involved in the evaluation of AGI-1067, a drug designed to reduce the level of fatty plaque deposits (atherosclerosis) in a person's arteries. The company that developed the compound, Atherogenics, predicted the drug would have positive effects on many different types of serious heart problems. But the original results were unclear. When Nissen did a re-analysis of the Atherogenics trials, AGI-1067 was suddenly a breakthrough. He told *Forbes* magazine, "It in fact is promising ... there is no other interpretation. But it's not the final word."[61] But when a 2007 study of AGI-1067 showed that the drug actually increased bad cholesterol levels, decreased good cholesterol, and was associated with a rise in the overall number of heart failures and strokes, Dr. Nissen's name was not among the authors.

Ultimately, Vioxx was not more dangerous than other drugs on the market; it was just in the wrong place at the wrong time. The scandal was created in part by the convergence of new trends in technology and changes in the way people in the scientific community and the public at large perceived medical innovation. Both helped make possible the rise of tabloid medicine. As we showed in the previous chapter, the online world allows everyone to promote their point of view, whatever its veracity or merit, and find a far wider readership than ever before. As more and more people turned to the Internet for health facts, the power of traditional sources of authority eroded and information was democratized. Misinformation also replicated and spread unchecked, becoming apparent truth through sheer repetition. The same trends we found when we analyzed Google results on Crestor and Avandia also occurred in the case of Vioxx; anti-pharma interest groups and legal sites largely dominated the real estate, all insisting that the drug was enormously dangerous.

The lasting effect of the scandal was the creation of a template for hyping future controversies and spreading fear in which the use of the Internet was a central component. Using inexpensive statistical tools and data found on Google, it is easy for critics to generate a scandal that fits the story line of Vioxx. With the help of a pharmaceutical industry that has failed to speak directly and plainly to the public, an eager media that relies on the sensational story line, and a coterie of biased sources, from members of Congress who scour the Web for hearing material to instant experts such as Steve Nissen, medicines for high blood pressure, diabetes, high cholesterol, sinus infections, children's coughs, and even cancer—medicines that help most people most of the time—are now being assailed as either ineffective or dangerous. And the science that supported their use is being attacked, not with more science but with political challenges to scientific authority.

In this climate, it has become more difficult for new drugs to win approval from the FDA. After the denigration of the agency in the media for not having forced a withdrawal of Vioxx as soon as suggestions of cardiovascular risk emerged, the FDA became much more risk adverse, unwilling even to chance that a new side effect would appear after approval and make it look bad. This was made worse by the fact that a large segment of the American population was no longer willing to accept the trade-off that is at the very heart of all medical treatment: no drug is without both benefits and risks. And their trust in the FDA's ability to judge the balance had been reduced significantly. Researchers have also become quicker to see the smallest suggestion of problems as a danger. Speaking on the results of a meta-analysis of Bextra, another COX-2 inhibitor, which indicated elevated risks of heart attack and stroke, Dr. Garrett FitzGerald explained that "before Vioxx, my reaction would be: this is interesting—is it real? But the landscape changed after Vioxx. Thus, the findings take on more significance."[62]

The changes that followed the end of Vioxx have not made arthritis patients better off, either. An increasing number of elderly users of NSAIDs may be at greater risk of serious gastrointestinal complications, according to research presented at the American College of Rheumatology Annual Scientific Meeting in Boston. The authors found the following:

> Increasing implementation of good gastroprotection strategies reached a peak in 2004 when the percent of patients not receiving gastroprotection (Gastroprotection Gap) reached 14 percent from 79 percent in 1997. However, this gap more than doubled, reaching approximately 35 percent in 2005, following a decline in selective COX-2 inhibitor use, without a commensurate increase in other gastroprotective therapies. As the gastroprotection gap increased in 2005, a sharp rise in serious GI complications was observed.[63]

New benefits of COX-2 inhibitors may also get lost in the worries now surrounding their use; studies indicate that they can prevent or mitigate the development of colon cancer (a finding from the APPROVe study that was shunted aside in the controversy), breast cancer, lung cancer, prostate cancer, and more.

The irony of the Vioxx scandal and its devastating aftereffects is that it came at time when new kinds of tests using genetic and chemical markers, by providing doctors with an easy way to determine which patients will benefit from a drug and which will be vulnerable to side effects, have raised the hope that such controversies over drugs may one day be a thing of the past. In January 2005, an article in *Bio-Century* argued that this new field of pharmacogenomics can help us "avoid throwing the baby out with the bathwater by finding a way to identify the very few patients who should not be taking the coxibs, which are safe for the majority of users and critically important to a core group for whom other drugs don't work."

Contrary to the actions of Graham and Nissen, two other players in the fight over Vioxx, Eric Topol and Garrett FitzGerald, have proved strong supporters of pharmacogenomics. FitzGerald's work on the mechanism by which COX-2 affects the circulatory system is vitally important to developing new tests, since it is only by understanding the workings of the enzyme that we can find markers that indicate which patients are vulnerable to ill effects. FitzGerald has told the scientific community that medical questions like those surrounding coxibs are "precipitating us into moving into personalized medicine faster than anticipated."

Topol recognized that research on coxibs has revealed significant benefits beyond just pain relief, especially in the prevention of cancer, and has made clear that the impression conveyed by the press that he wanted all COX-2s withdrawn was an erroneous one. Instead, he has called for change in the monitoring of drugs already approved, including giving the FDA more authority to make companies do more studies and be more cautious in their use of drug marketing. Topol has called pharmacogenomics "invaluable" since "[i]f you could ferret out who is likely to have the benefits or the risks that would make a big difference."[64] Unlike Nissen, he has not profited from his criticism of Merck. Indeed, Topol balked at trying to cash in on the Vioxx panic, instead leaving the Cleveland Clinic to focus on personalized medicine and steering clear of the Nissen publicity machine.

Unfortunately, Vioxx was just the beginning. Our drugs are not safer now than they were in 2004—perhaps the opposite—but they are certainly less numerous. We are more afraid of drugs and less willing to accept the reality of medicine: that 100 percent safety is impossible and that those who pretend otherwise are offering nothing but a chimera. As a result of the changes to the attitude of the FDA and the public alike toward new drugs, many drugs that make our lives better and longer have never made it onto the market, and innovation is slowed by worries that politics rather than science will determine whether money and time invested in research come to fruition. Existing drugs with important benefits are banned or restricted, denying some patients the only medication that has ever worked for them.

The bottom line is that the only winners in the Vioxx case are trial lawyers, politicians, pharma critics, and journalists bolstering their own reputation and readership at the expense of others. The losers? The rest of us. We are the ones who will lose as the drug companies are impeded from bringing new drugs to market (or given no incentive to do so), older drugs are attacked and restricted, and innovation becomes impossible.[65] We are constantly assailed by scare stories about some new dangerous drug until we no longer know which are safe or whom we can trust. Perhaps it is time for Vioxx to become a symbol of a different kind, not of industry greed and callousness or government incompetence, but of the dangers of letting medical questions be determined not by science but by politics and fear.

CHAPTER 5

Web of Fear: Vaccines, Autism, and the Emergence of "Instant Experts"

T HE INTERNET HAS NOT only placed before us a dizzying array of information, but it has also created a legion of "instant experts," whose only qualifications may be a strong opinion and followers willing to believe what they have to say. These "experts" are often imbued with heroism for their very lack of credentials and drape themselves in the mantle of the little guy standing up to the establishment. In other cases, Internet experts might be those with legitimate expertise and training, but who are using these credentials cynically and opportunistically.

These instant experts are not content to spread misinformation and fear, they seek to usurp the place of legitimate scientists and undermine established medical and scientific authority. They accuse doctors and researchers of being involved in an enormous conspiracy and claim that these experts derive monetary gain from perpetuating this cover-up. Meanwhile, they themselves have enormous conflicts of interest. And these instant experts react ruthlessly to those who disagree with them, launching disproportionate retaliation that takes the form of harassment and even threats.

The dangers posed by instant experts have been dramatically shown in the debate over whether autism is linked to vaccination. Science has come out conclusively against the theory that immunizations cause autism, but an empire of websites, foundations, and activist groups has been created to advance this belief and to promote a myriad of often bizarre and frequently risky treatments for autism. This anti-vaccine movement has only grown stronger over the past ten years, often shoving aside the leading experts in the United States and the world in favor of its own instant experts.

For the casual researcher, the Internet is dominated by the viewpoint that vaccines are dangerous, and the evidence can seem overwhelming. Such claims are all the more powerful because activists have tapped into the desire of parents and relatives of children diagnosed along the autism spectrum to believe that the condition has a clear, and preventable, cause and is reversible. Unfortunately, these contentions are untrue; autism is a disorder with complex genetic origins, and it is a lifelong condition, although most people with autism improve over time. The consequences of this potent misinformation are serious both for public health and for individual patients.

MALIGNING THE MMR

British researcher Dr. Andrew Wakefield is representative of the second kind of instant expert: a disaffected scientist whose training became a means to advance his own agenda and interests, whatever the cost to the public or the scientific community. In 1998, he ignited the controversy over the link between vaccines and autism when he announced that he had uncovered evidence that the measles, mumps, and rubella (MMR) vaccine inflamed and damaged the digestive systems of children, allowing toxins and chemicals to enter the bloodstream and damage the brain, leading to autism. Or at least that is what Wakefield told reporters when he called a press conference to promote his research. In fact, the conclusion of the paper, published in the prestigious journal *The Lancet*, admitted, "We did not prove an association between measles, mumps, and rubella vaccine and the syndrome described [autistic symptoms with bowel problems]."[1]

Wakefield's study was, in fact, riddled with problems. The sample was extremely small, only twelve children, making it impossible to determine whether any pattern was real or just coincidence.[2] In addition, when other scientists looked closely, they found that most of the children had intestinal issues prior to getting the vaccine and did not show evidence of the "leaky gut" claimed by Wakefield.[3] Finally, the theory was scientifically implausible for two reasons: first, wild measles is not correlated with autism, and second, only a small number of children with autism also have gastrointestinal issues, which eliminated the possibility that MMR was a major trigger of autism.[4]

None of this mattered to Wakefield. Characteristic of an instant expert, his goal was not science but celebrity, at whatever price, and the promotion of his own dubious research at the expense of his colleagues. This was not the first time Wakefield had tried to grab the spotlight, nor the first time that his research was flawed. In 1993, he blamed measles for Crohn's disease, only for his findings to prove impossible to replicate.[5] However, his strategy in using a press conference to announce a link between vaccinations and autism worked devastatingly well. The story was picked up throughout the British press and set off a panic that spread to the rest of Europe and the United States. Parents of children with autism thought they finally had an answer and a culprit. They began to organize around the belief that their children had been hurt by the vaccine.

Meanwhile, the vaccination rate for MMR fell precipitously in the United Kingdom in the aftermath of Wakefield's announcement, reaching 70 percent nationally, with uptake as low as 50 percent in some areas, down from 90 percent. Measles began to reemerge, with pockets of the disease appearing in communities with low vaccination rates. Wakefield had advised worried parents to have the MMR administered as three separate vaccines, but as this was not available in the United Kingdom, many children were not vaccinated at all. Doctors tried desperately to reassure the population that the MMR was safe, but they were often not heeded. On the other side of the Atlantic, U.S. representative Dan Burton, whose grandson is autistic, used his position as chairman of the House Government Reform Committee to initiate hearings on the safety of immunizations that would last from 1999 to 2002. Representatives of leading foreign and domestic scientific organizations were not allowed to participate, but Wakefield was among Burton's star witnesses during the highly biased proceedings.

The plunge in vaccine uptake in the United Kingdom did not come without a cost. In 2002, the resurgence of measles claimed its first victims, three children in Dublin, where more than one hundred children entered the hospital with measles complications. But Wakefield seemed unconcerned, especially since he seemed vindicated when pathologist John O'Leary announced that he had found measles in the guts of children with autism at a much higher rate than in normal children (82 versus 7 percent).[6] A second study in which O'Leary participated claimed to have identified the measles virus found in autistic children as the vaccine strain.[7] Wakefield was riding high, accepted around the globe as an expert on autism and a heroic doctor who had uncovered a danger menacing the world's children, even as other scientists were unable to duplicate his findings and questioned his results and methodology.

BETTER SAFE THAN SORRY?

Representative Dan Burton's hearings over autism and vaccines had already stirred up parents in the United States, who, like their counterparts in the United Kingdom, believed they had found an explanation for their children's autism in Wakefield's theory. But, in 1999, the flames of the debate were further fanned by worries about another vaccine component, the mercury-based preservative thimerosal, after an analysis found that children could get up to 187.5 micrograms (millionths of a gram) of mercury from vaccines in their first six months. That was above the EPA limit for methyl mercury (although within the guidelines from other sources) and, therefore, struck concern in some scientists.

Neal Halsey, a pediatrician advising the Centers for Disease Control and Prevention (CDC) on vaccines, pushed for an immediate removal of thimerosal. His conviction that this was the right course of action was strengthened after seeing signs on a fishing trip "warning people about eating fish with mercury," which made him wonder, "Does it make sense to allow it to be injected into infants?"[8] Others on the CDC's vaccine advisory committee believed, based on the available science, that thimerosal was safe at the levels found in vaccines and that suggesting that it was not would lead to a decline in immunization and, therefore, protection against infectious diseases. However, Halsey had threatened to go to the media and trial attorneys, so the advisory committee caved in. Invoking the Precautionary Principle, the CDC recommended removing thimerosal from vaccines even though there was no evidence that it was dangerous. Barely a week had elapsed between the time Halsey set off the scare and when vaccine makers agreed to remove thimerosal over the following two years.

At the same time, after a thorough investigation, the European Medicines Agency (EMEA) announced that there was "no evidence of harm to children caused by the level of thimerosal in vaccines currently being used and that it was imperative for vaccination to continue in accordance with national immunization schedules to prevent disease outbreaks." But the EMEA also said that thimerosal should be phased out to mitigate public concerns.[9]

From the beginning, there were two problems with the connection between thimerosal and autism. The first problem was that thimerosal, while about half mercury, contains *ethyl* mercury, for which there are no exposure guidelines. So the scientists used the ones for *methyl* mercury. However, ethyl mercury has different properties, including being processed out of the body more quickly.[10] The second problem was that children receive more mercury from breast milk in their first year then they do from vaccines. Scientists were divided on whether the use of thimerosal was even a potential problem, and many believed that the U.S. government had reacted to the issue too hastily, allowing political concerns to overwhelm scientific ones.

The worries that the withdrawal had been undertaken precipitously were quickly borne out. While the move to eliminate thimerosal from vaccines was intended to calm fears and reassure the public while scientists looked further into the issue, many people interpreted it as an admission of guilt. Why, they wondered, would thimerosal be taken out of vaccines if it were safe? And why would the government and the medical establishment keep reporting that there was no danger when this seemed belied by their actions? The next logical leap was that the scientists and doctors must be hiding something. Anti-vaccination activists, parents with autistic children who needed someone to blame, and others who saw an opportunity for profit began to coalesce into a movement that promoted the theory that immunizations caused autism. Using websites, they trumpeted the dangers of vaccines and the evil of doctors, scientists, and national health agencies, who, they claimed, were callously concealing a threat that was damaging millions of children.

With the waxing of this movement came the creation of a legion of anti-vaccination "experts" dispensing their dubious wisdom online and in the media. One was Barbara Loe Fisher, cofounder of the National Vaccine Information Center, an anti-vaccine crusader since the early 1980s, after her son supposedly sustained brain damage from the diphtheria, tetanus, pertussis (DTP) immunization. Despite having no medical scientific credentials, she was able to successfully portray herself as a vaccine expert in the media, in politics, and later on the Internet, which provided a new and highly effective medium for her message. This method of the media- and Web-savvy, if scientifically ignorant, "expert" would be repeated many times in the anti-vaccine movement.

Another "expert" who emerged during the early stages of the debate was another parent, Lyn Redwood. She was a nurse practitioner, but it was emotion rather than reason or experience that convinced her that thimerosal was behind her son's autism and made her a fervent convert to the anti-vaccine movement. In 2000, Redwood linked up with another parent of an autistic son, Sallie Bernard, who had never studied medicine, but who, as owner of a market research company, was well versed in promoting a message. Together they wrote and published an article in a low-circulation journal called *Medical Hypotheses* claiming that autism was actually mercury poisoning. The piece, "Autism: A Novel Form of Mercury Poisoning," continues to be frequently cited on the Internet by anti-vaccine activists. Bernard and Redwood concluded that the symptoms of the two conditions are identical and that, therefore, autism could be treated with chelators, drugs used to remove heavy metals from the body.

Subsequent study would contradict Bernard and Redwood's assertion that the symptoms of autism and mercury poisoning were exactly the same. In 2003, Karin B. Nelson and Margaret L. Bauman published a rebuttal in *Pediatrics* that noted that classic symptoms of mercury poisoning are reduced field of vision, ataxia (lack of muscle coordination), dysarthria (slow, poorly articulated speech), muscle weakness and spasticity, peripheral neuropathy (circulation problems in the extremities), and often toxic psychosis. None of these are characteristic of autism, nor do conditions known to be caused by mercury, such as Minamata disease, significantly resemble autism.[11]

None of this mattered a bit to the anti-vaccine movement. When their flawed article did not produce the desire results, Bernard and Redwood created a Web-based organization to spread their message. Called Sensible Action for Ending Mercury-Induced Neurological

Disorders, and known as SafeMinds, the organization would become one of the leading groups online and off in promoting the theory that thimerosal was implicated in autism—and a champion for a variety of bizarre and risky "cures." Like Barbara Loe Fisher, both women presented themselves, and were accepted, as experts in autism and were interviewed in print and on television, frequently with scientists or doctors excluded. When asked about the fact that many doctors doubted that there was a connection, the instant experts were dismissive: "Oh them," Fisher responded in one article, "They have been attacking parents who have been talking about vaccine safety concerns."[12] All three also used their legitimate-sounding organizations to lend apparent authority and weight to their message, leaving many parents believing that their claims were scientifically valid and accepted.

By 2002, in the United States, only some flu shots and a few rarely used vaccines still had more than a trace amount of thimerosal in them. By then, Neal Halsey had reason to regret his quick action. He spoke out repeatedly against the theory that vaccination led to autism, resisting the attempts of the anti-vaccine movement to co-opt him for their cause.[13] Unlike Wakefield, Halsey had stuck to the science in the years after the move toward thimerosal-free vaccines, instead of trying to use the controversy to enrich himself. But the public was no longer listening to him.

Instead, popular fears were reinforced by the work of two unscrupulous scientists, Mark and David Geier. The pair, a father and son, had already built their livelihoods on dubious medical research and lawsuits against drug companies, and they saw autism as a rich new frontier. In 2003, they published an article in the journal *Experimental Biology and Medicine* that concluded that the Vaccine Adverse Event Reporting System (VAERS) demonstrated that thimerosal was implicated in autism, mental retardation, and speech disorders.[14] It was soon followed by two more articles, including one that purported to show that autistic children treated with chelator drugs excreted greater amounts of mercury than nonautistic children, which appeared in the *Journal of American Physicians and Surgeons*, a credible-sounding new publication that in fact promoted a strong anti-vaccine and anti-government bias.[15] Both articles were deeply methodologically flawed. In particular, what parents who heard about these studies did not know is that anyone can send a report to Vaccine Adverse Event Reporting System, and such reports are not checked to remove duplicate submissions or to determine if they are true. And the Geiers were not about to tell them.

The Geiers were not the only scientists to jump on the "thimerosal causes autism" bandwagon. One of these nascent instant experts was University of Kentucky chemistry professor Boyd Haley, who became famous for a problematic paper about the reduced ability of autistic children to excrete mercury into their hair. One of his coauthors was Mark Blaxill, a member of the leadership of SafeMinds, the anti-vaccine organization founded by Lyn Redwood and Sallie Bernard.[16] Haley also made money from selling various tests and "cures," including chelators intended for animals, to the families of autistic children.

Another scientist to become involved in the anti-vaccine movement was Richard Deth, a professor of pharmacology at Northeastern University. In 2004, he was part of a team that published an article in *Molecular Psychiatry* alleging that nerve cells treated in the lab with thimerosal exhibited blockage of a metabolic pathway that, he alleged, reduced the ability of autistic children to excrete mercury.[17] Deth claimed that B12 shots would fix the problem. A third was Mady Hornig, who announced she had made mice autistic by giving them thimerosal. Her research proved not to be replicable and was subsequently disproved.[18] None of the scientific results of the anti-vaccine movement's scientific "experts" have withstood the scrutiny of their peers or been borne out by subsequent study.

In spite of these serious scientific shortcomings, during the first few years after the removal of thimerosal, the anti-vaccine instant experts dominated the landscape of the autism debate, taking over the online environment and insinuating themselves into the print and television media. As a result of an apparent proliferation of evidence against vaccines, at least to anyone running a Google search, more and more parents began to question—and even challenge—their doctors. Although the turn away from immunizations was less dramatic than in the United Kingdom because of immunization requirements to enter public schools, vaccine rates in some areas of the United States fell below the 90–95 percent needed for herd immunity, which prevents diseases from spreading if they are introduced in a community and protects those who are not vaccinated because they are too young or cannot get immunizations for medical reasons.

Instant experts dismissed the dangers of these illnesses and instead argued that catching the diseases was a good thing, allowing children to acquire immunity "naturally" and, therefore, ostensibly more safely. The very success of vaccination had become a weakness; few parents had ever seen the diseases that immunization had rendered rare or extinct, and, as a result, failed to comprehend their danger. In communities with high immunization rates, the unvaccinated can free ride in relative safety. However, vaccine-preventable diseases are not gone, and some parents have had to live with the serious consequences of listening to online charlatans. In 2000, Suzanne and Leonard Walther decided against vaccinating their daughter Mary Catherine after an online search turned up scaremongering sites that blamed vaccines for conditions ranging from allergies, to autism, to shaken baby syndrome. Not long after, Mary Catherine developed meningitis from a vaccine-preventable infection and ended up in the hospital at risk of death or brain damage.[19] Anti-vaccine crusaders risked the lives not only of their own children but those of others every day, and they made the danger greater every time they encouraged other parents to follow their example.

SCIENCE STRIKES BACK

The power of instant experts in determining public understanding of scientific issues is demonstrated by the way they continued to dominate the autism debate despite the influx of evidence in the early 2000s that indicated that vaccines played no role in causing autism. An analysis in Finland published in 2000 found that MMR was not correlated with autism,[20] and two years later a similar study concluded that among Danish children, "No matter how researchers analyzed the data, there was no difference in the autism rates of children who received the MMR vaccine and those who did not."[21]

As for mercury, in August 2003, epidemiologist Paul Stehr-Green, who had been a critic of Halsey's invocation of the Precautionary Principle, reported in the *American Journal of Preventive Medicine* that children in Sweden and Denmark born after thimerosal was discontinued there continued to show a rising incidence of autism.[22] In September, Kreesten Madsen of the University of Aarhus in Denmark published a study in *Pediatrics* that found the same thing.[23] In October, Ander Hviid at the Danish Epidemiological Center in Copenhagen announced an identical result in the *Journal of the American Medical Association*.[24] Over the next year, evidence that vaccines were not linked to autism continued to come in. In September 2004, two more articles were published, both from the United Kingdom, one in *Pediatrics* by John Heron of the University of Bristol, the other by Nick Andrews of the Communicable Disease Surveillance Center in London. Both found an interesting result: as the amount of thimerosal a child received went up, incidence of neurological problems actually went down. This was a strong blow against the idea that vaccines caused autism.

Finally, in response to a barrage of new science, the Institute of Medicine convened a blue-ribbon panel, which eventually announced, "The committee concludes that the evidence favors rejection of a causal relationship between thimerosal-containing vaccines and autism" and "concludes that the evidence favors rejection of a causal relationship between MMR vaccine and autism."[25] One member of the

IOM committee said that after examining hundreds of articles, "the evidence linking thimerosal to autism is purely theoretical at best."[26]

The instant experts responded by casting aspersions on the epidemiological methodology used by these new studies, claiming that it was not population data like that in the studies in Sweden and Denmark that mattered, but laboratory data such as in the studies by Hornig and Deth. On their websites and in interviews, they alleged that epidemiological data was unreliable. In fact, there are enormous problems inherent in generalizing from cells or animals to humans, as Hornig and Deth did. The population studies, however, which included tens of thousands of children, would have revealed even rare vaccine-related events. Yet anti-vaccine criticism of the new research was largely accepted outside of the scientific community. The average parent searching the Internet did not have the background to understand the debate over scientific methodologies, and neither did most members of the media covering the controversy.

Furthermore, these technical academic papers could hardly compete with the instant experts' heartstring-tugging stories of children "stolen" by vaccines and "recovered" through chelation, B_{12} shots, and other biomedical interventions. For the media, hyping the controversy over autism drew better ratings then merely presenting new scientific evidence, and the instant experts put all their PR savvy into presenting themselves as the people with the real answers, using emotionalism to counter dry scientific fact. Scientists had trouble finding forums that gave them a chance to explain that all the research showed no indication at all of a link between autism and vaccines.

DANGEROUS MEDICINE

The anti-vaccine movement's instant experts were successful in their attempts to take over the discussion of immunizations and autism because they used a one-two punch: first, they terrified patients with emotional anecdotes of vaccine-damaged children, and then they held out a solution, a cure, for autism. Many parents found themselves vulnerable to the testimony of a procession of parents who recounted stories of toddlers wracked by seizures, turned suddenly comatose, or afflicted with spiking fevers that sent them to the hospital. The punch line was always the same: "He/she was developing perfectly normally before, and then after the vaccine, all of a sudden, he/she was lost in another world." The instant experts also portrayed autism as hellish, even a fate worse than death and autistic children as "stolen," "lost," and victims of "mad child disease."

The truth is that studies have shown that parents tend to "misremember" the timing of events depending on their beliefs about what causes autism or because of other events, such as a move or a new baby, going on in their life at the same time.[27] In addition, they often miss, ignore, or forget subtle signs of autism that have been present since birth, as a number of scientists have demonstrated.[28] Finally, the time many vaccinations are given is also when autism is most likely to develop, and the "annals of autism research make it clear that a subset of autistic children suddenly regressed at this age long before the ... vaccine became available."[29]

Yet when doctors rejected the claims of parents and other family members that they "just knew" something was wrong or saw a change in the child after a vaccine, there was a visceral popular reaction against what was perceived as a dismissal of parents' knowledge of their child. The ordinary mothers and fathers were lionized by the anti-vaccine movement precisely because they were not trained scientists or doctors and, therefore, were easily identified with. At the same time, many families with children with autism or a related condition suddenly thought they had found the answer to the indefatigable "why?" that had plagued them—and now they also had someone to blame. The medical authorities were presented as blind and self-interested, caught up in the dictates of the establishment, beholden to the money of the vaccine manufacturers, unable to see the evidence right in front of them. "Won't you please just listen to the parents?" was the anti-vaccine movement's keening refrain, against which science was largely powerless. All the statistics about the probability of harm from immunizations paled against the personal story of someone online.

The other half of the instant experts' equation was the seductive promise that autism was curable. Instant experts promoted a litany of treatments for autism, each of them hailed as a miracle that would "recover" children and give parents back the sons and daughters that the condition had "stolen" from them. Many of these "cures" had been created by disaffected scientists who perceived themselves as brave mavericks uncovering the hidden truth—and they were handsomely paid for their efforts. Often, physicians peddling autism cures were DAN! doctors, so-called because they belonged to Defeat Autism Now!, an organization that had been set up in 1995 to promote alternative "biomedical" treatments for autism. A wide variety of bizarre treatments for the disorder have emerged over the last decade, some benign, some less so. They include "sonar depuration, cranial manipulation, laser therapy, camel's milk, magnetic clay and hyperbaric oxygen."[30] Others are gluten- and casein-free diets, urine injections, RNA drops, and, at one point, secretin, a hormone in the digestive system. More dangerously, the Geiers have advocated the so-called Lupron protocol, which uses "a synthetic hormone most often used to treat prostate cancer or to carry out the chemical castration of sex offenders."[31]

But perhaps the most prominent—and most controversial—of these "cures" was chelation. Bernard and Redwood sowed the first seeds of its use for autism by theorizing that autistic children were mercury-poisoned and would improve if the mercury in their bodies were removed. Soon those seeds grew exponentially. Chelation has never been scientifically shown to help autism in any way; the mechanism is not even biologically plausible. Even in cases of acute heavy metal poisoning, chelation is used right after exposure and for a relatively short period, not for years, as in some autistic children. Chelation is also dangerous, with strong warnings in the packaging,

especially about pediatric use, and can cause complications ranging from rashes and nausea to white blood cell suppression and liver
failure.[32] On August 23, 2005, the treatment claimed its first known
autism victim when five-year-old Tariq Nadama was killed by a heart
attack caused by chelation.[33]

Despite the problems that plagued the anti-vaccine movement's
research and the lack of demonstrated efficacy of the treatments it
touted, parents insisted, and continue to insist, that their children
improved dramatically as a result of these remedies. However, anecdotes are not facts, and these cures "work" because children with
autism are not static, as they are often portrayed by the instant
experts; their development is delayed but not stopped. Dr. Deborah
Fein has found that 20 percent of children with autism will eventually
no longer be classified as autistic but that no treatment can predictably produce this result.[34] Furthermore, instant experts have constructed a perfect "heads, I win; tails, you lose" scenario: If the child
gets better, it's the treatment. If the child does not get better, then
the parents did not try hard enough/use enough treatments/begin
the intervention early enough. But parents Googling for answers
should know that these charlatans have pages of testimonials and
that legitimate scientific and medical sites on autism are hard to find,
swamped by anti-vaccine pages.

THE AUTISM EPIDEMIC AND THE HIDDEN HORDE

One of the most consistently powerful weapons used by the instant
experts in the anti-vaccine movement to play on parents' fear has
been the myth of the autism epidemic, since it sounds and appears
to be true despite having been consistently disproved. Barbara Loe
Fisher insisted that before the 1990s, "you didn't see autistic children.
Autism was so rare. Most people had never heard of it," and it was only
recently that it had become ubiquitous.[35] The reason, the anti-vaccine
movement said, was too many immunizations and too much mercury.

Its proponents claimed that autism rates corresponded to the use of thimerosal and the number of required vaccines. In the anti-vaccine echo chambers of the Internet, this claim was repeated so many times that, for millions, it became true.

Thimerosal in vaccines was introduced around 1930, often taken as year zero of the autism epidemic, a tendency compounded by the "discovery" of autism in the 1940s. A scientist at Johns Hopkins University, Dr. Leo Kanner, is credited with first diagnosing and naming the disorder in a 1943 paper, after studying eleven children who he believed exhibited a new syndrome. However, what was new was only the name, not the condition. In the scientific literature, autism goes back at least as far as the 1870s, when a doctor in England reported a number of cases consistent with what we today call autism, children who were diagnosed with "dementia" or "dementia, congenital."[36] Other doctors also described autism-like conditions under a variety of terms throughout the late nineteenth and early twentieth centuries, often subsuming autism under schizophrenia, to which it was believed to be related until the 1970s.[37]

At the same time that Kanner was doing his research, an Austrian doctor in Vienna named Hans Asperger was studying a group of children with strikingly similar behavior. In the seldom-cited second section of his 1944 paper, "Die autistischen psychopathen im Kindersalter," Asperger described having seen more than two hundred patients with autistic behaviors during the previous ten years and said that he had studied some patients for two decades or more.[38] Of one he wrote, "we have followed for almost three decades the course of the life of a boy and young man, all of whose behavior shows the pronounced picture of autistic [psychopathology]. From child[hood] on into adulthood he had starkly autistic behavior."[39] But because he wrote in German, Asperger's work was unknown in the English-speaking world for decades, and translations are still rare.

The reason autistic people were rarely seen in the past is that until a few decades ago, most people with moderate or severe autism probably landed in institutions or special schools for the disabled. In 1904, two out of every one thousand Americans were institutionalized, a number that rose to three in one thousand (more than fifty thousand Americans) by 1950.[40] Families were often advised to relinquish their children to state custody and to forget they ever existed. At that time, the "refrigerator mother" theory of autism was also in ascendance, alleging that it was cold, unloving mothers who made children autistic. Subjected to many strange and cruel treatments, the children deteriorated the longer they were institutionalized.[41]

Other severely autistic children became "attic children—so called because they often have been kept hidden, damaged to life without hope."[42] They were allowed to remain at home but had little or no contact with the outside world. In Europe, some of Asperger's patients faced an even worse fate. The Nazi regime passed a law that declared disabled children had "life-unworthy lives" and should be sterilized or exterminated. Dr. Asperger had to work valiantly to save "his" children.[43]

Children with less severe autism spectrum disorders, although perceived as odd, were probably able to remain and even thrive in the mainstream, as was the case with many of Asperger's adult patients. Both Kanner and Asperger also found autistic traits in the parents of many of their original patients. Today more and more adults, including those who are now elderly, receive diagnoses on the autism spectrum, and many others have realized that they show autistic traits.[44] Research also has uncovered large numbers of adults with other diagnoses who instead, or also, fit the criteria for autism. The anti-vaccine movement, however, denies the existence of these adults with autism, the so-called "hidden horde" in the words of Mark Blaxill of SafeMinds, since they received fewer or no vaccines.

The source of the apparent autism "epidemic" lies not in changes in the percentage of children who have autism spectrum disorders (ASDs) but in how such children are classified and whether they are diagnosed. For decades, autism continued to be classified as an infantile version of schizophrenia, just as it had been in the 1910s. This was true in both the original *Diagnostic and Statistical Manual* (DSM-I) of 1952 and the 1968 DSM-II.[45] Autism did not get its own category until the DSM-III in 1980, which included only *infantile autism* and had strict criteria, all six of which had to be presently or previously met for a diagnosis to be made.[46] These early definitions covered only "classical," or Kanner, autism. Low-functioning autistic children may also have been diagnosed as mentally retarded, especially if they were nonverbal and therefore difficult to test. It was not until the 1994 DSM IV that the criteria for autistic disorder were loosened and entries for other conditions on the spectrum, including Asperger's syndrome and "pervasive developmental disorder not otherwise specified" (PDD-NOS), were added. Some researchers on autism believe that "50% to 75% of the increase in diagnoses is coming in these milder categories," so these additions have sweeping implications.[47]

Research has shown that as the criteria changed, so did the diagnoses children received. The March of Dimes found that in California, "the increase in autism diagnoses almost exactly matched a decline in cases of retardation: autism prevalence increased by 9.1 cases per 10,000 children, while mental retardation dropped by 9.3 per 10,000."[48] Doctors are also more able today to identify ASDs when they see them, and the disorders are more in the forefront of their consciousness. Despite assertions from vaccine critics that autistic children could not possibly be missed, Dr. Judith Miles of the University of Missouri medical school held, "Often you don't get a diagnosis because these kids don't jump out at you; some do, but the majority of diagnoses come from very exact questioning." She asserts that in the past, many doctors "didn't ask the questions and didn't come up with the diagnosis."[49]

Reporting of autism cases has increased also due to the educational aid provided for those with autism under the 1990 Americans with Disabilities Act.[50] Autism became a category for special education only in 1991–1992, and the resulting explosion in the number of autistic children in the databases is comparable to that seen in other diagnoses added that year. Parents are also more likely to seek a diagnosis on the autism spectrum because of the services that come with it, especially as the stigmas once surrounding autism have lessened, and doctors are more likely to comply. One doctor said she would "call a kid a zebra if it will get him the educational services ... he needs."[51] This is dramatically shown in data on schoolchildren in Minnesota entering developmental programs. The autism rate was thirteen per ten thousand among six-year-olds in 1995/1996, but five years later, the autism rate for eleven-year-olds was thirty-three per ten thousand. So "[b]etween the ages of 6 and 11, they'd suddenly 'become' nearly three times as autistic—or rather, doctors, parents, and school counselors were enrolling them in programs more aggressively."[52]

THE ANTI-VACCINE PARADOX

At the end of 2004, following the Institute of Medicine report, the debate was essentially over for the medical and scientific community: vaccines did not cause autism. But a strange paradox occurred: the more the science disproved the link, the stronger the anti-vaccine movement became. For vaccine critics, 2005 was a banner year. The vaccine critics did not have science on their side, but they now had celebrity in the form of Jenny McCarthy, and later, from her one-time boyfriend, Jim Carrey. A former Playboy model, McCarthy has an autistic son named Evan, who she claims "recovered" through biomedical treatments.

After Evan was diagnosed in 2005, Jenny McCarthy found her way to, and subsequently became a spokesperson for, Talk About Curing Autism (TACA), which blames mercury and encourages biomedical interventions. She also joined Generation Rescue, which now bills itself as "Jenny McCarthy's autism organization." Although McCarthy never even finished college, she has awarded herself a "Google PhD." Based on these credentials, she believes that she is more qualified to speak about autism than doctors and scientists who have been studying the condition for decades. She has explicitly dismissed any evidence that she is wrong, telling Oprah Winfrey, "My science is Evan, and he's at home. That's my science."[53]

Unfortunately, thousands of Americans have bought into this equation of celebrity with expertise and eschewed the advice of their doctors in favor of unvetted information disseminated on the Internet and the *Oprah* show. McCarthy is a paradigm of how fame has been allowed to eclipse knowledge, lending instant credibility to lies and misinformation. Like the other instant experts championing the thimerosal hypothesis, she has taken refuge in personal experience and anecdote, shouting down anyone who tries to disagree with her. Using her celebrity, McCarthy was able to gain substantial and continued media attention for the anti-vaccine movement, reinforcing the idea that there was still a debate and energizing parents who continued to believe vaccines were responsible and that their children had benefited from various autism "cures." In her two autism-related books, *Louder Than Words: A Mother's Journey in Healing Autism*, and *Mother Warriors: A Nation of Parents Healing Autism Against All Odds*, McCarthy continued to allege that she, and many other parents, cured their children of autism through biomedical interventions, despite the lack of scientific evidence for such treatments and the inconsistencies in McCarthy's contentions about even her own son.

The paradoxical success of the anti-vaccine movement was also fueled by the publication of what would become one of the holy books of the vaccines-cause-autism movement, *Evidence of Harm*, which took its name from the conclusion of the CDC's 1999 report on thimerosal, which said that current study had shown "no evidence of harm."[54] The book's author, journalist David Kirby, was apparently commissioned to write it by Lyn Redwood of SafeMinds, although he had never written on science before and had a history of misrepresenting and exaggerating his credentials. The book presented a script as old as history, a tale of David versus Goliath, the parents versus the uncaring establishment, in which the truth was being concealed or ignored. Kirby, in turn, presented himself as a maverick reporter uncovering the truth hidden by the people in power. His position as a crusader has been amplified by his position as a science reporter for the Huffington Post, which has become a leading and widely read online source of pseudoscience regarding issues ranging from vaccines to antidepressants and medication for ADHD, reflecting the views of its publisher, Arianna Huffington.

Caught up by his portrayal of himself as a crusading journalist and taken in by his claims, the media embraced Kirby and trumpeted his disingenuous and deceptive message. It continued to offer him and others like him as experts, in spite of the science showing that they were wrong. The population, having seen the claims of these "experts" on the news or in the paper, all too often took them for truth, especially when a Google search turned up a panoply of anti-vaccination websites. Kirby wrote on his blog about the reception to his book: "From the media not ONE NEGATIVE WORD so far. Not one. Only from the Quackwatch bloggers, the pediatricians, the National Network for Immunization Information, the CDC, and for some reason, the state of Minnesota." In other words, from the people in a position to know his lies for what they were. And to Kirby and his supporters, these were exactly the people who did not matter.

Not only did *Evidence of Harm* bring the anti-vaccine message to a new and wider audience, but it also exemplified the way the instant experts had tapped into a fear deep within their audience that science by its very nature could not quell. Kirby wrote in the book's introduction, "The CDC has been unable to definitively prove or disprove the theory that thimerosal causes autism," and furthermore, "'no evidence of harm' is not the same as proof of safety. No evidence of harm is not a definitive answer."[55] The problem is that science can *never* prove a negative 100 percent. It can only indicate that something is very unlikely. Yet people yearn for certainty and have trouble accepting the idea that an absolute answer may be impossible. The public hears not the overwhelming evidence but the doubt, not the 99.999999 percent but the 0.000001. They walk away believing that science does not really know—or that scientists are covering their backs if they are wrong. It is the harnessing of this desire that gives instant experts their power; they can promise anything and everything because their promises are based on belief and not data.

It is to play to such popular worries that, despite the extensive research on the issue, anti-vaccine zealots still repeat that "studies have not been done" and "there is not enough research" to determine whether vaccines are tied to autism. In particular, they have become fixated on the absence of a controlled study of vaccinated versus unvaccinated children, which is unfeasible for ethical, logistical, and mathematical reasons, and is also unnecessary, since the many epidemiological studies that have already been carried out have included vaccinated, unvaccinated, and partially vaccinated children and have found no indications of any divergences between them.[56] Of course, to the instant experts, no amount of research or data will ever be enough so long as it does not support their beliefs. Still, it is an effective tactic, because to those not intimately familiar with the vaccine-autism debate, it seems both credible and reasonable, and it has allowed the anti-vaccination movement to claim that all they want is more study. In fact, they are working to steal the mantle of authority from doctors and scientists, neutralizing credentials and study by claiming that such authorities have failed us and only the instant experts, ordinary but driven, can provide the answer.

CONSPIRACY!

The anti-vaccine movement uses another classic tactic of instant experts of all kinds: they accuse their opponents of having conflicts of interest that taint their work, and they allege that those opponents are deliberately hiding the truth. It is a well-worn strategy but all the more effective as a result, since it has produced a familiar story that casts pharmaceutical companies manufacturing vaccines in the role of the villain, heartlessly selling unsafe products to fill their own coffers. (In fact, vaccines make up only a very small amount of such companies' revenues.) Government agencies such as the FDA and CDC, the anti-vaccine movement has said, are complicit in these actions, either because they are too cowed to stand up to industry or because they are likewise getting rich off the suffering of children. The narrative portrays doctors as paid off by drug companies to push vaccines and never to question their dangers or necessity. The instant experts and their followers then assume the position of crusaders uncovering the great corporate conspiracy and fighting for the lives of their children.

This story of conspiracy and conflict of interest has been nowhere more clearly articulated than in Robert F. Kennedy, Jr.'s, article "Deadly Immunity," published simultaneously online on Salon.com and in *Rolling Stone* in June 2005. He chose as his rallying cry Simpsonwood, the name of a government scientific retreat held five years earlier to review a new analysis of the role of vaccines in autism rates.[57] Early data collected by Thomas Verstraeten had shown a connection between immunizations and several neurological problems, including tics, speech delays, and attention deficit disorder (but not autism). So Walter Orenstein, head of the CDC National Immunization Program and the man who had commissioned the study, invited around fifty doctors and scientists to Simpsonwood, a retreat and conference center in Georgia, to discuss the findings. At the meeting, several questions were raised about the accuracy of Verstraeten's data, and when these concerns were taken into account, the correlations disappeared. In November 2003, Verstraeten published the final analysis in *Pediatrics*, concluding, "No significant associations were found."[58]

The Simpsonwood conference in 2000 had attracted almost no notice in the press at the time, but now, five years after the event, Kennedy was using it as the center of a conspiracy theory that alleged that the medical establishment was in collusion to hurt children by hiding the truth about vaccines. In a typical instant expert tactic, he misleadingly and selectively quoted from the transcript of the actual meeting, the quotes shorn of any context, to produce the impression that the conference indeed centered on creating a cover-up.[59] The article was riddled with gross errors, and numerous corrections had to be issued by both Salon and *Rolling Stone*. But many of the readers never saw the retractions, or did not heed them. Kennedy's scare tactics were wildly successful and helped expand the panic over vaccines just when the science should have put it to rest.

The irony of the instant experts' attack on scientists and doctors for being conflicted was that they were themselves beholden to lawyers and interest groups, a fact that went largely undiscussed and unnoticed. In 2004, British journalist Brian Deer discovered that Andrew Wakefield had possessed not one but two financial incentives to reach the conclusion that MMR caused autism. First, the parents of at least five of the autistic children he was studying were in the process of suing drug companies for vaccine-related injury. Deer reported that their lawyer, Richard Barr, was affiliated with the British anti-vaccine organization JABS and had paid Wakefield over $100,000 to create science to back up their case.[60]

Further research would show that the actual sum was more than seven times that, totaling £435,643, or well over $700,000. Second, "Wakefield hoped to profit from the panic he created, having filed to patent his own 'safer' vaccine product," which he claimed would mitigate or eliminate the risk of autism, and he had started two companies to offer autism diagnosis kits.[61] Deer also discovered that during his study, Wakefield had carried out harmful procedures on the children that were not authorized by the hospital's Ethical Practices Committee of the Royal Free Hospital, where he practiced. Finally, Dr. Nicholas Chadwick, who had worked for Wakefield, revealed that his tests of the biopsy samples were all negative, and the few positives were false positives. But Wakefield had presented all the results as positive. Chadwick had therefore asked for his name to be taken off the 1998 paper.[62]

The other scientists who had collaborated with Wakefield on the *Lancet* article were apparently shocked at the allegations. Ten of the twelve contributors quickly renounced it, and the journal apologized for publishing the piece, saying it contained "fatal conflicts of interest" on the part of Dr. Wakefield.[63] Also professing to be "shocked and disappointed" by Wakefield's behavior was John O'Leary, whose lab had seemed to vindicate Wakefield in 2002. However, Deer would discover in 2006 that O'Leary had gotten over $1 million from the same lawyer as Wakefield, Richard Barr.[64] Dr. Stephen Bustin, who had investigated O'Leary's lab, revealed in 2007 that O'Leary had likewise used contaminated samples that produced false positives.[65] The work of several other scientists who had seemingly supported Wakefield's hypothesis also had been funded by Barr.[66]

The media was not anxious to admit that they had been mistaken about Wakefield, and gave far less coverage to the truth than they had to the lie. The devious doctor made for excellent television: he seemed the very picture of the young, charismatic physician, and his controversial allegations created top ratings. Also, by the time the perfidy of Wakefield and his accomplices was exposed, the backlash against the MMR was too far gone to be easily stopped, and thousands of parents could not be convinced that the immunization was safe after all.

In the United States, the picture was very much the same. SafeMinds had paid Richard Deth $60,000 to carry out his research alleging that autistic children are unable to excrete mercury, and had given Mady Hornig $35,000 for her "autistic mice" study. Both had stacked the deck in their experiments to ensure that the outcome would be what they wanted. Many of the instant experts also had become well-paid mainstays of court cases against vaccine manufacturers, and of proceedings before the National Vaccine Injury Compensation Program, set up in 1986 to hear cases of alleged damage caused by immunization and to provide compensation where appropriate. However, their knowledge and research would be repeatedly discredited by legitimate scientists. One judge labeled Dr. Mark Geier "a professional witness in areas for which he has no training, expertise and experience" and called him "intellectually dishonest."[67]

TERRORISTS AND PROSTITUTES

But while the instant experts continued to push aside scientific evidence in favor of their own narrative, the real experts were still pushing back with new studies from around the world, all of which showed the same thing: that autism is not correlated with vaccines of any kind. In 2005, a study in Japan, where the use of the combined MMR had been stopped after Wakefield's *Lancet* paper, found no difference in the autism rate of children who had received the MMR and those who had received single vaccines.[68] This was no surprise, since Wakefield had never been able to provide a credible reason that single vaccines were superior to the MMR in the first place.

The thimerosal hypothesis fared no better. A study in July 2006 in *Pediatrics* by Eric Fombonne of McGill University found that autism rates continued to go up in Canada despite the absence of thimerosal in vaccines; in fact, the group with the highest autism incidence had the lowest mercury exposure.[69] And an extensive analysis by the CDC, led by Bill Thompson, which conducted more than forty tests and combed the data meticulously for possible patterns, announced in September 2007 in the *New England Journal of Medicine* that there was no correlation.[70] As a sop to the anti-vaccine movement, the CDC had even allowed Sallie Bernard of SafeMinds to be involved in the design of the study, and she promoted the research until the results failed to conform to her biases.

As the results from scientific studies challenging their position continued to come in, the anti-vaccine movement stepped up its attacks on pro-vaccine scientists and doctors, attacks that escalated into violence and threats of physical harm. One of the biggest targets has been Dr. Paul Offit, medical director of the Vaccine Education Center at the Children's Hospital of Philadelphia and the holder of a chair at the University of Pennsylvania Medical School. Offit is a prominent and outspoken advocate for vaccination and an equally open critic of the vaccine hypothesis. To anti-vaccine crusaders, he is the Dark Lord of immunizations. Offit is also hated because he developed a vaccine against rotavirus, now licensed to Merck. Despite the fact that he no longer stands to gain financially from the vaccine, his development of it is seen as proof that he is in the pocket of drug companies and being paid off to allow children to be hurt or killed.

As a result, he has received anonymous phone calls from people who have listed his children's names and schools, implicitly threatening them, and he had to hire security guards. Offit has written that he has been called "a prostitute"; has been asked, "How in the world can you put money before the health of someone's baby?" and "Why did you sell your soul to the devil?" and has been accused of being "directly responsible for the death and damage of hundreds of children."[71]

As he went into a June 2006 session of the Advisory Committee on Immunization Practices in Atlanta, more than a hundred protesters stood before the U.S. Centers for Disease Control and Prevention shouting epithets at him. One of the protestors, carrying a megaphone, yelled, "The devil! It's the devil!" Another brandished a poster with "TERRORIST" and a photo of Offit's face on it. As he was about to enter the building, a man in prison garb took hold of his jacket but let go when asked to do so. "It was harrowing," Dr. Offit recalls.[72]

Since then, however, Dr. Offit has remained a vociferous supporter of vaccines and an unfailing opponent of efforts to undermine their use. As a result, he remains "enemy number one" of the anti-vaccine movement. He has been repeatedly sued for libel as a result of his unflattering portrayals of prominent anti-vaccine leaders in his 2008 book *Autism's False Prophets*, one of several books he has written on the history of immunizations and anti-vaccine movements. In it, he attacks head-on the role of anti-vaccine crusaders in creating and perpetuating the controversy over autism and immunizations. Two things seem certain: Dr. Offit will never pipe down and stop standing up to these instant experts and their supporters, and they will never stop trying to silence him through harassment and intimidation.

But Dr. Offit is far from the only physician who has ended up in the crosshairs of the anti-vaccine movement. Another pro-vaccine doctor, Dr. Gregory Poland of the Mayo Vaccine Research Group, part of the Mayo Clinic, told ABC News in 2008, "Among the most egregious things—I got a letter once railing against my involvement in vaccines and hoping that something serious would happen to me and hoping that something serious would happen to one of my children ... I had people come to the door of my home and harass my wife and kids, so I no longer have my address listed in the phone book." He also had to get extra security for his lab after an intruder tried to get into his work computers.

The goal is clear, and unfortunately it has been achieved in some cases. Poland admitted that he "know[s] a lot of colleagues who have decided to write something slightly different or say something slightly different because they are afraid of inciting anti-vaccine groups." Some doctors have preferred to take up other areas of research rather than continue to subject themselves to the anger of anti-vaccine ideologues. In general, says Dr. William Schaffner of the Vanderbilt University School of Medicine, "threats certainly—as well as the anticipation of heated 'feedback'—clearly has inhibited colleagues from engaging in the public discussion of contentious issues."[73]

Even those who are not doctors find themselves harassed. Prominent bloggers have threatening comments posted to their pages and "trolls" regularly invading their posts, sometimes preventing dialogue and even overloading the sites. A few have shut down or curtailed their blogging because of vitriolic, nasty comments about them and their families. In 2008, a prominent blogger on autism, Kathleen Seidel, was served with a subpoena by lawyer Cliff Shoemaker in a vaccine case against a drug company and asked to hand over almost all paperwork related to her site, Neurodiversity.com, including all correspondence. When she countered, Shoemaker accused her of being paid by pharmaceutical companies. The subpoena was finally quashed, but not until Seidel had spent considerable time and energy fighting it.

Such examples abound. Not only are such tactics unacceptable, but they also reduce scientific progress when scientists are afraid to carry out studies of vaccines out of concern that doing so will place them and those around them in peril. That is precisely what the instant experts want; their purpose is to destroy or muzzle true experts and take their place, and in so doing to twist scientific inquiry to conform to their personal beliefs. The vaccine controversy is not a debate over science anymore—and has not been for years—and the anti-vaccine movement is determined to continue the fight until they get what they want, science and public health be damned.

THE NEVER-ENDING VACCINE DEBATE?

Despite the efforts of the instant experts and their followers, there is some hope that science may yet surmount ideology and anecdote. Slowly the media has started to catch on that the accumulated evidence stands starkly against vaccines being implicated in autism. A number of news outlets have finally made clear that the science shows no connection between immunizations and autism. Doctors and scientists are beginning to get equal time in the media without being shouted down by members of the anti-vaccine movement, and new books and articles have helped to expose the lies of vaccine opponents. Websites and blogs countering the autism-vaccine link have increased, providing clear, detailed analyses that debunk the instant expert's claims and reinforce the science. Finally, proponents of neurodiversity, who believe that autism can produce assets as well as deficits and who oppose "cures," are finally starting to be heard. But members of the media have already been subjected to the same types of personal and legal attacks as scientists when they crossed the anti-vaccine movement.

Both epidemiological and laboratory studies continue to vindicate science's conclusion. In early 2008, the data from California for 2007 showed that autism cases were still rising, more than five years after thimerosal had been phased out. Then, in the fall of 2008, an attempt to replicate Wakefield's original MMR study found no connection. Surprisingly, two participants were former defenders of the vaccine-autism connection, Mady Hornig, who had run the 2004 autistic mice study, and Wakefield's one-time accomplice John O'Leary.[74] New epidemiological evidence from Italy agrees that the number of vaccinations children receive is not correlated with autism rates.[75] Jenny McCarthy even has a celebrity rival: actress Amanda Peet, a spokesperson for the pro-vaccine group Every Child By Two. More and more data now point to a strong genetic component for autism, if a complex one involving multiple genes. It is a start, but there is still a long way to go before the influence of the instant experts is broken.

The goalposts of the autism debate are infinitely moveable as far as instant experts are concerned; as one theory is knocked down by science, these "experts" come up with another. Some are bizarre, such as claims that mercury plumes from China are making California kids autistic. Others require a heavy measure of doublethink, such as claims that the flu vaccine is still driving autism rates even though the amount of thimerosal children receive has dropped tremendously. The instant experts now demand that we "Green Our Vaccines" and say, "I'm not *anti*-vaccine; I'm *pro*-safe vaccine." They shift the blame to other vaccine ingredients, particularly aluminum, which is an adjuvant that allows vaccines to generate stronger and longer-lasting immunity. They also scare parents with distorted claims that vaccines contain antifreeze, ether, formaldehyde, and aborted fetuses, or they simply speak ominously of unnamed toxins.

Others claim that children get "too many [vaccines], too soon" and advocate selective vaccination or spacing out immunizations, ignoring that the vaccine schedule is carefully constructed for maximum effectiveness and, contrary to claims, is tested to prevent harmful interactions. They also fail to understand that there are many fewer immunologic components in today's vaccines than in previous versions, and vaccines generate far fewer antibodies than having the actual illness. Worse, despite their avowals, these instant experts *are* anti-vaccine, often admitting they would not vaccinate their future children. The truth is simple: as long as there are vulnerable parents, there will always be a new anti-vaccine theory.

In March of 2008, the instant experts also began to link autism to mitochondrial disease after the Vaccine Injury Compensation Program court compensated a young girl named Hannah Poling after her mitochondrial disorder worsened following a vaccine, producing some autistic symptoms. In fact, Hannah was diagnosed with the brain disease encephalopathy, and only some of her symptoms matched those of autism. Nor do instant experts appear to be correct that mitochondrial disease is common in people with autism, and current research on the topic is still very scanty.[76] Furthermore, because mitochondrial disorders can be exacerbated by illness, especially fever, people affected are urged to be vaccinated. Finally, the standard of proof in the Vaccine Injury Compensation Program court is much lower than in regular court, and its judges, or Special Masters, do not have scientific backgrounds.

Despite its shortfalls, the VICP has mostly come down on the side of science. As a result of the thousands of cases brought before the court, test cases were designated for the various theories of causation. In February 2009, the outcomes of the first three test cases, those arguing that the MMR alone or in combination with thimerosal produced autism were announced. None of the three families involved, the Cedillos, Hazlehursts, and Snyders, received compensation, and the three decisions were strikingly similar and quite scathing when it came to the evidence for the theories being presented.

George L. Hastings, Jr., the Special Master for the Cedillo case, said that the data were "overwhelmingly contrary" to the family's theory and that the Cedillos had been "misled by physicians who are guilty, in my view, of gross medical misjudgment."[77] Meanwhile, the Special Master in the Snyder case opined, "[t]o conclude that Colten [Snyder]'s condition was the result of his MMR vaccine, an objective observer would have to emulate Lewis Carroll's White Queen and be able to believe six impossible (or, at least, highly improbable) things before breakfast."[78] The Special Masters also made clear that they found the government's experts far more qualified than those of the families.

The anti-vaccine forces would lose again a year later, on a second set of three cases, which argued that thimerosal on its own was responsible for rendering children autistic. In the decision, one of the Special Masters wrote that the witnesses testifying for the families "were outclassed in every respect by the impressive assembly of true experts in their respective fields who testified on behalf of respondent [that thimerosal does not cause autism]."[79] And yet the battle rages on, played out on talk shows, news programs, and especially the forums, blogs, and websites of the Internet.

TRUTH AND CONSEQUENCES

Today in the United States, at least 90 percent of children receive many of the recommended vaccines, but vaccination rates are still below herd immunity in some communities, and many children are missing one or more vaccines.[80] The number of children with exemptions that allow them to attend school without being vaccinated is higher than ever before, and still going up. In 2007, the *Journal of the American Medical Association* found that 55 percent of doctors reported at least one parent refusing to vaccinate their child at all in the past year, and 85 percent said a parent refused one or more shots.

As a result, the first six months of 2008 saw the highest incidence of measles in twelve years, with 131 cases and fifteen people landing in the hospital, most of them unvaccinated.[81] The United Kingdom, likewise, has had repeated measles outbreaks and several deaths. In 2006–2007, an epidemic produced 1,726 cases, more than in the previous ten years combined, and another outbreak in 2008–2009 showed cases at a thirteen-year high.[82] Measles also popped up in Israel, Switzerland, Germany, Austria, Italy, and other countries.

Measles is not the only vaccine-preventable disease that is returning. Cases of pertussis, or whooping cough, which is especially dangerous for infants, are also going up dramatically in the United States.[83] Mumps is coming back in the United States, the United Kingdom, and Canada, including outbreaks in New Jersey, New York, and Quebec in 2009–2010.[84] Cases of *Haemophilus influenzae* type B (Hib) have sent a rising number of babies to the hospital with meningitis, in some cases producing permanent damage. Even chicken pox, deemed a mild childhood illness by many parents, can produce long-term problems and even kill.[85] A number of the recent outbreaks of vaccine-preventable disease have been caused by unimmunized people who contracted the illness abroad, indicating that even diseases that vaccination has made rare in the developed world remain threats in this age of global travel.

Yet those who brought about this result have not been forced to truly answer for their actions. Evidence of Andrew Wakefield's misconduct grew in 2009, when journalist Brian Deer showed that the medical records of almost all of Wakefield's original subjects did not match what had been written in Wakefield's *Lancet* article. Colon biopsy results on most of the children were normal and later reclassified abnormal. In one case, three outside labs found no measles in the biopsy, indicating once again that Wakefield's positive results were false. Furthermore, several children showed signs of autism before the MMR, while others did not develop autism until long afterward. Lastly, the cases were not the random sample claimed; rather, many of the parents had sought out Wakefield.[86]

In part as a result of all the evidence against Wakefield that Deer has compiled over the years, he, along with two colleagues and co-authors on the *Lancet* article, was subjected to investigation by the United Kingdom's General Medical Council (GMC) for misconduct and his license to practice eventually revoked. The result, in early 2010, was gratifying for those who had watched him produce misleading research and rhetoric for more than a decade with apparent impunity: the panel deemed him guilty of offenses that "include those of dishonesty and misleading conduct [and] would not be insufficient to support a finding of serious professional misconduct." Similar verdicts were handed down on the other two accused scientists, including findings that they had acted contrary to the medical interests of the research subjects.[87]

The following week, on the heels of a *British Medical Journal* commentary calling on the journal to do so, *The Lancet* totally retracted Wakefield's 1998 article and acknowledged that its conclusions were "false."[88] Another study Wakefield had published, this one in *Neurotoxicology*, was also withdrawn.[89] Wakefield soon after left his position at Thoughtful House, a biomedical facility in Austin, Texas, where he had taken refuge from the GMC proceedings despite the fact he is not licensed to practice medicine in the United States.[90] While it was claimed that he resigned voluntarily, observers widely believed he had been pushed out. Nonetheless, the punishment is not only late in coming but mild, considering the damage Wakefield caused. Further, it has only made him all the more a martyr of the anti-vaccine movement, seen as the conspiracy-uncovering physician pilloried for publicizing what the establishment was supposedly hiding. Worse, none of the other instant experts have faced any consequences at all for promoting dangerous and false theories.

Over the last ten years, the autism debate has provided a platform for dozens of instant experts, ranging from doctors seeking fortune and fame by selling their science, to crusading parents who want someone to blame for their child's autism, to politicians who use their position to advance their agenda. A movement has emerged that has antipathy toward all science that does not support its view and that has succeeded in exploiting the Internet and our new reliance on online information to spread its message more effectively than its predecessors could ever have dreamed. Journalist Amy Wallace nailed it in an article in *Wired* when she wrote:

> [I]f you need a new factoid to support your belief system, it has never been easier to find one. The Internet offers a treasure trove of undifferentiated information, data, research, speculation, half-truths, anecdotes, and conjecture about health and medicine. It is also a democratizing force that tends to undermine authority, cut out the middleman, and empower individuals. In a world where anyone can attend what [Jenny] McCarthy calls the "University of Google," boning up on immunology before getting your child vaccinated seems like good, responsible parenting. Thanks to the Internet, everyone can be their own medical investigator.[91]

Science has spoken, but the instant experts and their followers refuse to hear.

CHAPTER 6

The Suicide Crisis: Sowing Fear about Antidepressants

M EGAN MCMANUS SEEMED TO have it all. An apparently happy student at Palatine High School in Illinois, she had top grades and lots of friends. Yet she had been struggling with clinical depression since she was thirteen. Back then, she was prescribed Zoloft and responded well. But in 2004, as a result of news reports claiming that antidepressants such as Zoloft were linked to or caused suicide, her mother, Kathleen, removed her from the medication. At the time, Kathleen recalls thinking, "It wasn't worth taking that risk that she would commit suicide or have suicidal thoughts."

Yet the decision to discontinue Megan's medication had the opposite effect: instead of making her safer, it placed her more at risk. After losing a good friend to suicide, Megan launched an online group called Students Overcoming Suicide, with the hope of preventing other teens from killing themselves. Yet Megan's own depression came back in 2007, and she tried to commit suicide. She was again prescribed drugs to control her depression, but it was already too late. In July 2007, at just eighteen years old, she took her life. Kathleen now wonders if taking Megan off Zoloft led to her death, and she told the press, "I always ask myself why ... why, why, why did this happen? I do really regret it, and I wish that she was still on it."[1]

Kathleen is not responsible for her daughter's suicide. The blame can and should be placed on those who spread warnings about the risks of antidepressants in an effort to panic millions of parents and induce them to take their children off these medications, as Kathleen did. We have seen how supposedly science-based government agencies reacted to the spurious connection between vaccines and autism by taking action against alleged dangers "just in case," and thereby allowing immunization rates to fall and diseases to reemerge. Even more starkly, the addition by the FDA in 2004 of a black box warning on the antidepressants called selective serotonin reuptake inhibitors (SSRIs) contributed in part to the largest jump in teen suicide in twenty-five years. Not only was it the largest and fastest U.S. increase in decades, but suicide rates rose internationally as other countries took similar actions.

The FDA warning was merely the culmination of years of scaremongering and misinformation that had already begun to send suicide rates rising even before the FDA decided to take action. The controversy was driven by instant experts, led by British psychiatrist Dr. David Healy, who sought to undermine the use of SSRIs for all patients. Mostly unsuccessful in their attempts to link the drugs to suicide and violent behavior in adults, they then turned their attention to pediatric use, combining doubts that SSRIs worked in children with trial data showing a slightly higher risk of "suicidality" in young patients being treated with the drugs. But suicidality itself is an elastic and scientifically invalid measure, one that was created specifically to support these efforts to indict SSRIs by allowing critics to classify events in a way that supported their point of view.

As a result, scared parents, beset by reports online and in the media of children and teenagers killed by SSRIs, not only stopped their sons and daughters from taking the drugs, but also put pressure on agencies such as the FDA to ban or restrict them. Afraid that the price for skepticism about these claims would be more suicides, regulators gave in to the instant experts who had so adroitly manipulated the data and the debate. The result was yet another case of the dangers of the Precautionary Principle and the perils of acting too quickly on incomplete information.

NO BETTER THAN A PLACEBO?

To understand the SSRI controversy, you first have to go back to the debate over whether antidepressants work at all, especially for children and adolescents. Like other tabloid medicine examples, the campaign to undermine trust in SSRIs began with an effort to demonstrate that they were unnatural products that caused the death and emotional destruction of children.

Consequently, many critics of SSRIs assert that antidepressants have no benefits for people under eighteen, and therefore there is nothing to offset their risks. First, they claim that there are few randomized controlled trials in this age group. Second, they argue that the vast majority of studies show that SSRIs are no more effective at treating depression than a sugar pill and that, indeed, most clinical trials show a large benefit from a placebo—sometimes larger than for the drug tested. To them, the rapid increase in the use of these drugs, for any age, is due to industry marketing, not clinical value.

The critics are right about the fact that many clinical trials for antidepressants show a large placebo effect. In fact, significant placebo response has been found in studies for *every* treatment for depression, whether it was a drug, therapy, or exercise. This may be in part because treatment is more than the pill that patients take every day. Dr. Walter Brown suggested in *Psychiatric Times* that the "treatment situation" includes other essential elements associated with healing, such as counseling, evaluation, and prognosis, and these are common to both the placebo and treatment groups.[2] Making patients feel that their problem has been identified and can be controlled and improved is itself part of making them feel better, and this effect is especially strong when it comes to psychiatric conditions.

The placebo response has been a big problem in clinical trials for all types of mental illness and has been widely studied. Scientists attribute it to misdiagnosing patients, poor recordkeeping, the fact that mental illness can worsen and subside spontaneously, or even the reality that many people who are enrolled in studies drop out before the studies are over. It is also an artifact of a tendency for the greatest improvement to occur in the first two weeks of treatment, before a medication has had a chance to fully work.

These issues are compounded by the use of big studies with multiple trial sites, even as such research is proposed as a solution to the uncertainties that continue to surround SSRI use. As found by a large study of children with major depression, the bigger the study and the more sites involved, the bigger the placebo response, which may be true in part because "studies with many sites recruited participants with less severe illness, suggesting that screening for participants may be less stringent in trials with more sites."[3]

But the fact that many patients get better on a placebo doesn't mean that the drugs do nothing, and in fact, for many patients, medication is not only helpful but essential. While patients who improve on the sugar pill usually reach a plateau after a few weeks of treatment, those receiving the actual drug can continue to get better slowly. There is also strong population data that show that higher rates of SSRI use are associated with lower rates of suicide.

The most unequivocal evidence of benefits in children and adolescents is for Prozac, the only SSRI to be specially tested for use in this age group and which was discovered to reduce depression by almost 30 percent in one trial. The study concluded that a combination of medication and cognitive behavioral therapy was the optimal treatment for pediatric depression, with 71 percent of the patients getting better on the dual regime. Drugs alone helped 60.6 percent, and therapy alone, 43.2 percent. Suicides went down for all patients.[4] Similarly, in an earlier study, 56 percent of patients taking Prozac were in the "much better" or "very much better" categories, compared to 33 percent on a placebo.[5] A third trial saw more than twice as many depressed pediatric patients fit the definition of remission (41 percent versus 20 percent).[6] Positive results have been obtained for OCD and anxiety as well as depression.[7]

Zoloft was also found to be more effective than a placebo in a study conducted from 1999 to 2000, in which researchers found that "69 percent of the subjects who took the drug improved significantly, compared with 59 percent of those who took a dummy pill." Some doctors believe that the ten-point difference is "modest," but it is nonetheless a clear demonstration of the benefit of SSRI.[8] In total, of eight studies completed through 2004, two found benefits for SSRIs of more than 20 percent, three of 10 percent or more, and the last three of lower percentages.[9] Subsequent studies have remained mixed, but a significant proportion of them continue to find substantial benefit.

A study that evaluated the existing literature on the efficacy and safety of pediatric use of all SSRIs, for not only depression but also obsessive-compulsive disorder (OCD) and other anxiety disorders, concluded that pediatric patients in all three categories did better on the drugs. Overall, patients on SSRIs had an 11 percent higher response rate for major depressive disorder (MDD), 20 percent for OCD, and 37 percent for other anxiety disorders. The authors judged that in all three categories, SSRIs helped patients sufficiently to offset the potential for negative side effects. More importantly, differences in suicidal thinking and behavior between the active and placebo groups were minimal in all but one of the twenty-seven included trials.[10]

FROM SUICIDE TO SUICIDALITY

Convincing the public that SSRIs don't work in children (or at all) was only one facet of the critics' strategy. The second facet was spreading the belief that use of the drugs led to suicide. Lacking the data to prove such a connection, they did the next best thing: they invented a condition called suicidality, which was not only easily confused with completed suicide but which also could be endlessly redefined.

The shift from the use of the word *suicide* to *suicidality* began not in the United States but in the United Kingdom, where, in 2001 and 2002, Dr. David Healy was leading the effort to determine whether SSRIs caused suicides. In many ways, Healy followed the crusading path of fellow Briton Andrew Wakefield and, likewise, conducted his research while being retained by law firms suing makers of medicines. In this case, Healy was an expert witness who testified that SSRIs caused the new disease of suicidality, and he was used extensively in successful litigation against Eli Lilly, in which he testified that a man who murdered his family did so because he was on Paxil.

Like Wakefield, Healy was lionized in the British media for courageously standing up to industry for pushing harmful drugs for the sake of profits. He became a cause célèbre when an offer to teach and conduct research at the University of Toronto's Centre for Addiction and Mental Health was rescinded days before he was to take the job. The reason was CAMH's concern about the science behind opposition to SSRIs, fueled by a speech Healy had recently given in which he leveled a variety of strong and unfounded accusations against the drugs. But Healy alleged in an interview with the Canadian Broadcasting Corporation that Eli Lilly, which had provided CAMH with a $1.5 million grant the previous year, had pressured the center to drop him. Although there was no proof to support his contention, this version of events was widely accepted and publicized in the media and online.

The truth was that CAMH was only one of many institutions and individuals with reservations about the quality of Dr. Healy's science. Thoroughly convinced that SSRIs were more dangerous than the pharmaceutical industry was willing to admit, he had carried out several studies that claimed to link antidepressants to suicidality and suicide but that used questionable methodologies and assumptions and twisted the data to suit the predetermined conclusion. One of the biggest problems was the conflation of suicidality (which includes suicidal thinking and ideation and is often very broadly defined) and suicide. Healy did nothing to establish the difference between suicidality and suicide and indeed actively treated them as interchangeable. He told the press, "Doctors have been getting the mantra from the drug companies for twelve years that it is the disease [causing the suicide] and not the drug. It does provide a nice way out for GPs who just don't want to contemplate the possibility that a drug they prescribe could cause death."[11]

Suicidality, a condition created by Healy and other SSRI opponents, represented but the latest chapter in an assault on SSRIs that began with the development and release of Prozac in 1986. Prozac was never "just any drug. Soon after arriving on drugstore shelves ... Eli Lilly's antidepressant transcended simple pilldom, becoming instead a cultural icon. Hailed as a wonder drug one minute, cast as evil incarnate the next, the green and white capsule has generated multitudes of lawsuits, and garnered more attention than some presidential candidates."[12]

Over the subsequent quarter century, many more SSRIs have joined Prozac. While many of these medications differ only slightly in how they work and are formulated, the fact is that most people suffering from a mental illness, particularly major depression, do not respond to the first medicine they are prescribed and need to try several before finding one that is effective. In fact, fully 60 percent of all people treated for depression with SSRIs have to try more than one medication. Individual differences in response to medications depend on many factors, including age, diagnosis, dosing, compliance with treatment, and biological factors.

Much like the fear generated about vaccines, the reframing of Prozac, and subsequently other antidepressants, started with anecdotes involving the medication's hidden dangers. Tales of strange behavior and suicides on SSRIs had been in the press and trickling onto the Internet for some time. In the 1990s, defense attorneys representing murderers and violent criminals tried to pin the blame on their clients' use of Prozac—efforts that, for the most part, failed. But of all the issues raised by Prozac skeptics, the most difficult for many people to sort out was the contention that the drug was linked to suicide, an association that began in 1990, when a Harvard University researcher, Dr. Martin Teicher, reported on six patients who "developed intense, violent suicidal preoccupation" shortly after starting the drug.[13]

By the mid-1990s, however, most scientists had lost interest in the issue. Several larger studies concluded that subjects on Prozac showed no increase in suicidal acts or feelings, and some actually reported that the drug reduced suicide risk. In 1991, an FDA advisory committee concluded that there was no persuasive evidence for a suicide link, allaying many people's fears. Scientists and physicians generally agreed that "disentangling the effects of the antidepressants from the effects of depression itself, a disease that has a high rate of suicide, was difficult or impossible."[14]

But the critics of Prozac and its counterparts were not going to give up so easily. As they abandoned the suicide-drug connection, they created a whole new syndrome that could be associated with antidepressant medications. Literally out of nowhere, a condition called suicidality appeared. It was meant to be considered a surrogate measure, or marker, for a change in behavior or disease. But to be a reliable surrogate measure, there has to agreement on what is being measured, and the surrogate has to be a fairly good predictor of a specific set of outcomes. So, for instance, measuring blood pressure is useful only because there is a common approach to taking such readings, and because it has been demonstrated that the level of one's blood pressure can predict a specific disease and be correlated with health improvement.

What's more, a surrogate measure, or marker, should ideally be something that occurs frequently enough to be measured accurately.

If the outcome it measures is rare, it is especially important that the marker's relationship to a change in health be well established through lots of observations that confirm that every time someone uses the marker, the same thing is being measured with the same methodology. The most common way to test whether a marker is actually predicting an event (cause and effect), as opposed to being statistically associated with some result, is to compare patients with a specific condition to those that don't have the condition and see if the marker appears in the former group but not the latter.

Suicidality has none of these features. Indeed, it has never been clearly defined but, rather, is a moving target subject to enormous latitude for interpretation—and manipulation. Even the data used to develop a measure of suicidality were inconsistent, imprecise, and vague. As Dr. Donald Klein, who pioneered the use of medication to treat depression, notes, the "composite variable, termed 'suicidality'... incorporates not only actions evaluated as suicide attempts (often in the absence of articulated intent, plan, or injury) but also 'ideation,' which cannot yield firm inferences about lethal intent."[15] Suicidality is a spectrum, including not only serious behaviors but many minor ones, identified without a standard procedure or format. Events that could be interpreted as self-destructive, even when the intent is unclear, also tend simply to be placed in the category of suicidality, especially if the patient has a past history of self-harm or violent behavior.

Thus, suicidality was a creation of tabloid medicine entrepreneurs, designed to provide a tool for reframing SSRIs as dangerous, even deadly, medicine. Lacking scientific validity for its supposed purpose (predicting possible suicides), it has instead been used to generate studies, press releases, op-eds, and websites stating that SSRIs are associated with suicide and to spark concerns about the safety of SSRIs both in the United States and abroad, beginning well before the decision in 2004 to place a black box on the labels.

CATALYZING THE CONTROVERSY

Despite his efforts opposing SSRIs, until late 2002, Dr. Healy had not yet assembled all the elements for this tabloid medicine campaign. This changed thanks to a BBC report called *The Secrets of Seroxat*, which featured Dr. Healy and alleged that the drug Seroxat (called Paxil in the United States) had a hidden potential to cause self-harm and suicide. The show triggered an outpouring of public commentary and, with it, demands for greater scrutiny of Paxil and other SSRIs for serious side effects—especially because the program ran just as the United Kingdom's Medicines and Healthcare products Regulatory Agency (MHRA) was reviewing data from a study by GlaxoSmithKline of pediatric patients on Paxil. While reviewing the data, the British drug regulators found what they called a "signal" of more suicidal thoughts and behavior among children taking Paxil than those on a placebo. As a result, they asked the company for additional data and for explanations of what the company thought the trial results meant. The MHRA shared their concerns with the FDA, which in turn also requested further data.

Healy and his ilk had done their work well in pushing for the acceptance of suicidality as the operative measure for judging events uncovered by clinical trials. Now events labeled in the study as hostility, emotional instability, and conduct problems were being relabeled by regulators as either "possibly suicide-related" or "suicide attempts." Yet, the published results of the study had specifically discussed that an adverse event "was defined as serious if it resulted in hospitalization, was associated with suicidal gestures, or was described by the treating physician as serious," and the researchers conducting the study had found that only one of the eleven serious adverse events was related to Paxil.

The decision of the MHRA and the FDA to reclassify more of these serious events as "suicide-related" had the effect of drawing a closer connection between taking Paxil and suicide, even though there were no suicides in the study.[16] As a result, the new analysis claimed that six of the ninety-three patients taking Paxil had a possibly suicide-related event, compared with only one of the eighty-eight patients taking the placebo, making it appear that the drug was associated with a sixfold greater risk of suicidal thoughts and behaviors. This stood in contrast to two other trials of SSRIs examined by U.S. and UK regulators, in which "the risk of a suicide-related event or attempt was nearly equal for both the active-drug group and placebo."[17]

Then, a month before the MHRA was to decide on Paxil use in people younger than eighteen, the BBC's *Panorama* ran another report, *Emails from the Edge*. It revealed the phenomenal response (sixty-seven thousand phone calls and fourteen hundred emails) it had received in response to its October documentary. Viewers had also reported sixteen suicides, eleven of them in the previous two years, that apparently had never been disclosed to regulators and which were attributed to SSRIs. The resulting media and public outcry was predictable. Headlines and articles in the British press blared, "Antidepressants Linked to Child Suicides," "Drug 'Carries Risk of Suicide in Children,'" "Doctors Warned Not to Prescribe Anti-depressant to Under-18s," and "Seroxat ... Could Cause Young People Under 18 to Kill or Harm Themselves."

In this environment, UK regulators issued strongly worded warnings to doctors not to prescribe Paxil to anyone under eighteen, arguing that "in light of little or no evidence that [the drug] had any efficacy in child and adolescent depression, the risk outweighed any potential benefit."[18] A week after the MHRA action, the FDA also urged doctors to be on the lookout for indications of suicidality in pediatric patients on SSRIs but never explained that increased thinking and talking about suicide were not associated with suicide itself.

If the FDA thought that would be the end of the controversy, it was very, very wrong. The *New York Times* fanned the flames further when it ran a story about the UK ban that claimed that "[t]he FDA is investigating whether the data support a link between suicide and the SSRIs ... in children and adolescents," and the Associated Press also reported, "FDA Cites Possible Suicide Link in Paxil."[19] While the *New York Times* account did make a distinction between suicidal actions and suicide, noting that no one in the Paxil study had taken their life, many news accounts did not, and other media outlets then ran with the same incorrect information.[20]

Surrounded by headlines warning of danger and suicide, the FDA expanded its review of antidepressants to include twenty-three studies on a variety of SSRIs. The agency commissioned outside reviewers from Columbia University to look at the data because, as Dr. Thomas Laughren, Director of FDA's Division of Psychiatry Products, noted, "We did not have the level of detail in these cases that one would have liked to do a rational classification."[21] Like the British review, the U.S. scientists defined suicidality very broadly in order to capture all events that could possibly fit in this category. For most of the SSRIs the FDA studied, the danger of suicidality was not highly elevated in patients in the drug group, and there was substantial variation between trials.

The overall relative risk for suicidality found in the agency's analysis was 1.78—or, in other terms, an increase of a couple of points in the percentage of patients showing suicidality on the drug compared to on the placebo (2.1 percent for the placebo and 3.8 percent for the drug). Most statisticians and scientists do not consider a relative risk below 3 to be indicative of a substantial added risk. (By comparison, the relative risk of getting lung cancer for a smoker is more than 20.) This finding was consistent with previous studies that had either found relative risks between 1.5 and 2 or no increased incidence of suicidality at all.[22]

When it came to clear suicide attempts or completed suicides, there was no difference. Not one single child in any of studies on SSRIs evaluated by the FDA committed suicide. Once again, suicidality had proven to be an artificial measure, unrelated to suicide itself. The Columbia University analysis was also consistent with large-scale studies in the United States and Europe that had found that increased use of antidepressants is associated with reduced suicide rates across all age groups.

In the United States, beginning in the 1950s, suicide rates were on an unbroken upward trajectory. But in 1987, the year after Prozac was introduced, suicides began suddenly to go down. Furthermore, the data indicated that the rates fell much more quickly for women, who are two times as likely as men to be placed on SSRIs, and that regions with the highest SSRI prescription rates were also those experiencing the biggest declines in suicides.[23] Another study, published in the October 2003 issue of *Archives of General Psychiatry*, shows that the same correlation can be found in pediatric patients. The authors reviewed 588 case files of kids aged 10 to 19 and found that a 1 percent increase in antidepressant use was associated with a decrease of 0.23 suicides per 100,000 adolescents per year.[24]

At the same time, extensive research has shown that people with depression who go untreated are the most likely to commit suicide. According to Dr. Matthew V. Rudorfer, a panel member from the National Institute of Mental Health, the suicide rate among adolescents who receive no help for their depression is 15 percent.[25] Not only is this far higher than the suicide rate for those on SSRIs, but it also clearly shows the potential for harm if antidepressants are denied to children. This fact is reinforced by another analysis, in which "[r]esearchers found blood antidepressant levels in less than 20 percent of suicide cases," suggesting that "the vast majority of suicide victims never received treatment for their depression."[26] The risk of denying drugs to pediatric patients is especially great because SSRIs cannot be easily replaced by other treatments. Cognitive behavioral therapy (CBT) has shown promise in some studies, but research suggests that the most effective treatment is a dual approach involving both CBT and medication.[27]

Last, there was evidence, ignored by the FDA and left out of the debate, that showed that simply watching children on SSRIs carefully during the early stages of treatment can reduce or prevent problems.

One reason, according to Dr. Boris Birmaher of the Western Psychiatric Institute and Clinic at the University of Pittsburgh, is that "[k]ids at high risk of suicide are the ones seeking treatment. Once treatment begins, suicidality begins to decrease ... This is an important message for the public. If you are not aware of this, you can mix up the cause of suicide—depression—with the effect of treatment."[28]

Furthermore, there can be a paradoxical relationship between improvement on SSRIs and suicide, as one psychiatrist indicated:

> Sometimes when people begin to get better ... not all their symptoms will remit at the same time. We often see suicides occurring because a depressed person with intentions to commit suicide had previously lacked the energy to do so. Sometimes, after going on an SSRI drug, that patient's energy levels will shoot up, but the intention to commit suicide is slower to remit, leading to an apparent connection between the treatment and suicide.[29]

Close monitoring can also address two other problems linked to SSRIs: akathisia, a condition causing acute restlessness and anxiety that sometimes leads to suicide, and activation syndrome, another temporary side effect that may manifest in a similar way. Both are most likely to appear in the first weeks of treatment, which may help explain why children who take SSRIs for more than six months have lower suicide rates than those taking them for less than two months.[30]

NOT-SO-SMOKING GUNS

Of course, the press simply ran the headline that SSRIs nearly doubled suicidality and hinted that this translated into actual suicides. When the FDA held its first hearing on the suicidality issue in February 2004, the *Washington Post* reported, "Federal regulators said for the first time yesterday that clinical trials of popular antidepressants such as

Prozac, Paxil and Zoloft show a greater risk of suicide among children taking the drugs compared with those taking dummy pills."[31] Suicidality may not be the same as suicide, but groups who already had a bias against the drug, and the public and the press—both of whom largely lacked the background to understand the distinction—failed to see a difference. When scientists tried to set the record straight, they seemed pedantic, interested in quibbling about semantics while children might be in mortal danger.

In covering the issues surrounding pediatric use of antidepressants, the media avidly repeated the anecdotes and the arguments of critics, and in so doing played a central role in shaping, wrongly, popular perception and use of SSRIs. As an article called "Antidepressants and Increased Suicidality: The Media Portrayal of Controversy" in *The Scientific Review of Mental Health Practice* argues, it is important to look at the coverage of the controversy in the press because "most people (including those taking or who have children who are taking antidepressants) acquire information through newspapers, television, and the Internet."

The authors' analysis shows that the media coverage was biased and incomplete, spreading fear rather than facts. A review of ten randomly selected articles from the mainstream media published between February and March 2004 found that only in two did "the article's headline present a reasonably balanced description of the potential link between antidepressants and suicide," and only five covered both sides of the debate in the article. Half omitted "the potential risks associated with not treating depression," and none talked about "the availability of alternative empirically supported interventions for depression."[32] These articles appeared not only in the pages of the morning paper but also were posted on the newspaper websites and then reposted and linked by other sites, multiplying the reach of their incomplete information. Websites set up to spotlight the supposed dangers of drugs compiled long lists of articles apparently supporting their point of view, feeding users who landed on their site a steady diet of half-truths.

Even academic journals joined the clamor. In March 2004, with the controversy still at a simmer, the *Canadian Medical Association Journal* published an article claiming to have secret, smoking-gun documents. The authors alleged that "[a]n internal document advised staff at the international drug giant GlaxoSmithKline (GSK) to withhold clinical trial findings in 1998 that indicated the antidepressant paroxetine [Paxil] ... had no beneficial effect in treating adolescents." The *CMAJ* alleged that GSK decided to withhold the results of two trials, studies 329 and 377, in which they say the drug showed no efficacy or was outperformed by a placebo.[33]

The claim that the placebo outperformed the drug in either trial is transparently false, and the journal clearly hoped that no one would bother actually to obtain the studies in question. In study 329, the Paxil group failed to show statistically significant improvement on the primary measures but produced significant results on four secondary endpoints.[34] In study 377, there was no statistically significant difference from the placebo, in either direction.[35] Both studies showed that the drug showed adverse effects statistically similar to the placebo; indeed, the company mulled using them as a proof of safety, if not efficacy.[36]

As for withholding the results, well, that isn't quite true either. Study 329 was the original study that ignited such scrutiny from both British and American regulators, and it was published in 2001 in the *Journal of American Academy of Child and Adolescent Psychiatry* (a fact the *CMAJ* piece had to acknowledge). Furthermore, both studies can be found with a few clicks on GSK's website.[37] The same is true for two other GSK studies, 511 and 453, which a consumer safety advocacy group would subsequently accuse the company of hiding.[38] Some smoking guns those turned out to be.

But perhaps most important is what the GSK document actually says. The cover letter describes the situation: "The results of the studies were disappointing in that we did not reach statistical significance on the primary end points and thus the data do not support a label claim for the treatment of Adolescent Depression." The company had carried out the studies hoping for an outcome that would encourage the FDA to add "adolescent depression" to official approved indications for the drug, but it had not succeeded. There is no indication that the data were to be hidden, only that they weren't going to be sent to the FDA as part of a new application. Study 329 was already to be presented and published; for study 377, "there [were] no plans to publish data," but there is nothing in the report to indicate this was to be prevented.[39]

Nonetheless, for opponents of SSRI use, from Dr. Healy, to groups such as the Alliance for Human Research Protection, to natural health entrepreneur Joseph Mercola, the refusal of the FDA to follow the United Kingdom in banning pediatric use of Paxil was yet another example of an industry-influenced cover-up. Parent groups were quick to pick up on the controversy, although they were divided between those who believed SSRIs were beneficial and those who thought they were dangerous. All of these actors made liberal use of personal stories, privileging personal experience over data, and flooding the Internet with claims that SSRIs caused suicide and the FDA and industry were covering up the danger.

Politicians got into the act as well. Senator Charles Grassley took the allegations of Healy and other critics and ran with them, claiming the FDA was trying to hide the real dangers of drugs for depression. He and Representative Bart Stupak held hearings to promote their conspiracy theory and even threatened to legislate that patients under eighteen could not be given SSRIs at all. So high were tensions during FDA meetings to discuss the data on SSRIs that the chairman of the committee wore a bulletproof vest during the proceedings. Scientists on both sides, as well as safety groups, representatives of pharmaceutical firms, and alternative medicine proponents, all turned out to express their points of view. Irate parents of children both apparently helped and supposedly hurt by SSRIs made impassioned statements.

It was these emotional accounts that produced the most lasting effect on those attending the FDA hearings. But the government scientists were able to do little to defuse the fear and anger. The panel members, who were picked to weigh in on whether medicines can be used effectively and safely in the real world, ignored the fact that, in many cases, medications had been prescribed by primary care physicians who had failed to advise parents on possible adverse effects and who did not provide adequate follow-up care. Parents whose children experienced problems while on the drugs or who did not see results felt betrayed, while others were upset simply because they had been blindsided by the uproar over the potential for suicidality and felt that information had been withheld from them. As a result, they were primed to believe the allegations of increased suicides in kids and adolescents on SSRIs and ready to vent their rage on the FDA.

Amid the growing uproar over SSRIs, studies demonstrating a benefit were dismissed as being the work of researchers on the take from industry. With rare exceptions, research and clinical experience evaluating the balance of risk and benefits of SSRIs in treating mental illness were ignored in the debate, and the media and Web coverage offered little nuance, only fear and hyperbole.

Under pressure from all sides and surrounded by fear and recriminations, the FDA announced, in March 2004, that labels on ten SSRIs would now be required to bear a warning that patients of all ages needed to be watched for suicidality. That fall, the agency went one step farther and, in October, released the news that a black box warning on pediatric use would be mandated, with the new label to be introduced in early 2005. A member of the FDA's Psychopharmacologic Drugs Advisory Committee, Dr. Andrew Leon, underscored how the Precautionary Principle had influenced the agency's actions when he explained that the studies the FDA examined "did not provide definitive evidence of risk, *yet they failed to demonstrate an absolute absence of risk* [emphasis mine]."[40]

THE CONSEQUENCES OF THE BLACK BOX

In 2005, with the black box added and SSRI prescriptions dropping not only for teens and children but for adults as well, the crusaders who had fought to save society from antidepressants basked in their victory. They told the press and wrote on their websites that the truth had won out and a blow had been dealt to both perfidious drug companies and a modern culture that encouraged the popping of happy pills. However, not everyone was so sanguine. Many physicians and researchers who believed in the benefits of SSRIs for children and teenagers were alarmed by the attacks on the drugs and by the changes made by government regulators in response. Some scientists were "concerned that the available research findings do not support a warning that may be misinterpreted by some practitioners or parents to mean that antidepressant medications actually cause children and adolescents to commit suicide."[41]

They also feared that pediatric patients who would benefit from these antidepressants would be less likely to receive a prescription. It wasn't long before evidence proved that their fears were well founded. Later that same year, health website Medscape reported:

Data from Medco Health Solutions showed that at the end of the first quarter of 2004, the number of persons younger than 18 receiving antidepressants declined by 18% compared with the fourth quarter of 2003; the number dropped another 5% in the second quarter of 2004. This decline contrasts sharply with what had been a 77% increase in the number of filled prescriptions for antidepressants and other psychotropic medications for children and adolescents from 2000 to 2003.[42]

Partially driving this drop was the fact that many doctors had become reluctant to prescribe SSRIs to children. Some of this shift was not necessarily negative; primary care doctors were more likely to refer patients to specialists rather than offer medication themselves, but prescriptions continued to fall overall.

The trend had begun before the black box warning, driven by increasingly strong warnings from the FDA, but now it accelerated. Previously, the percentage of pediatric patients with depression who were prescribed an SSRI had averaged above 60 percent, but that figure began to drop in the second half of 2004, and fell precipitously to land below 30 percent by October 2005. The number of patients taking no antidepressant at all rose from around 20 percent to well above 60 percent, following a mirror image trajectory to that seen for SSRI prescriptions. In 2004 alone, the number of prescriptions of SSRIs among children dropped 22 percent, according to a study in the *American Journal of Psychiatry* in September 2007. Among those age fourteen and under, it was a 20 percent reduction for prescriptions in general and 30 percent for new ones.

Not only were prescriptions down, diagnoses of major depressive disorder were, too, especially by pediatricians and primary care physicians. After having risen significantly over the last five years from three to five in one thousand, the rate of diagnosis now returned in 2005 to what it was in 1999. This was approximately 32 percent lower than would be anticipated from the prior trend, and it brought the number of diagnoses below the estimated population rate of depression for children and teens that had been established from other research, suggesting that some pediatric patients were not getting the help they needed.[43]

But the most disturbing developments were in the incidence of suicide, already the third leading cause of death for the pediatric population. Suicides rose 14 percent, by far the largest single-year difference since at least 1979, when data on the national suicide rate were first gathered.[44] Of special concern was the fact that the suicide rate for girls between ten and nineteen years old went up by a third, from 2.66 per 100,000 to 3.52 per 100,000, while it increased only 8 percent among boys of the same age. Isolating just girls age ten to fourteen, the increase was a worrying 76 percent, as the rate jumped from 0.54 per 100,000 to 0.95 per 100,000.[45] And it wasn't a one-year anomaly; suicides remained elevated in 2005 as well, before beginning to go down again.[46]

Dr. Boris Birmaher, of the University of Pittsburgh, opined, "Years ago we speculated that suicides—not suicidal thoughts or suicide attempts but real deaths—were going down because a lot of doctors, not just psychiatrists, were prescribing SSRI antidepressants ... Then comes the black box, and without any other specific reason there was a huge increase in the number of kids dying from suicide. This is not proof, just a statistical association. But it is suspicious."[47]

Furthermore, contrary to expectations, other treatments did not increase sufficiently to fill the gap. There was increased use of psychotherapy, and slightly more patients were given prescriptions for older tricyclic antidepressants (which are considerably more dangerous than SSRIs), but this could hardly make up for the fact that the percentage of patients given no antidepressant had sky-rocketed more than 200 percent.[48] Nor did prescription rates rise for Prozac, which has been specifically demonstrated to be beneficial to depressed children, or for anti-psychotic drugs that can also be used for depression.[49]

Children were being left without proper treatment, and the decrease in diagnoses of major depression suggests that many children with depression and similar disorders were going without help of any kind—and therefore were at high risk for suicide. This was especially dangerous because one million children and teenagers in the United States are being treated for depression, about 3 to 5 percent of all young people, and depression rates increase with age within this group. Furthermore, 10 percent of teenagers have tried to commit suicide at least once by the time they are eighteen, and 30 percent of children with depression attempt suicide.[50]

Finally, the ripple effect of the black box labeling expanded beyond children and teenagers. There were declines in the diagnosis and treatment of adults, and concerns about SSRIs spread far beyond the actual warning issued by the FDA and took on a life of its own. By May 2007, diagnoses had dropped 29 percent for adults and 37 percent for young adults (as well as 44 percent for children).[51]

Despite the scientific realities, the years that followed the addition of the black box label have been filled with continuing hyperbolic rhetoric of drug opponents who rely on indignation to carry their point when the data do not. Alternative medicine practitioners have had a field day with the SSRI controversy because they perceive it as a vindication of their belief that conventional drugs are both inefficacious and dangerous. One, Dr. Joseph Mercola, wrote that there is "damning evidence of the drug companies' patent disregard for the safety of humans and focus on profits."[52] But continue reading and you will find Dr. Mercola's cure for depression: dietary changes and, oh, buying a copy of his book. This is representative of many alternative health websites devoted to discrediting drugs, and the companies that manufacture them, in order to promote their own remedies, which range from the absurd to the downright dangerous. Nonetheless, they possess email lists with thousands of subscribers and an interconnected network of sites that often pop up prominently on Google searches.

But alternative medicine advocates are only one of the forces intent on continuing to discourage the prescribing of SSRIs to pediatric patients. Websites linked, openly or covertly, to law firms are common. Like other opposition sites, they spotlight anecdotes of children who hurt or killed themselves or others while on SSRIs, and they also play up legal cases against antidepressant manufacturers by families that blame the pills for a loved one's death. Trials where the companies lost are presented as proof that the families were right and that the drug was at fault, even though such court proceedings do not turn on science or data but on emotional appeals. What is most insidious about these sites is that many searchers who land on them are not aware that legal firms are behind the content and therefore are not alerted to the obvious bias.

As in other cases, consumer advocacy and parents' organizations have also played important roles in promoting reduced use of antidepressants in children. Both types of groups have made prominent use of terrifying and upsetting stories of children and teenagers who, within days of beginning treatment with an SSRI, suddenly underwent profound behavioral changes and became suicidal. Often, they include not only suicides but also homicides and attacks for which antidepressants are judged responsible. The presumption is that any suicide or other violent act that took place while someone was on antidepressants or had recently stopped taking them was caused by the medication. It is extremely difficult to counter the emotional account of a parent who lost a child to suicide with dry scientific data and statistics. But that doesn't mean that the drug was at fault.

And while many of these safety advocates are genuinely trying to protect the public, that doesn't make them correct. From a medical perspective, many of these stories are implausible or inconsistent, or they skip over the fact that the patients had a prior history of self-harm and suicidal behavior. One story blames an SSRI for a suicide that took place only three *hours* after the patient's first dose, inconceivably quickly for the drug to have caused the suicide, given the fact that SSRIs often take weeks to show any kind of effect. The websites created by these groups often take pains to appear objective and rational, adopting a reasonable tone, making token acknowledgments of the benefits of antidepressants, and citing various studies (which tend to be selectively chosen, out of date, or misrepresented). However, the general content of the sites is clearly driven by a particular agenda and point of view, with the amount of content indicting SSRIs far outweighing the disclaimers and "balanced" material. Frequently, long lists of cases are used to scare readers and reinforce accusations that very serious adverse reactions to SSRIs are being concealed. Nonetheless, the overall impression left for an Internet user is that the site is credible and authoritative.

INTERNATIONAL TRENDS

The United States and the United Kingdom were not the only two countries that became caught up in the conflict over pediatric SSRI prescriptions. Indeed, the controversy took hold in many different countries at approximately the same time, driven by the same hyperbolic interpretations of the existing scientific data and spread by media stories and Internet sites. In an interconnected world, our debates and fears are interconnected as well. Thanks to the Internet, there is no separation anymore between press in one country and press in another, between sites created by Brits or Americans or any other nationality.

Back in Britain, where the scare began, regulators soon decided that Prozac was the only SSRI that should be prescribed to children.[53] European drug regulators had also told doctors in December 2003 that SSRIs were not indicated for use in children, and they discouraged doctors from prescribing the drugs to those under eighteen. Prescriptions dropped 33 percent over the next two years in the United Kingdom, with the unsurprising exception of Prozac prescriptions, which went up 60 percent.[54] While suicide rates didn't show an increase, neither did they go down, and the fact that Prozac continued to be allowed—and, indeed, was promoted—may have played a role in preventing a rise like that seen in the United States.[55]

In the Netherlands, a similar warning was issued against the use of antidepressants in children, leading to a 22 percent decrease in prescriptions, and the country subsequently saw, from 2003 to 2005, an increase of 49 percent in the suicide rate for patients nineteen years old and under. In boys younger than fifteen, the suicide rate went up massively: 446 percent.[56]

In Canada, a 2004 advisory regarding pediatric use of antidepressants was also followed in the subsequent two years by a decrease in prescriptions for all antidepressants. The U.S. warning also showed cross-border effects. Researchers found that of the 72 percent of Canadian psychiatrists who had heard about the FDA's action in the United

States, 80 percent altered how they chose and evaluated treatments for their patients.[57] For newer antidepressants, of which SSRIs are the largest part, prescriptions declined up to 40 percent, with the exception of Prozac prescriptions, which went up 10 percent. Prescriptions for young adults also went down 10 percent as a result of the warning on pediatric use.[58] Data from Manitoba show that prescriptions in the province fell 14 percent, and suicides there rose 25 percent. Overall, suicide data for Canada show that suicides in children age ten to fourteen went from 1.3 per 100,000 in 2004 to 2.0 per 100,000 in 2005.[59] One doctor opined, "Our best explanation is that a warning that was intended to protect people in essence has probably harmed people."[60]

ADMITTING ERROR

More than five years have passed since the black box first began appearing on drug labels. The coverage has largely disappeared, and the consumer safety groups have mostly moved on. There are new issues on their front burners these days. But the residue remains. News stories continue to tell readers that SSRIs are believed to be dangerous. Advocacy groups have added antidepressants to the list of perils they have uncovered. Websites opposing the drugs provide endless compilations of supposed cases of harm and spotlight emotional anecdotes. Parents and teenagers looking for information or help online continue to find misleading or disingenuous accounts rather than facts and reasoned risk-benefit analyses. For those desperate for information and aid, the University of Google still provides an education designed to scare people to death. Literally.

So far, the FDA has not admitted that it erred at all in adding the black box, nor has it acknowledged the impact the change had on suicide rates. Dr. Robert Gibbons, who voted against the black box, said in 2007, "The FDA has made a very serious mistake. It should lift its black-box warning because all it's doing is killing kids." A colleague of his on the panel, Gail Griffith, now regrets voting for the warning and says had she "known how much the label would rattle parents, [she] wouldn't have voted for it."[61] It is not too late to correct that mistake, and the FDA should do so immediately. So far, however, it has only compounded the error by adding a black box warning on SSRI in young adults in December 2006, leading the media to once again falsely report that the warning was occasioned by a "suicide risk" from the drugs.[62]

As a result of our news cycle culture and our ambivalent relationship with science, once the initial hype about the newest danger recedes, it no longer captures our attention. The verdict is handed down in those first days and weeks of saturation and outrage, and it is not reassessed as we learn more, new science comes in, and the consequences make themselves felt. The news networks seldom run a new program to tell us that our former fears were unfounded; after all, who wants to watch the *60 Minutes* program on the dangers that turned out to be nothing more than hype or a breaking news segment on the data disproving the one-time controversy? At the same time, Internet sites keeps scare stories alive forever, adding new developments only if they support the sites' agendas. Many websites don't even post the date that their content was last updated.

The impact of the black box is still being tallied. The last year for which data is currently available, 2007, shows that the suicide rates may have stabilized again after the rise occasioned by the FDA's action and the controversy that helped precipitate it, but it is too early to tell whether in the long term suicide rates will resume the downward trajectory they maintained for decades before the SSRI furor. No matter what the eventual answer to these questions, the damage already done cannot ever be entirely reversed: children have died and public trust has been eroded.

It is seductive to give in to the calls to be safe rather than sorry and to take action even before a danger is clearly proven. After all, wouldn't it be terrible if the risk were real and we didn't do something until it was already too late? But there may be an equivalent or greater risk in denying treatment as a result of dangers that are nonexistent or exaggerated. This is what happened with SSRIs. In 2004, we knew that SSRIs were correlated in pediatric, especially adolescent, patients with somewhat elevated rates of something called suicidality. But suicidality was also found in people who did not receive SSRIs, and it failed as a measure to predict suicide or even major depression for that matter. What we did know is that studies had repeatedly shown that areas with higher rates of SSRI use had lower suicide rates and that as the levels of SSRI prescribing fell, suicides increased.

Instead of proceeding judiciously, the FDA (and government agencies in other countries) reacted precipitously and excessively. Egged on by "safety advocates," parents who believed their children had been hurt by SSRIs, grandstanding politicians, scaremongering websites, and news coverage that promoted and perpetuated fear, they gave in to political pressure rather than making their choice based on data and scientific analysis. Predictably, the public became fearful as a result, doctors worried that they were putting themselves at legal risk if they kept prescribing SSRIs, and some patients and their families became reluctant to fill or take prescriptions for antidepressants.

Since then, we have learned more about both the efficacy and the risk of antidepressants, and population data continue to tie higher SSRI use to fewer suicides. Doctors have reinforced the notion that careful monitoring can mitigate and control the danger. Research is under way to determine how to individualize treatment with existing medications (but one all of which are now in generic form), including by combining them with some form of talk therapy. What's more, a new study indicates that two genes may make SSRI users more likely to display suicidality, which could soon allow doctors to identify those who should not be given the drugs or who need extra monitoring.[63]

But what we have really learned since 2004 is the risk of *not* prescribing SSRIs. We have undergone a grand experiment, not only in the United States but also in Europe and Canada, as policies and popular opinion governing SSRI use were changed by political demands and ideological lobbying. The results are in. Antidepressants are fickle subjects of controlled trials, but epidemiology has spoken all the louder as a result. When SSRI prescriptions drop, suicides go up. Nonetheless, just as those who maintain that vaccines cause all sorts of brain damage in infants evince an unshakeable belief in the face of overwhelming contrary evidence, many opponents of SSRI use still maintain that they just "know" they are right.

It would be disturbing enough if this were an isolated case, but it is only a particularly damaging example of what goes on all the time. Regulatory decisions are not being made on the basis of scientific data and opinion but as a result of media hype and popular fear. The Internet has strengthened this phenomenon and made it both borderless and timeless, allowing misinformation to reproduce itself a thousandfold and remain powerful long after it is disproved. The ultimate goal of those who have learned to turn the Internet so effectively to their purposes goes beyond any single drug or apparent danger, however. Their attacks are ultimately aimed at discrediting the scientific establishment itself and all those who align themselves with it. How they have often succeeded will be the subject of the next chapter.

CHAPTER 7

Assault on Scientists: The Conflict-of-Interest Canard

D R. NEAL S. YOUNG is the chief of the Hematology Branch of the National Heart, Lung and Blood Institute at the National Institutes of Health. Over the past two decades, he has been responsible for pioneering treatments for rare blood diseases, including aplastic anemia, a condition that shuts down the ability of bone marrow to produce sufficient red cells, white blood cells, and platelets and which affects mostly children. His discovery that many blood disorders are caused by a malfunction of the immune system led to immunosuppressive therapies that have increased survival rates for aplastic anemia from less than 10 percent to more than 70 percent. Literally thousands of children's lives have been saved by Dr. Young, who has treated more young people with blood disorders than any other doctor in the world.

A sought-after speaker, Dr. Young gave a lecture in 2004 for a pharmaceutical company and was paid for his time. In accordance with the NIH rules governing conflict of interest, he asked for and received permission from the agency before delivering the speech. And that should have been the end of the story. But then, one day, he suddenly found his life under the microscope, one of dozens of NIH researchers who were being accused of having violated the agency's conflict-of-interest policy. The news that he was being investigated was followed by weeks of demands that he hand over ever more documentation related to the lecture. For eight months, Dr. Young was carefully scrutinized before finally being found innocent. He told the *Washington Post* that it was a "very intrusive, time-consuming and anxiety-provoking experience."

Dr. Young was the victim of a witch hunt set off when a *Los Angeles Times* article accused the National Institutes of Health of being corrupt and endangering the lives of millions because many of its scientists had consulting arrangements with industry. The thrust of the article, entitled "Stealth Merger: Drug Companies and Government Medical Research," focused on Stephen I. Katz, who was and still is director of the NIH National Institute of Arthritis and Musculoskeletal and Skin Diseases. The article recounted the events surrounding the death of a patient who was enrolled in an NIH clinical trial.[1] It did not directly accuse Dr. Katz of killing the patient because a drug manufacturer gave him money. But it didn't have to.

The *LA Times* article was spread quickly through the Internet by groups such as the Center for Science in the Public Interest and by bloggers staunchly critical of private companies. Other newspapers and major television networks soon picked up on the story. So it was only a matter of time before politicians got in on the act. A congressional investigation was launched to determine the extent of the conflict-of-interest problem. The subcommittee looking into the issue subsequently found discrepancies between two lists detailing interactions between companies and the NIH, one created using data supplied by the pharmaceutical firms, the other generated by the agency. When the lists were placed side by side, some 130 entries were absent from the latter document. Swiftly, the committee concluded that dozens of NIH researchers had failed to conform to the agency's disclosure policy.

The public reaction was predictable. The media published spates of articles concluding that government scientists were being corrupted by industry. The consumer safety groups put the story on the home page of their websites and issued press releases on the supposed scandal. Anti-industry blogs posted that they weren't surprised and that they had warned about this all along. Meanwhile, the congressional subcommittee at the center of the affair hyped its findings, and other politicians chimed in with their own statements. The *Washington Post* editorial page concluded: "It's a legitimate question whether any outside consulting at all should be allowed."[2] To all who feared that conflicts of interest were compromising American medical research, this was just one more piece of proof.

The discovery of the discrepancies between the two lists sent NIH director Elias A. Zerhouni from defending work between government researchers and drug companies to searching the agency for the culprits. He imposed draconian new limits on relationships, compensated or not, between NIH scientists and industry, as well as restrictions on how NIH employees could invest their money. The new rules also limited the ability of researchers to work with universities and other organizations and sought to restrict which awards researchers could accept based on whether those awards were considered to be legitimate. Even support staff—including secretaries and lab technicians—were required to sell any stock they might have had in a drug company. In the wake of the new rules, the agency struggled to recruit new scientists and physicians, who feared getting caught up in the controversy.

But it turns out that as many as 80 percent of the supposed discrepancies between the two lists were due to simple administrative error. Many of the entries were missing because the information collected from the drug companies extended into 2004, while the NIH list stopped at the end of 2003. Other supposed cases of malfeasance were actually cases of mistaken identity. And still other cases were not included in the NIH list because they were not coded as "consulting," the only type of interaction the committee had asked the agency about. Of course, the fact that the vast majority of the accusations turned out to be false received little coverage or commentary in the same media, blogs, and websites that had initially jumped on the story so eagerly. No one in Congress, the media, or advocacy groups apologized to Dr. Young or others scientists who had been investigated.[3]

Such witch hunts are now standard operating procedure. Indeed, at the core of tabloid medicine is a grand conspiracy narrative in which the truth is being hidden by a cabal of the self-interested that includes drug companies, government agencies, doctors, scientific researchers, and anyone else who disagrees with its orthodoxy. Its adherents know that if they discredit and marginalize the existing medical and scientific establishment, their own instant experts will be able to fill the gap. And they have been all too successful because they have tapped into the deep and fundamental distrust of many Americans of the existing elites and of scientific and medical research in general.

Fifty or sixty years ago, for most people, scientists and doctors were heroes who held all the potential of the future in their hands, and working for or with a drug company wasn't a stigma. But slowly, our reverence has faded and been replaced by uncertainty and suspicion. Skepticism of large corporations and institutions that were established to centralize authority has been one strong impulse shaping our nation's political environment throughout its history. In some cases, this has led to greater openness, accountability, and a growth in individual rights. At the same time, movements to cut the evil influence of institutions can undermine the ability of such institutions to promote trust by weakening their capacity to create consensus and to encourage deliberation instead of conflict.

There are deep political and cultural disagreements over the level of risks society should take. Ultimately, the fight over statistics is really a battle to redefine commercialization as inherently dangerous. Rather than engage in debate and discussion, anti-industry advocates seek to discredit their critics. And they do so by alleging that the thoughts and actions of those they disagree with perpetuate and support industry's efforts to hide the truth about technologies.

As a result of this campaign, we have begun to wonder whether these researchers and physicians really have our best interests at heart, and this narrative of conflict and secrecy influences legislation and regulation. It is now a truism that medicine in the United States is rife with conflicts of interest caused by blatant attempts by pharmaceutical companies to buy doctors and scientists. The upshot is apparently a clear and simple one: America's doctors and medical researchers, whatever the validity of their research or the positive contribution they make, cannot be trusted if they receive industry support or work with industry in any way.

Type *conflict of interest* into Google or your favorite search engine (go ahead, I'll wait) and you get back a list of sites denouncing physician malfeasance; copies of disclosure policies from academia, government, and scientific journals; and links to articles on how conflicts are endangering Americans. Even the most cursory of Internet searches on the issue are likely to yield dozens of articles about the huge honoraria paid to physicians, trips to the Caribbean sponsored by drug manufacturers, ghostwritten articles, and the dangers of drug-logo emblazoned pens. If you're lucky, you might get a hit or two offering another point of view, but since the average Internet user looks at only ten sites, he or she probably never even runs across a dissenting Web page.

Individual cases are sensationalized, and most evidence takes the form of stories about doctors or overinterpretation of prescribing patterns and trial outcomes, all embellished by commentary that seldom attempts to hide its bias. The beauty and the danger of anecdotes is that you can almost always find a few to illustrate your belief. Science deals in the aggregation of many, many data points and the testing of a particular hypothesis. But people aren't programmed to respond to this kind of information; we are made to be moved by the individual and the identifiable and to generalize from the single to the many. Just as we may fear a drug because we heard one story of a terrible adverse event, so we may condemn all doctors for the misdeeds of a few.

The media and, even more so, the Internet offer us with an endless supply of these anecdotes. They even tell us what they mean. And in the process, these stories acquire extraordinary power to affect the choices Internet users make, how research is carried out and disseminated, and even the careers of individual doctors and scientists. Controversies over conflicts of interest are no longer battles fought in the closed circles of the scientific community, in letters and articles in journals, or in contretemps at conferences and meetings. We are all experts now, all "informed" and "empowered" and "educated." In this environment, conflict-of-interest accusations have become an effective and wide-reaching weapon wielded by industry opponents and aggrieved patients and a means to attempt to shut down discussion, undermine research, and attack doctors and scientists who produce undesirable or controversial results.

A NOT-SO-NEW WORLD

Marcia Angell encapsulated the core belief shaping tabloid medicine's pursuit of supposed conflicts of interest when she wrote, "It is simply no longer possible to believe much of the clinical research that is published or to rely on the judgment of trusted physicians or authoritative medical guidelines."[4] Angell's comment reflects an extremist view of science that fails to be confirmed by the facts. If the clinical research of the last two decades cannot be trusted, why have so many of its products given us longer and improved lives? Are the recent treatments for cancer, depression, HIV, and many other illnesses that have been derived from industry-supported clinical research in fact inferior to earlier ones? Angell's assertion reflects a bias against industry support of research that has as profound an impact on her work as any financial conflict might create. But moreover, it is a way of framing risk, of quickly determining what institutions are dangerous or evil and which individuals and movements are pure.

But consider a few of the leading scientists who made vital medical breakthroughs thanks to their work with pharmaceutical companies. Gertrude Elion, who won the Nobel Prize in 1988 for physiology and medicine, conducted most of her award-winning research while head of the Department of Experimental Therapy at Burroughs Wellcome (now GlaxoSmithKline) and also served on numerous NIH committees and panels. By the criteria of Angell and others, the work Elion did to identify the difference between healthy cells and cells taken over by viruses, which was used to develop the first treatments for HIV, leukemia, and organ transplant rejection, should be considered suspect.

The same standard can be applied to Sir James Black, who discovered how to find and use disease receptors to block the progression of ulcers, arthritis, and cancer; National Medal of Science winner Herbert Boyer, who used his basic research on recombinant DNA to found Genentech; Nobel Prize winner Lee Hartwell, who is seeking to commercialize his discoveries about how cancer cells evolve; or Judah Folkman, whose work on stopping cancer from progressing by cutting off its blood supply spawned Avastin and many other medicines. By Angell's litmus test, the work of these individuals should be discredited, and the clinical research evaluating the benefits of the medicines developed as a result should be considered suspect as well.

Angell's analysis also illustrates another common contention of conflict-of-interest vigilantes: the belief that "once upon a time," scientists were neither corrupt nor corruptible and pursued science for science's sake and for the greater good. They believe it is the fall from Nature, the polluting of a pristine time. But while there has indeed been growth in the amount of collaboration and financial support that university-based researchers receive from drug companies, academia working with industry is hardly a new trend. It has been the policy of the U.S. government since Franklin Roosevelt established the forerunner to the NIH precisely to encourage such involvement.

In the report recommending the creation of the National Science Foundation and what would become the NIH, Vannevar Bush, FDR's science adviser, wrote:

> Discovery of new therapeutic agents and methods usually results from basic studies in medicine and the underlying sciences. The development of such materials and methods to the point at which they become available to medical practitioners requires teamwork involving the medical schools, the science departments of universities, Government and the pharmaceutical industry. Government initiative, support, and coordination can be very effective in this development phase.[5]

And this policy paid high dividends in the form of fast and wide-ranging innovation that continue to impact our lives and our world. As Susan Hockfield, the president of MIT, explained:

> To meet the battlefield demand for a host of new technologies, in the early 1940s the federal government invested aggressively in innovation. Research and development funding exploded, large-scale research sprang up at universities, new federal agencies emerged and academic researchers worked with industry to swiftly deploy the latest ideas. By war's end, the modern research university and institutionalized federal funding of early-stage research had been launched. Half a decade of wartime training, amplified by the GI Bill, supplied a huge pool of skilled engineers and scientists. Together, these developments powered successive innovation waves ... that drove decades of post-war prosperity.[6]

Hence to equate the absence of industry involvement with the "good old days" of science is to rewrite history. Indeed, support of scientific innovators by companies can be clearly traced at least to the nineteenth century. But to Angell and others like her, the increase in industry support for the commercialization of biomedical research is an ominous and unwelcome development.

However, suspicion of pharmaceutical companies isn't entirely a new trend either. It has been around in the United States at least since the 1950s, when Senator Estes Kefauver held a series of hearings to demonstrate that these firms were making obscene profits by establishing a monopoly for their products and marketing them even if they didn't work, a narrative that is no different from the story advanced by tabloid medicine.[7] But the systematic effort to create suspicion about the integrity of medical researchers and physicians is fairly new and became more pronounced in the 1970s, when scientists involved in the environmental movement began to attempt to link cancer with even small amounts of chemicals in the environment. As use of the Precautionary Principle rose and tabloid medicine was born, accusations of conflict of interest increasingly became one of the weapons of choice of the principle's proponents against those who supported and participated in cooperation with industry.

POSITIVE, NEGATIVE, NEUTRAL

There are several types of supposed conflicts of interest of which scientists are often accused. The first is in published scientific trials. Those concerned about conflicts allege that when research is sponsored or conducted by industry, the results are inevitably positive, with negative information hidden or spun. However, research on the subject is inconsistent and questionable. A large number of studies correlate for-profit funding with positive reported trial outcomes, but they often draw conclusions about what is "tainted" without considering the results of research conducted by others without industry support.

These self-styled medical muckrakers rely on meta-analysis to combine selected trials to establish a statistical connection between industry support of researchers and studies that show particular drugs and devices as effective. The problem is that in meta-analysis the included trials can be chosen to influence the results, and data can be reinterpreted or reclassified in order to create a larger or more meaningful association. Because of the potential to cherry-pick studies and data, meta-analyses were originally used to generate new questions for further research. Meta-analyses are also quick to produce, since they require nothing more than a computer and some statistical software, and medical journals are eager to publish such controversial, and therefore high-impact, studies.

Further, meta-analysis is susceptible to a phenomenon called Simpson's Paradox, in which other variables skew the research so that the answer given by the aggregate data is different than the one that appears when you look at component subgroups. Sometimes just one group impacts the data in a way that alters the overall impression. So if one type of patient is especially susceptible to a dangerous side effect, it can make the drug look risky for everyone.

Simpson's Paradox also occurs when two things are being compared that are different in ways other than the variable being measured. That's what can happen when looking at positive studies produced by industry- versus nonprofit-funded ones. Dr. Xiao-Li Meng, chairman of Harvard University's Statistics Department, has argued that "medical studies are replete with examples of Simpson's Paradox, often identified because such research attracts great interest," and he believes that such cases are so prevalent because "[w]hen you find data that go with your theory, then you don't dig deeper."[8]

What's more, how you classify the studies can make a big difference. Critics try to bolster their argument that industry-sponsored trials are always positive by listing studies as positive if any benefit at all is found, even if that benefit is not statistically significant. Trials with mixed or inconclusive results are deemed negative or positive depending on the preference of the person carrying out the meta-analysis. The category of positive trials may even include studies that support two or more competing drugs.

When care is taken to avoid these traps, the association between industry funding and positive results often disappears. Perhaps the best example is a study by Tammy J. Clifford, Nicholas J. Barrowman, and David Moher that considered articles from the *Annals of Internal Medicine, British Medical Journal, Journal of the American Medical Association, The Lancet,* and the *New England Journal of Medicine.* The authors "failed to document any association between funding source, trial outcome and reporting quality among a sample of RCTs [randomized controlled trials] that were recently published in the top five general medical journals." The article found no correlation between type of financial backing and whether the conclusion was positive, negative, or neutral.[9]

Furthermore, positive studies are more likely to be published in general, regardless of where the money to conduct them came from, and this is not only because of the researchers involved but also the preferences of journals. Negative results are often less interesting and less useful to scientists, because studies are designed to disprove a hypothesis. Whether it is a private company or an academic researcher in a "publish or perish" environment, the positive study is a key to success. In fact, a recent review tested the hypothesis that "if publication pressures increase scientific bias, the frequency of 'positive' results in the literature should be higher in the more competitive and 'productive' academic environment." Indeed, the analysis confirmed that when the main author came from a state that had a high number of journal articles per capita, there was a higher frequency of positive studies.[10]

Conflict-of-interest vigilantes also seldom attempt to show that studies conducted or funded by industry are incorrect or use low-quality research or study designs. And for good reason. A number of studies have found that trials paid for in whole or part by drug companies are of equivalent, or superior, quality to those sponsored by other sources, providing strong evidence against the accusation that company-sponsored research uses poor or fixed methodology to produce a desired outcome. In fact, as one study noted, "Trials funded by for-profit organizations had better methodological quality than trials funded by nonprofit organizations regarding allocation concealment and double blinding" and also "reported a significantly higher number of adverse events in the experimental arm. This might reflect differences in the quality of reporting."[11]

Likewise, Lexchin et al. examined thirteen studies looking at the correlation between methodological rigor and funding source and concluded that none of them produced results suggesting that industry-sponsored trials were of lower quality than those carried out using money from government or other sources. Four studies scored the quality of the company-sponsored research above that of the other articles, and nine held that the quality was comparable.[12] Similar trends have been found in a number of other articles, even ones that are otherwise critical of the impact of company support on research.[13]

Finally, unsurprisingly, companies choose the trials and products they feel are most likely to show positive results, and prefer methodologies that show off their product to its full advantage. Even if most people think of the pharmaceutical industry as having almost unlimited funds, drug development is extraordinarily expensive, and the money must be used in both the pre- and postapproval phases in the most effective way possible. Given that both patent life and research dollars are limited, it often makes more sense for a company to direct their funds into studying new uses for their products rather than in running trials that place their therapy head to head against the competitor's drug. Furthermore, since the standard for a drug's FDA approval is performing better than a placebo comparator, many studies use this design, a fact that has been presented as an indication of malfeasance and yet is perfectly logical.[14] Those who feel that demonstrating efficacy against a placebo is not enough evidence for approval and that a stronger standard is therefore needed should pursue these concerns with the FDA, not malign drug companies for doing only what is required of them.

Simpson's Paradox rears its head once more when it comes to the second common contention of critics: that, whatever the source of the funding for the trial, if the researchers involved have relationships with the companies who made the drug in question, then they may manipulate the results, consciously or unconsciously, to favor the firms to which they are beholden. Yet factors other than just industry relationships may partially determine whether a researcher's work is likely to end up in the positive, neutral, or negative category. Most notably, those who are adamant about *refusing* to work with pharmaceutical concerns may also be those who are cynical about drugs and their makers in general and are more likely to interpret data in a critical light. They may also insist on study designs or populations that favor the therapy they want to win, often the older or less expensive drug.

And often they have their own points of view, intellectual bias, or consulting relationship that could be regarded as a conflict of interest. Think, for instance, of Steve Nissen or David Graham, whose negative analyses of Vioxx may not have been driven by the data but by an ax to grind with the drug, with Merck, and with the pharmaceutical industry. They created their methodologies to achieve this objective and interpreted the information in a strongly ideological manner. Or consider critics, such as Curt Furberg, who have testified as expert witnesses in lawsuits against drugs and for whom cementing their role as anti-industry gadflies enhances their ability to make money testifying for tort lawyers. So it is not surprising that their publications focus on the dangers of drugs.

Many researchers and experts design and conduct clinical trials for more than one company and often come up with conclusions at odds with the firm they carried research for in the past. This is exemplified by one of the most commonly cited studies on physician conflict of interest, which examined journal articles on calcium-channel antagonists. It concluded that "[a]uthors who supported the use of cal-cium-channel antagonists were significantly more likely than neutral or critical authors to have financial relationships with manufacturers of calcium-channel antagonists" and "more likely ... to have financial relationships with any pharmaceutical manufacturer, irrespective of the product." Therefore, the authors imply, relationships between researchers and companies must taint scientific results.

But the data show something interesting: 96 percent of positive authors had monetary ties to a company that made calcium-channel antagonists, but in this group, 88 percent also had a relationship with a "manufacturer of [a] competing product." Similarly, among neutral authors, 60 percent had links to makers of calcium-channel antago-nists, 53 percent to makers of competitors.[15] But if doctors slanted their conclusions to please their sponsors, we would expect that the doctors in the first group would be reluctant to come out strongly in favor of calcium-channel antagonists and would rather be more neutral so as not to alienate companies on either side of the debate. The forces of tabloid medicine ignore this important issue because they believe that any industry support is corrupting.

Despite the shortcomings of existing research on conflicts of interest that call into question the apparent consensus that trials and researchers tied to the pharmaceutical industry are irremediably biased, the public hears and reads only the conclusion that such fund-ing inevitably and riskily undermines research and—more importantly, when it comes to mobilizing the population—their own health. Some promoters of this point of view are scientists whose agenda is ending or curtailing industry backing for scientific trials and eliminating all or most relationships between doctors and researchers and the com-panies that make drugs or medical devices. Others are members of advocacy groups who cast their agenda as ensuring consumer safety, such as Public Citizen or the Prescription Project, which crusade on behalf of generic drug use. (Never mind that the generic drugs were originally developed by the very industry they are criticizing.)

The framing of industry research as corrupt is increasingly easy because of the role the Web plays in spreading the tabloid medicine narrative. Scientists critical of work with industry know how to use journalists without science backgrounds who are looking for a good story and whose words now extend far beyond the printed page to be reproduced and linked on a wide variety of websites. Publishing on the Web also saves researchers time and money, and journals' need for online content encourages the submission and acceptance of review articles and meta-analyses by industry critics. In fact, Drs. Neal Young and John Ioannidis argue that the Web has changed the incentives to publish to favor review articles that will contradict previous findings or have a sensational conclusion.[16]

But, as previous chapters have shown, some of the most zealous of those using tabloid medicine to gain attention and advance their point of view are amateurs who do not conduct peer-reviewed primary research, but who are instead empowered by the Internet to participate in such debates in a way that was previously impossible. At times, these critiques are based on nothing more than emotion and ideology, an evocation of belief rather than evidence. But even more dangerous are those who have taken advantage of the access the Internet has given them to scientific papers and information. As journals are increasingly available online, laypeople with prejudices are using scientists' and doctors' own words and data as weapons against them, twisting the information until it suits their fantasy and glomming on to any journal article that can be construed to support their beliefs.

The Internet also facilitates the consumption of only the information that bolsters our beliefs. We can now run Google searches until we find people who share our views, link to like-minded sites, and set up RSS feeds that give us a steady diet of information that supports our convictions. It is before this tribunal and within this bubble of strenuously enforced ideological conformity that scientists and doctors accused of conflict of interest, or simply the authors of controversial research, find themselves. They get trapped in an online Wonderland where the denizens are all too eager to cut off their heads.

The instant experts and their followers know their opponents have been slow to fight back on the Internet turf. This is because science, with its foundation in data, mathematics, and careful analysis, doesn't lend itself to the rough-and-ready, say-what-you-want, ubiquity-equals-truth world of the Internet and because the scientific and medical community has taken too long to see the danger and the power of the Web.

LITTLE GIFTS, BIG INFLUENCE?

Other fights over conflict of interest center not on research but on physician prescribing behavior and whether it is affected by contact with industry representatives. When you read articles on the issue, whether online or off, whether in the mainstream press or in an academic journal, you almost always get the impression that there is no question that such conflicts are not only rampant but dangerous. Drug critics claim that doctors do not prescribe drugs based on what is best for the patient but on whom they received a gift from recently and that in so doing, they endanger the health and lives, not to mention the pocketbooks, of patients. But there is not a single study demonstrating this supposed causality chain linking physician-industry interaction, prescribing pattern changes, and poor clinical outcomes.

The giveaways of island vacations and sporting event tickets so prominent in online stories are no longer, so critics now focus on small gifts such as pens, refrigerator magnets, or food, simply asserting that sandwiches and pens have the same corrupting impact on physicians as trips to Maui. The contention is that even tokens create a sense of debt and, therefore, the need to repay the rep in some way. However, there are no real data showing that this is true or that such a feeling of obligation would extend any farther than a willingness to listen to the rep's spiel.

Even Anthony DeMaria, editor in chief of the *Journal of the American College of Cardiology* and an opponent of some of the over-the-top perks given to doctors, said that he "question[s] whether a pen, note pad, or sandwich for a lunch or ... conference renders it impossible to make evidence-based decisions in the patient's interest." Furthermore, since almost every pharmaceutical concern gives out pens (and other similar minor gifts), he held that "[i]t seems hard to believe that any individual company could gain much influence by providing the same tokens as everyone else."[17]

The same applies to drug samples. If you want to know why you receive fewer of them, thank tabloid medicine. Samples to doctors were used regularly to give doctors a chance to see if new medications had a benefit, and it isn't a surprise that companies hoped this would lead to new prescriptions. Critics object to samples on the grounds that they undermine the use of cheaper and equally effective better generics, a fine goal—but a disingenuous one. Once again, they are pretending that generics are not only available for every indication but also really just as good.

But generics are not right for every patient, a fact some studies try to obfuscate by comparing branded and generic drugs that are not equivalent and claiming that they are comparable in efficacy and applicability. There are also many medicines for chronic illnesses that have not come off patent, so there is no generic available to use. Finally, there are a number of other practical and financial reasons why sample use makes sense, for instance, to make sure a medication works before the patient invests in a full prescription, to tide a patient over until he or she can get to the pharmacy, or because the patient needs the branded drug but cannot afford it.

Often, the criticism leveled at interactions between doctors and industry center, at their core, on information. Many doctors see contacts with companies as a source of new knowledge about the latest studies and developments on drugs, while critics see these same conversations as merely a tool to increase sales of products without any benefit. While many articles track supposed influence by whether a doctor prescribes medications he or she learned about from drug reps or industry-sponsored programs, they just assume a priori that these drugs are being used inappropriately and don't consider whether they are a good fit for patients.

Consistent with the tactic of stifling debate and competition rather than engaging it, groups such as the Prescription Project, Consumers Union, and the Institute on Medicine as a Profession want to replace industry marketing with something called "academic detailing," which is nothing more than tabloid medicine's pharmaceutical "reeducation." Ostensibly, it "combines the interactive, one-on-one communication approach of industry detailers with the evidence-based, noncommercial information of academia" and replaces information "designed with commercial objectives in mind, regardless of whether more effective, safer or less expensive options exist."[18]

But, not surprisingly, the academic detailing movement excludes or discounts research conducted by those who are "tainted" by industry and seeks to restrict the use of branded drugs. Academic detailing is tabloid medicine in action, designed to promote the drugs that its practitioners think physicians should be prescribing and unwilling to admit or discuss studies demonstrating that other medications work better in many patients.[19] In the world of tabloid medicine, cheaper is always better because it means fewer new drugs are used. Defining all other research as corrupted allows the academic detailers to make clinical recommendations based on whether other studies are conducted by researchers who are "independent."

BRIGHT LINES AND BERLIN WALLS

As a result of efforts to portray industry support as inherently corrupting, disclosure policies to control interactions with industry have been put in place by medical schools, government agencies, scientific journals, and other institutions. There are two commonly touted solutions to the supposed problem of conflicts of interest: disclosure and outright bans on various (or all) types of interaction between doctors or scientists and pharmaceutical company representatives. Both solutions, however, are flawed, because there is no evidence that such regulations improve the quality of health care or promote better research. What the new conflict-of-interest rules actually do is allow those who push tabloid medicine to get more control over the institutions they believe are corrupt.

Nonetheless, such regulations are almost ubiquitous. In a survey published in 2000 in the *New England Journal of Medicine*, of 297 journals, medical schools, federal agencies, and other research organizations, a mere 6 percent of respondent institutions had no conflict-of-interest policy, and in the intervening decade, this percentage has dropped further as scrutiny has only grown.[20] Proposed guidelines come from many sources, including both the government and scientific and medical organizations such as the Association of American Medical Colleges and the Association of American Universities. The Pharmaceutical Research and Manufacturers of America (PhRMA) has also created suggested rules governing researcher interactions with industry.

But the stringency of policies varies considerably. Many scientific journals now operate under the Uniform Requirements for Manuscripts Submitted to Biomedical Journals, which includes requiring authors to disclose any source of income that may be regarded as a conflict.[21] Such transparency is necessary and welcome. But increasingly, academic medical centers, medical schools, and journals are imposing even more restrictive policies, requiring researchers to reveal extensive details of all aspects of their finances, from the amounts and sources of all their income to their investing decisions. Many scientists and doctors consider these too restrictive and warn that they will negatively impact research. Meanwhile, at the other end of the spectrum are vague policies that offer oversight but no specifics.

At particular issue are certain types of articles, such as editorials and reviews, that are construed as having an especially powerful impact on practice; these often have more stringent disclosure rules.

However, insisting that only those authors with no real or perceived conflicts of interest can write such pieces can often exclude the best and most knowledgeable doctors in the field, who have the most relevant and authoritative information to give their fellow physicians. These doctors are asked to consult or lecture on behalf of industry precisely because they are at the top of their fields and therefore their services and insights are in demand.

Furthermore, a properly written piece such as an editorial or a review is transparent; the writer lays out the rationale and studies that inform his opinion, and therefore such a piece is open to analysis and critique by the reader. The *New England Journal of Medicine* partially acknowledged this when it eliminated a rule that said those with conflicts could not write reviews or editorials and instead set the figure of $10,000 from any one pharmaceutical company as the limit for those who authored such articles. The editor in chief of the journal said, "[t]his change will allow us to recruit the best authors, the people who have experience with new treatments to write these editorials and review articles."[22]

The same is true of physicians involved in creating medical guidelines, another area of research that has been targeted for particular conflict-of-interest scrutiny. Critics professed to be shocked when a 2002 study found that 87 percent of doctors involved in creating medical guidelines have a link to a drug company, including receiving money for their research. It said also that 58 percent "had financial ties to companies whose drugs were either considered or recommended in the guidelines." But these results aren't really either surprising or disturbing. First, there were issues with the sample, since it was based on voluntary response and only half of those asked to participate agreed to do so. Second, I would hope that those preparing the guidelines looked at all the relevant drugs, which would almost inevitably mean that doctors with any relationship with a pharmaceutical manufacturer would include drugs made by that company in their analysis.

Furthermore, the doctors who worked with industry had ties to many different drug manufacturers, making any sort of systematic bias on their part for or against a given company unlikely. As five of the doctors included in the study argued, "it may be neither possible nor desirable to exclude authors who are involved with industry since the 'experts' who write guidelines are the same individuals who are most likely to receive financial support to conduct research."[23]

Since most doctors come into contact with companies at some point in their work, the available pool of physicians allowed to do research or publish would be tiny if only those without industry relationships were allowed to do so. But for the supporters of tabloid medicine, this is precisely the point: by knocking out all possible competition, all that would be left would be their own experts. Disclosure policies, especially highly stringent ones, have the effect of judging all scientists guilty of being corrupt until proven innocent. As Lynn A. Jansen and Daniel P. Sulmasy argue, bioethics is founded upon the belief "that good arguments can come from any quarter and that no argument should be dismissed or discounted simply because of its source."[24] Using industry affiliation to limit those who can publish or speak not only risks not allowing the best experts to write on the subject but also "dispatches the pretext that a work should be judged on its merits, since the work is deemed unfit for publication solely on the basis of the identity of the author."[25]

Conflict-of-interest vigilantes hold that a conflict of interest "exists *not only* when judgment has been clearly influenced" but also "when judgment *might* or might be *perceived* to be influenced."[26] They have successfully pushed the idea that doctors cannot judge whether they have been corrupted and, therefore, we should assume that they have been. This leaves no possible defense; if the physician tries to argue that he has done nothing wrong, he is lying or in denial. In other words, he is not just guilty until proven innocent; he is guilty, period, with no proof of misconduct needed. Just as the Precautionary Principle places new technologies before the court and demands the defense prove them innocent, so the same is being done to physicians. I can think of no other industry or context in which such a policy would be tolerated. Refusing to publish important research because of industry support is intellectually oppressive, breeding ignorance and narrow-mindedness and impeding scientific debate and progress.

(JOE) McCARTHY STRIKES AGAIN!

Accusations of conflicts of interest are a strong weapon to render suspect unpopular results and undermine the reputation of doctors and scientists. The supporters of tabloid medicine know this all too well and use it all too effectively, especially because such claims of bias are even more effective with the public than within the scientific community. The Internet has spread far and wide the presumption that contact with pharmaceutical companies equals bias. Period. No exceptions. With every hit and every link, this belief has insinuated itself ever deeper into the fabric of the public debate over medicine. It pops up in online newspaper articles and on the websites of consumer groups. It is also declaimed fervently in patient Web communities.

Tarred and feathered in the court of public opinion, "conflicted" researchers and physicians find that their views and work cease to matter—at least in the eyes of those who buy into the equation of industry ties equal dishonesty. This is the ultimate objective of leveling conflict-of-interest charges: to invalidate research and researchers with whom the accuser disagrees. Today, "the label of conflict of interest is so commonly used with the intent to discredit a person or a work that it is disingenuous for anyone to claim that no accusation is intended."[27]

Earlier, we showed how the anti-vaccine movement has leveled charges of bias at researchers who have spoken out defending vaccines or who have simply carried out studies that failed to support the spurious connection between immunizations and autism. Paul Offit has impeccable medical credentials, has devoted decades of his career to the prevention of rotavirus (a disease that used to hospitalize tens of thousands of children in the United States and that kills hundreds of thousands annually in the developing world), and has never hidden the fact that he cooperated with Merck to bring the vaccine to market. But vaccine opponents seek to discredit Offit, not on scientific grounds, or merely with the charge that he allows children to be injected with a product that is unsafe, but by leveling charges of corruption and conflict. He is known on many anti-vaccine websites as "Dr. Proffit." Angry patients have demanded to know, "How in the world can you put money before the health of someone's baby?" Yet the leaders of the anti-vaccine movement are up to their necks in conflicts, whether it's Mark Geier, who makes his money as an expert witness in lawsuits against vaccine manufacturers; Andrew Wakefield, whose original research was paid for by a lawyer before Wakefield went to work for Thoughtful House, a "biomedical" facility in Texas; or David Kirby, whose income comes from his work as an anti-vaccine blogger and writer.

This kind of concerted character assassination has been facilitated by the Internet. Pharma scolds and "safety advocates" and interest groups manipulate the public debate by producing "proof," taken out of context or drawn out of thin air, against their opponents and their enemies and whipping up the resulting anger and outrage. Then they lean in close and promise the hidden truth, delivered by their own experts and for their own benefit, financial and otherwise. This little palace coup takes place every day, bit by bit, person by person, and the Internet is its most potent tool because it captures people who are often already vulnerable, concerned about symptoms, or seeking more information about a condition affecting them or someone close to them.

Furthermore, this situation is constructed to be self-reinforcing through links to other sites offering the same information and beliefs. An accusation made by one person can quickly get picked up by dozens more and repeated over and over. For those who want to believe it, the reality does not matter. The charge is simply accepted as truth and then repeated, spread onward from one site to another in articles, post, comments, and emails. Rendered anonymous by the Web, contributors are no longer constrained by the mores that hold in face-to-face conversations; their criticisms grow ever larger, their language ever more hyperbolic, and their positions ever more radical and hardened.

Over time, it becomes difficult to trace the original source of a claim, so the allegation acquires a patina of respectability, no matter its reliability. After enough repetition, a newcomer stumbling on such information on this or that website has no way of knowing that the indictment is even debatable. Because society has already gone a long way down the road of eroding trust in the scientific and medical communities, conflict-of-interest accusations often feel plausible, and that is enough for them to be taken unquestioningly. Even those who are skeptical will find that checking the veracity of such charges is often difficult or impossible with the resources available. This leaves those who doubt the truth of the claim on the defensive, caught up in a he said, she said situation where the outcome rests not on evidence but on who can tap into the emotions and biases of the onlookers more effectively. It isn't about science; it's about solidarity—about recruiting, keeping, and energizing followers.

To the public watching from the sidelines, getting their information in bits and pieces from news stories, Google searches, blogs, and the websites of interested individuals and groups, the story is presented as a fait accompli. The case is considered closed by readers and writers alike, and no new evidence or decision is allowed to threaten the foregone conclusion.

One of the most gratuitous examples of the character assassination of two scientists—and the public and media firestorm that ensued—can be found in what has gone down in scientific history as the "Baltimore case." In 1986, Nobel Prize–winning biologist David

Baltimore found himself at the center of a case of alleged fraud that stemmed from a paper he'd coauthored with a researcher named Dr. Thereza Imanishi-Kari and four other scientists. The controversy was set off when Dr. Margot O'Toole, a postdoctoral fellow in Dr. Imanishi-Kari's lab, unable to replicate some of the experiments, claimed that the data used in the paper were manufactured.

The result was an academic storm in which other researchers took sides. Baltimore forcefully defended his coauthor and refused to withdraw the article. While he was never suspected of having himself committed fraud, his support for his pilloried colleague was perceived as a failure to react appropriately to the allegations. Two investigations were quickly launched, one at MIT, where Baltimore and Imanishi-Kari were then teaching, and another at Tufts, where she was due to move. Both found that although some of the scientific work in the study had been less than precise, there was no evidence of active fabrication.

The damage to both scientists' careers might have been bad enough it if had stopped there, but what started as a scientific debate soon became a scandal on a national scale. On Capitol Hill, Representative John Dingell was on the prowl for conflicts of interest in scientific and medical research and he decided to make an example of Dr. Imanishi-Kari. Called to testify before Congress as part of the federal probe of his colleague, Baltimore vociferously insisted that she was innocent. Contrary to Dingell's expectations, Baltimore fought back against the investigators' claims, arguing that those without a scientific background lacked the grounding to interpret a case that was, at its heart, a conflict over scientific arcana about how the experiments were conducted and whether they worked as described. Some saw his refusal to bow before the representative as a stand for science against political persecution, but many more considered it an act of arrogance and a demonstration of how out of touch scientists were. Journalists were almost exclusively in the latter camp, which also had tremendous influence on public opinion on the case.

Not to be outdone by the House committee, the Office of Scientific Integrity at the NIH, which had sponsored the disputed research, opened an investigation. The inquiry included giving Dr. Imanishi-Kari's lab notebooks to the Secret Service, who tested the ink to determine when the data had been written down and whether they had been later changed. From these tests, they concluded that the information had been falsified. In 1991, the OSI wrote to Dr. Imanishi-Kari, "Acts of deliberate misrepresentation, falsification and fabrication described, constitute a pattern of conduct extending over a four-year period that establishes a lack of integrity and honesty on your part." The verdict rendered her ineligible for federal research money for ten years. The NIH dubbed Dr. O'Toole "a hero" for launching the inquiry.

But even the *New York Times*, otherwise highly critical of Dr. Imanishi-Kari and her defenders, admitted later that those targeted by the OSI had "had no right to see the evidence against them, to cross-examine witnesses, to bring their own witnesses or even to get a list of the charges against them, which tended to change as the investigation wound on. There was also no right of appeal." Despite the determination that she had committed fraud, the embattled Dr. Imanishi-Kari continued to protest her innocence and told the scientific community, "When there is a little money and a lot of fight, you start to do this kind of witch hunt and find some guy corrupt."

Throughout the controversy, the press pilloried both scientists, never wavering for a moment in concluding that the data had been concocted by Dr. Imanishi-Kari or that Dr. Baltimore had cynically and arrogantly tried to whitewash his colleague's fraud. After the OSI report was made public, thanks to a leak by someone working for Representative Dingell, almost all news sources came out viciously against the two scientists. Margot O'Toole was widely interviewed in television, radio, and print media, with nary a critical question. In the aftermath, the original article was retracted and the controversy forced Baltimore to step down as president of Rockefeller University due to fears that the ongoing scrutiny was hurting the university's ability to attract talent and acquire funding.

But the case didn't stop there. Another office devoted to scrutinizing scientific misconduct, the Office of Research Integrity (ORI) at the Department of Health and Human Services, using the findings from the Secret Service examination of Dr. Imanishi-Kari's lab books, convicted her of nineteen counts of research misconduct in October 1994. Dr. Imanishi-Kari then appealed her case to the Research Integrity Adjudication Panel of the Federal Department of Health and Human Services. The appeal was her last hope of keeping her job and clearing her name.

When the panel reached a decision in June 1996, it held that none of the charges were supported by the evidence and said that "much of what ORI presented was irrelevant, had limited probative value, was internally inconsistent, lacked reliability or foundation, was not credible or not corroborated, or was based on unwarranted assumptions." The panel also criticized the Secret Service probe, saying "although the Secret Service examiners knew at the time of their work that they were preparing for litigation (unlike Dr. Imanishi-Kari), their records contain alterations of the results and omissions of important information." The embattled researcher and her supporters had been vindicated at last. But Dr. Baltimore told the press, "after ten years taken out of [Dr. Imanishi-Kari's] life and all the travail I've been through, I feel a sense of relief but no accomplishment."

For ten years, two scientists were relentlessly pursued by politicians, government agencies, the press, and even their peers, vilified as corrupt and arrogant and portrayed as symbols of the overall deterioration in scientific standards and morality. And they turned out to be innocent, just as they had always maintained. The controversial paper was flawed, but the charges of fabricating data and altering records were resoundingly false. Yet the damage to the careers of those involved, especially Dr. Imanishi-Kari, can never be erased. Despite her unambiguous exoneration, her opponents have made no secret of the fact that they still think she is guilty, and no verdict or evidence can ever change their minds. Even more worrying, the incident seems not to be an aberration: of the first four cases appealed to the Research Integrity Adjudications Panel, three were overturned.[28]

The Baltimore case took place before the Internet had started to play the role in the medical debate that it does today. Yet during the decade the case lasted, the world was already changing—rapidly. When the controversy began, the Internet was not yet available to the public, but by the time it ended, the availability online of news and commentary via websites, online communities, nascent news sites, and even the forerunners of today's blogs was already beginning to impact how people obtained and disseminated information. In today's world, such a scandal would have been yet larger and nastier, and its repercussions even greater and longer lasting.

The media convicted Imanishi-Kari and Baltimore almost from the beginning, and the public went along with hardly a question. But the reach of the press was not nearly as wide or as pervasive as it is now, with the information not yet free to all or consistently reprinted and relinked. Nor were the two scientists subjected to the accusations of the blogosphere and the message boards. No one Twittered the Dingell hearings or started a website supporting the heroism of Margot O'Toole.

Nonetheless, the Baltimore case has found its place on the Internet. The news articles and programs that drove it are now uploaded and available on media websites and in online news archives. New articles, and the occasional blog, continue to reference the case as a paradigm of scientific controversy, dryly and skeptically noting that the charges were eventually dismissed. Some continue to accuse Baltimore of causing "damage to science's image" by not throwing his colleague under the bus.[29] The publications available on Google Books include not only the seminal work on the controversy, which reaffirmed the innocence of Baltimore and Imanishi-Kari, but also several books that continue to insist that fraud was committed—damn the evidence to the contrary.

The angry and hyperbolic reactions we have seen in recent years to alleged conflicts of interest or misconduct offer us a taste of what the

Baltimore case might have looked like had it taken place even a decade later. The damage it did—to the scientists at its heart, to public trust in science, to the barriers between science and politics—was immense. Now imagine turning up the volume a hundredfold, a thousandfold, and giving everyone with a belief and a computer the ability to disseminate that belief to the world. That is the potential of the Internet age, and it is a scary and dangerous prospect—as Paul Offit and those like him have found out—not only to researchers but to all of us, who risk losing new knowledge and new discoveries in the process.

JUST SAY NO!

Almost inevitably, those arguing that contact with the pharmaceutical industry is bad for research believe that doctors should just make the right decision and stop taking industry money. Yet medical research cannot be done without funds, and eliminating the money received from pharmaceutical companies would mean that many studies would never be done—and that therefore both benefits and risks might never be found. There is simply not enough other funding out there to make up the difference. Government agencies are stretched thin as it is, so having the state fill the gap is untenable; it has neither the money nor the resources to allocate so many more research grants. Meanwhile, foundations and nonprofit organizations have very limited resources.

In 2003, the NIH gave out $26.4 billion for biomedical research, while other federal agencies spent $6.9 billion, 28 and 7 percent, respectively, of total funding. State and local government monies were $4.3 billion, or 5 percent. Pharmaceutical companies, on the other hand, provided $27 billion (29 percent); biotechnology companies, $17.9 billion (19 percent); and medical device manufacturers, $9.2 billion (10 percent). That amounts to 58 percent of all funding, representing a huge rise from the 32 percent it was twenty years earlier. Only 3 percent of research dollars, or $2.5 billion, came from "foundations, charities, and other private funds."[30]

The picture hasn't changed much since then. Between 2003 and 2008, the NIH budget stayed at almost the same level. Although the agency received an extra $10 billion for 2009 and 2010 as a result of the American Recovery and Reinvestment Act, this represents a temporary windfall, not a permanent increase.[31] Many scientists are worried about the future of biomedical research and innovation in the United States, as young scientists have little incentive to become or remain clinical researchers due to the difficulty of obtaining federal grants. While the NIH still pays for most university research, the federal percentage has been declining, and the amount from industry rising, since the 1990s.

The central problem is that people believe that it is possible to have both innovative medicine and no pharmaceutical funding. For instance, at Harvard, two members of a committee on conflict of interest held both that "the public deserves to know that the biomedical research they support will be a search for truth uncontaminated even by a perception of bias" and "[t]hey deserve to expect that discoveries with the potential to improve health are rapidly translated in practice to clinical trials."[32]

You cannot achieve the latter without the money and logistical resources to carry out the very large and extremely expensive studies required. Until pharma critics explain how to make up close to $55 billion annually, constituting nearly 60 percent of total funding, insisting that researchers refuse funding from companies is unrealistic and naïve. In the real world, "scientists don't often have the luxury of saying, 'No thanks, I'll get my money from the NIH instead.'"[33]

THERE'S NO SUCH THING AS UNBIASED FUNDING

It is a fallacy that any kind of funding comes without expectations or beliefs. While companies have been singled out as the sole culprits of creating conflicts of interest in medicine, this is far from the reality. If we are determined to evaluate the potential biases introduced into scientific research, then we must cast a wider net than simply looking at whether a trial is industry backed or asking whether the doctors and scientists involved derive income from drugmakers. Chances are good that a researcher didn't choose his field because he thought it would make him rich, but "very few can adequately go about their scientific business without funding of some sort. And most of that funding will come with some sort of agenda."[34]

Advocacy organizations that help back medical research almost always have a particular point of view, and they often funnel their dollars to researchers who share and will produce results validating their beliefs, whether about the cause of a disease or the best treatment for it or some other aspect. For instance, research by "consumer safety" groups—surprise!—always finds that their threat of the day is a colossal danger. No drug ever turns out to be safer than originally thought; no chemical is ever discovered to have few ill effects.

Similarly, for alternative medicine organizations, whatever modality is being tested inevitably works, and not just a little but spectacularly, even when it lacks all biological plausibility. Or think of anti-vaccine groups such as Generation Rescue or SafeMinds, which are willing to pump considerable money into studies, however shoddy, that show that vaccines are linked to autism or that any one of dozens of dubious and perhaps dangerous "biomedical" treatments can reverse autism. Most organizations don't go this far, and many fund important and valuable research, but they do have points of view and sacred cows. Yet no one seems to blink an eye if they give money only to those likely to generate results that will back up their perspective.

In addition, patient organizations are often among the first to back studies of new and novel treatments, thus playing an important role in understanding whether and why such treatments work and potentially making them available more widely. But they also may be grasping at straws, searching for a cure or a way to mitigate the illness, and are deeply emotionally invested in finding one, whether or not it follows the data. Foundations, too, can have missions that reveal the type of results they seek from the research they fund, and they often provide money to a particular type of project likely to advance these ends. Research is not just about knowledge but about membership and media attention, influence and finances, and above all hope, even if it is misplaced.

Furthermore, government monies do not come without the same sorts of implied strings as pharmaceutical company funds. As Paul J. Friedman of the University of California—San Diego School of Medicine argued, "No one seems to recognize that National Institute of Health (NIH) money can have as much of an influence in inducing bias as any drug company money, and for much the same reasons."[35] This has become especially true in recent years with the burgeoning government interest in comparative effective studies that purport to identify the best treatment for a given condition, with the goal of shifting practice and reimbursement toward the drug or procedure crowned by the trial and away from others. This trend also subtly shades into cost-effectiveness, and as you might expect, the government is very keen for cheaper, older treatments to win such contests.

One example is the government-funded Antihypertensive and Lipid-Lowering Treatment to Prevent Heart Attack Trial (ALLHAT), which claimed to have proved older diuretic medicines just as efficacious in bringing down blood pressure as new types of drugs, including ACE inhibitors, calcium channel blockers, and alpha blockers. But the trial's methodology rigged the results. First, the design allowed patients in all groups to also take beta-blockers, which "clearly helped chlorthalidone [a diuretic], the eventual 'winner,' since administration of a diuretic and a [beta]-blocker provides a logical and effective blood pressure–lowering combination. Even the addition of a [beta]-blocker to a calcium channel blocker would be useful. The logical addition to an ACE inhibitor, however, would be a diuretic or a calcium channel blocker, neither of which was permitted in the trial."

Second, the study population favored the diuretic because it included a large percentage of African American patients, in whom neither ACE inhibitors nor beta-blockers are very effective—and for whom a combination of the two was "absolutely inappropriate." As a result, there was a 40 percent excess stroke rate in black patients randomized to lisinopril (an ACE inhibitor).[36]

These defects made the study very controversial, and many doctors failed to switch to diuretics because they did not feel the study results were accurate. Cardiologist Michael Weber explained, "ALL-HAT was from the very beginning to be a political and economic clinical trial. The hope for the study was to show that an older, cheaper drug, a generic diuretic, would be at least as good as newer expensive drugs."[37] Yet the study's supporters continue to complain that doctors have not uniformly switched to diuretics.

A similar case can be found in the NIH-backed Clinical Antipsychotic Trials of Intervention Effectiveness (CATIE), which were portrayed by anti-industry groups, as well as the media, as proof that new medications for schizophrenia were no more efficacious than old ones, and therefore should not be used. But schizophrenia patients, like those with depression, often try several drugs before uncovering one that works, and the study's results were far from simple, showing a complex mixture of benefits and side effects for each drug. Again, the trial was extremely controversial among doctors, and following its recommendations made it more difficult to effectively treat patients.

In both cases, politics became involved with science. And these are not anomalies; as science journalist Matt Herper of *Forbes* observed, "Every time there's a government study, it always seems to show no difference between the treatments."[38] Those who have to pay for treatments, the government included, have a vested interest in creating justification not to pay for more expensive treatments, and therefore for concluding that those do not work better than older, less pricey ones.

WE'RE ALL CONFLICTED

Last, but far from least, financial conflicts are only one of many potential sources of bias. Researchers may be motivated by the hope of gaining further grants or other money for their research, the ambition to win tenure, or the desire simply to obtain respect and admiration from peers. They might be influenced by pressure from family, friends, or colleagues; rivalries and conflicts with other scientists; or just wanting to confirm a deeply held belief. On the institutional level, medical and scientific facilities encourage studies that help fulfill their goal of "enhancing their reputations as research centers."[39] None of these motivations is financial in nature, and yet all are powerful, arguably even more so than those driven by expectation of monetary profit.

Yet those who are so zealous to crack down on every intimation that a researcher might have received funding from industry hardly ever mention other types of biases—and then, only as an afterthought. One journal argued that "nonfinancial conflicts are inherent to research," but "financial conflicts are not inherent to research—they are optional. Researchers are not forced to have financial conflicts, and restrictions based on them do not violate academic freedom." But as I have shown earlier, this is simply not so. The real reason for the emphasis on disclosure of monetary interests is that "[t]he public cares little about academic conflicts, but is alarmed by financial conflicts."[40] This is perhaps because financial support for research is easier to identify than intellectual or ideological bias. It is easier to put these preferences on trial than other factors that influence what is studied and how.

Yet if those who advocate disclosure truly want to help readers see all potential biases, they must go far beyond asking contributors to reveal the contents of their bank accounts and stock portfolios. But should scientists have to disclose their religious beliefs, their political affiliations, or their sexual orientations? All contain the potential for bias, and, indeed, there are precedents for scientists being asked such questions. What about cases where researchers focus on a particular disease or condition because they or someone close to them has it? As one scientist pointed out, "If you study Alzheimer's disease because your grandmother has Alzheimer's, you also have a personal interest."[41] Or think about the autism debate. Many of the people on both sides are involved in autism research and study because they have family members with an autism spectrum disorder.

But while a personal stake can lead to bias, it can also create motivation to do everything possible to undercover new information or find a cure. Treatments for many diseases, especially rare or obscure ones, have come about because someone became deeply invested in finding an answer or because of a single-minded researcher who believed deeply in his hypothesis, someone who would be correctly defined as having a bias, refused to give up. Thus, "science is advanced by the determined, committed, even the obsessed individual, not by the doubting peers."[42]

Moreover, tabloid medicine applies a double standard when attacking researchers for conflict of interest: The same conflicts that supposedly corrupt other researchers are ignored in those who take an anti-industry stance. One example is Dr. Steven Nissen, who has said that "the appearance of bias can damage trust as much as actual impropriety" and claimed in 2007 that he donated all "drug industry consulting fees ... to a philanthropic charity run by the American College of Cardiology." Yet, the charity was the Steven E. Nissen Healthy Heart Fund, and it subsidized such philanthropic activities as gym memberships for the staff of the American College of Cardiology. Further, in 2005, the $1 million in the Healthy Heart Fund was folded into the ACC Foundation which, the following year, elected a new president, Dr. Steven Nissen.[43]

Ultimately, does the obsession with rooting out conflicts allow us to have better, more innovative research or to be more informed patients? I don't think so. The bottom line is not that financial conflicts of interest are never a problem. There have certainly been doctors and scientists who behaved improperly, and there have been cases of pharmaceutical reps and companies who chased profit at the expense of patients. But a few bad examples shouldn't be used to justify damaging blanket rules. Funding by pharmaceutical companies may have the potential for conflicts, but the collaboration between academia and industry is not only intrinsic to scientific research as it now exists but has also been responsible for many important innovations over the years. Biases, financial and not, are enmeshed in the lives and work of every scientist and every doctor—indeed, of every person.

British health policy consultant Michael Tremblay expressed it well when he wrote:

> [W]ho is without conflict, who is without a sponsor, who is immune from the pressures to publish, to perform on committees ... ? Are we to stop sharing our experience for fear of opporbrium [*sic*] from colleagues who have little of interest to say as they sit in their tiny conflict-free worlds? ... The interesting people are all conflicted—they are engaged in the real world, with all its faults. The world is not neat and tidy, it is messy and complex, and better we learn to understand the conflicts, than naively believe we can avoid them.[44]

Or, as one journalist insightfully said of the furor over whether vaccines cause autism, "If every conflict of interest was ground for disqualification in the thimerosal debate, it wouldn't be possible to have a debate ... And that pretty much goes for any scientific discussion, unless it's being held by people who have no prior assumptions about anything."[45]

We can throw up our hands and trade the future of medicine for the knowledge that every effort is being made to ensure that scientists and drug companies never collaborate or do so only under highly scrutinized and monitored conditions. Or we can punish malfeasance when we find it, accept that not everyone will do the right thing every time (after all, we do so in just about every other sphere of society), and know that this is a small price to pay for new and accessible medicines that will make our lives longer and better. Tabloid medicine wants to choose not only what we know and think about medical technologies but also what treatments we develop and receive. Are we going to let it?

CHAPTER 8

Tabloid Medicine's Victims:
Public Health and Medical Progress

OR DECADES, HORMONE REPLACEMENT therapy was billed practically as a wonder cure, credited with extraordinary and wide-ranging benefits. Then, in 2002, the Women's Health Initiative (WHI) trial reported increased risks of breast cancer, heart attack, stroke, and blood clots in women taking the drugs. In a flash, the study radically altered thinking about hormone replacement therapy (HRT) and turned it into a Precautionary Principle poster child. Nearly a decade later, the WHI trial, with its repercussions for the use of HRT, remains one of the most misunderstood recent medical revelations.

The almost universal reaction to the news of the WHI's findings was first panic and then recrimination. Women attacked makers of hormone replacement therapies online and in the press for having deliberately lied about the benefits and dangers of the drugs, and they accused doctors of having been in the thrall of big pharma. Safety groups and women's organizations joined in with press releases and blog entries blasting hormone manufacturers. The safety crusaders, the media, Congress, and even some of the scientists involved in the study worked shrewdly and consistently to hype the dangers and to silence criticism. Lost in all this outrage, anger, and fear was what the data really showed and how the methodology of the study offered a false picture of HRT.

The risks of HRT were not only overstated; they were also presented in a way designed to elicit fear, emphasizing the number of extra cases of cancer, stroke, and heart attack but not making clear that the risks all were higher by less than 1 percent, which in most cases could not be considered statistically significant. Yet women continued to be told that HRT use resulted in a 24 percent higher danger of having a heart attack.[1] Furthermore, the danger is tied to the patient's underlying danger of developing various conditions; for those with low existing risks, the potential for serious side effects is minimal. The fact that women on HRT had reduced incidence of colorectal cancer and bone loss and osteoporosis was also given short shrift or omitted altogether.

Further, key mistakes were made in the early design of the WHI trial. First, the average woman in the trial was sixty-three, and most women in the study started taking hormones at least ten years past menopause. Today, the typical woman who is considering hormone therapy is in her late forties or early fifties. She's just beginning to experience the hormonal turmoil—the hot flashes, mood swings, and other changes—associated with the menopausal transition. Although few women in this age group were studied in the WHI, these are the women who have been most frightened and affected by the research.

This fundamental flaw in the study design means the data are of limited use in trying to understand the full range of risks and benefits to the typical user of menopause hormones because age plays a critical role in the risks and benefits of HRT. The data show that hormone therapy is highly beneficial for many women within ten years from the start of menopause or under age sixty-five, but it offers correspondingly higher risks for older women or those more than ten years beyond the beginning of menopause.

When the results of the WHI were separated out by age group, women age fifty to fifty-nine on HRT had a nearly 40 percent lower risk of cardiovascular problems than women the same age who were not. Women sixty to sixty-nine years old had a slightly lower risk than counterparts not taking the drugs, and only those age seventy to seventy-nine had an increased risk, about 11 percent higher than women not on HRT.[2] Even in the last group, research has indicated that the increased danger of heart problems may depend on how long the drug has been taken and can be mitigated by limiting the duration of HRT use. Yet Dr. Jacques Rossouw, at the time acting director of the WHI, told a roomful of reporters, "The results have broad applicability. The study found no differences in risk by prior health status, age, or ethnicity."[3] That simply wasn't true.

Second, the rise in the incidence of cancer, stroke, and heart attack depends on what kind of HRT the woman is taking. Only one arm of WHI, the one looking at combined estrogen-progestin, was stopped in 2002, and this combination is known to have higher risks than estrogen alone. A second part of WHI looked at women on estrogen only, and by the time it was halted in 2004, it had found a small increase in the incidence of stroke but no change for heart problems and a reduced breast cancer risk. This type of HRT also demonstrated the same beneficial effects for hip and other fractures.

Yet, as journalist Tara Parker-Pope noted in her book *The Hormone Decision*, "When the estrogen-only study showed the good news that estrogen might lower breast cancer risk by 20 percent, the NHLBI [National Heart, Lung, and Blood Institute, which sponsored the study] didn't tout the finding. Instead, the headline on the government press release said only that there was 'no increased risk of breast cancer with estrogen alone.' The NHLBI seemed to have a different standard for bad hormone news than it did for good hormone news."[4] Furthermore, the WHI trial tested only one formulation of HRT, a steroid pill form that was common when the study began but is less used today.

There are also considerations beyond simple calculations of risk and life expectancy. For many women on HRT, the treatment improves, often significantly, their quality of life, and that benefit must be included when weighing potential risks. In a study published in *Archives of Internal Medicine*, short-term HRT was found to slightly increase quality-adjusted life expectancy (QALE) for women with mild to severe menopausal symptoms. There was a decrease only in women who did not have any menopause symptoms, and even then it was very small: one to three months.[5] Many women insisted on continuing HRT despite the publicity about its risks, because of the immense difference for the better it made in their lives. However, half of women prescribed hormones in the aftermath of the controversy never filled the prescription, and many more were confused and unsure what to do.[6]

The scary and incomplete picture of the WHI's results offered by the study's leaders—light on careful analysis and context and heavy on hype—was no accident, but rather, a deliberate strategy. Tara Parker-Pope reported:

> The NIH wanted to make a splash. The NHLBI, which oversaw the WHI, worked hard to get media attention for the WHI study. Dr. Rossouw, the physician in charge of the WHI when the results were first announced, has since told me that the NHLBI was intentionally going for "high impact" when it called the press conference in Washington, DC. Dr. Rossouw and other NIH officials knew that important health announcements could get lost in the shuffle of daily news events, but they didn't want this study ignored. The goal, says Dr. Rossouw, was to shake up the medical establishment and change the thinking about hormones.[7]

The work of the scaremongers has unfortunately been highly successful. Across the Web, stories of supposed harm by HRT abound, and despite the balanced information put forth by reputable health sites, the dominant picture is one of danger and conspiracy. Although many studies have contradicted or modified the conclusions of WHI and similar studies, millions of women have stopped HRT since 2002 and many more remain terrified of the consequences of hormone use. Thousands of others are left with limited or no access to HRT because their doctors are afraid of the potential for recrimination and even litigation if their patients get sick and believe the drug is responsible.[8] It is a rational fear given that some patients who were once prescribed HRT have sued the makers of the hormones, claiming that the treatment was responsible for their cancer, heart attacks, or other ailments.

Other women have turned to so-called bio-identical hormones, derived from soy and other plants, and sold by alternative health advocates, often online. Promoted by instant experts such as Suzanne Somers, they have been touted as not only absolutely safe but also the key to renewed youth and well-being. But bio-identical hormones do not undergo the tests required for FDA-approved HRT products, and Dr. Vanessa Barnabei, a WHI investigator, explained, "Just because something is derived from a plant does not necessarily mean it's safe ... We have even less data on herbal remedies ... than we do on HRT."[9] Testing of bio-identical hormones has so far failed to show that they are even effective.[10]

Despite subsequent analyses and studies that have reaffirmed that HRT can be safely used and that it offers substantial benefits to many women, the controversy shows no signs of being extinguished. It is still considered by safety crusaders, consumer groups, and the population at large to be a perfect example of why patients cannot trust physicians and of the dirty tactics companies engage in to make profits. As Judith Reichman of UCLA and Cedars-Sinai Medical Center told colleagues at the Eighth Annual Congress on Women's Health and Gender-Based Medicine, "What we're facing now is a huge credibility gap."[11]

In many ways, the WHI trial was and remains the gold standard for what proponents of tabloid medicine want all medical research to be: government-funded research highlighting risks and making the case that drugs developed and marketed by pharmaceutical companies were being widely prescribed thanks to researchers who were conflicted or corrupt. Those who conducted the WHI and packaged its results for maximum effect knew exactly what they were doing and believed it was essential to make a splash. In the process, the WHI leadership deliberately sought to downplay benefits, inflate risks, and silence opponents who claimed that the data did not lead to a one-size-fits-all conclusion and could instead be used to personalize treatment for patients.

H. L. Mencken wrote of politics that its goal "is to keep the populace in a continual state of alarm (and hence clamorous to be led to safety) by menacing them with an endless series of hobgoblins, all of them imaginary." But he might well have said the same of those who today continually assail science and medicine. Instant experts and their followers have launched an assault on science in the name of safety, but they have left us more endangered and more afraid. As the example of HRT illustrates, we are so terrified by the scary headlines and the parade of clamorous warnings from websites that greet all new supposed risks that we don't understand what the data really indicate or what they really mean. We question the recommendations of our doctors due to something we've found online and are reluctant to accept the physicians' explanation of why what we've read is not true. We are wary of taking the pills prescribed and decide we're better off not taking them at all.

Encouraged by the forces of tabloid medicine, we demand perfect safety and vilify those who (inevitably) fail to provide it, impeding the work of researchers, companies, and government agencies. As a consequence, fewer new drugs are developed and approved each year, and we also fail to understand the implications of new information about drugs already on the market, instead becoming consumed by fear. The costs of replacing real science with tabloid medicine are many and widespread: fewer people taking medicines that work or following sound medical advice, a reduction in valuable research, and a continuing decline in biomedical innovation.

The divide between what science can do and what political and cultural forces seek to accomplish has never been greater. On the one hand, science and researchers—together with companies—are creating scientific advances that can and will predict and control our individual response to disease and treatments, making possible tests and medicines that deliver the right drug to the right patient well before an illness sets in, with greater benefits and fewer risks. Breakthroughs in the treatment and prevention of cancer are but one product of this individualization of risk and benefit. On the other hand, a well-organized and defiant movement insists that deliberate danger is not only a common feature of medical innovation but also a hidden threat and that researchers and companies are guilty in this state of affairs until proven innocent. There is no evidence to support this view, only someone's insistence that it happened that way, but that may be enough to make it so to millions.

LOSING SIGHT OF RISK AND BENEFIT

Tabloid medicine has also affected the number of new drugs developed and approved. As the Vioxx example demonstrates, the successful effort to build a lower risk tolerance for adverse events, coupled with greater demand for conflict-free research and evaluation of new drugs and devices, means that patients who could have lived longer or had a better quality of life because of these treatments are not receiving them. In some cases, medications denied by the FDA are available elsewhere in the world, leaving American patients out in the cold or forced to resort to dubious schemes to get a hold of them. Other patients are hurt by relying instead on other medicines that don't work as well or at all, or by choosing alternative remedies that at best act as placebos and at worse can have fatal consequences. By selecting alternatives, patients don't reduce the dangers from medical technologies; they just change them—and often increase them.

Researchers studying human behavior have found that when we believe we are protecting ourselves, we change our behavior in other ways that put us at risk. For instance, according to British research, wearing a helmet makes bicyclists ride in a riskier manner and also leads people in cars to drive less carefully around them.[12] At other times, we fail to recognize or accept that even the best safety measures may come with dangers of their own. Think of air bags: they save countless lives, but they do carry risks and don't always work perfectly. *Safe* and *unsafe* aren't a dichotomy, but rather a continuum, and our place on it is determined by the risks *and* the benefits. Only through weighing all sides of the choices before us can we pick the one that really makes us healthier. Yet the effect of tabloid medicine has been not only to change what our society defines and views as health risks but also to use government and public policy to limit the choice of medical technologies that may emerge in the future.

The pharmaceutical companies themselves have a measure of blame in the rise of tabloid medicine. They have sometimes oversold their wares, in terms not simply of efficacy but also of safety. The names and uses of medications are more familiar to us than ever, thanks to the increasingly ubiquitous advertising that pops up in print, online, and on television, making big promises and leaving contraindications and risk information for fine print and disclaimers delivered at high speed. As Dr. Marc Siegel said of patients' fear, "Part of the problem is the way the drug industry hypes its products, setting them up as some kind of panacea ... if it's sold as a magic elixir, the discovery of any flaw rings alarm bells."[13] By failing to be transparent about the benefits and risks, companies have handed power to the instant experts and the self-interested "safety" advocates and implicitly backed the same belief their opponents use so adroitly: that total safety is possible. It is unpalatable to be too open about the fact that one's products have the potential to be dangerous, but it is nonetheless imperative if the public is ever to be disabused of the notion that the existence of any risk is a sign of gross negligence. Companies and scientists need to describe how products are developed and to be more proactive in telling people, in terms that the majority of people understand, rather than in scientific jargon, about changes or advances in scientific understanding impacting both efficacy and safety.

Government regulatory agencies, too, have bent over too far backward to placate fearmongers and the worried public they create. The FDA now issues preliminary warnings about the possible risks of drugs based on a cursory review of patient reports and media accounts. Increasingly, the agency is forced to pull scientists off of reviewing new drug approvals to testify on Capitol Hill and respond to the latest headlines about potential dangers, almost always false or overblown. Already the FDA is understaffed and underfunded, despite additions to it in the last couple of years. In 2009, the agency was finally able to hire more staff, but the number of employees is now only what it was in 1994. Nonetheless, critics accuse the FDA of being a puppet of industry, willing to approve dangerous drugs and withhold evidence of new risks in order to curry companies' favor. Similar charges are leveled against other organizations that regulate and fund scientific research, and these attempts to control or prohibit interactions with industry are impeding the work of scientists both in government and in the private sphere.[14]

Meanwhile, the efforts of private companies, the FDA, and university medical centers to come up with tools to promote personalized medicine have been attacked and thwarted by grandstanding politicians, backed by the rest of the usual suspects. One member of Congress, Rosa DeLauro (D-CT), has continually denied $1.5 million for the Reagan-Udall Foundation, which Congress established in 2007 as part of the FDA Modernization Action "to identify and address unmet scientific needs in the development, manufacture and evaluation of the safety and effectiveness of FDA-regulated products, including post-market evaluation." The private, nonprofit foundation's mission is to support scientific projects and programs that the FDA itself has identified as important to its regulatory mission and consistent with the Critical Path Institute, an organization set up to facilitate cooperation between government and industry in translating medical research into marketable products.

DeLauro chairs the Agriculture Subcommittee of the House Appropriations Committee and, therefore, controls not only the FDA's budget but also the purse strings of many other agencies and congressional earmarks. She refuses to appropriate funds for Reagan-Udall because she insists that it will lead to industry control over FDA approval standards. DeLauro holds that genetic-based markers really don't measure outcomes and will lead the FDA to endorse the approval of drugs based on a lower standard. Consequently, she insists that "the FDA should postpone activities related to the foundation until it can assure the pharmaceutical and device industries will not have undue influence."[15] But this will never be achieved to her satisfaction until she and her fellow tabloid medicine advocates have control over such institutions.

THE PRICE OF PURITY

Demanding a firewall between researchers, scientists, and doctors on one side and industry on the other impedes the development and availability of new drugs. When the Bayh-Dole Act was passed in 1980, allowing academic discoveries to be commercialized although they had been funded with money from the government, its goal was to facilitate bringing the breakthroughs made by university researchers to patients. At that time, discoveries in the academic realm were not being translated quickly enough into drugs or other technologies that were available to the public. Three decades later, Bayh-Dole has succeeded brilliantly; prior to the act, the number of patents given each year to American institutions of higher education was below 250, but by 1999, that figure was 3,914. Translation of university finds into marketable products shot up, and many important medications and technologies that save or prolong lives came out of this process.[16] You'd never know it, though, if you ran a Google search. Rather, you'd probably be quickly convinced that doctors and scientists in academia have filled their pockets to the tune of millions, paid off by a pharmaceutical industry that reaps enormous profits by selling the fruit of universities' hard work to the public at huge markups.

Bayh-Dole was necessary because, while researchers at universities have made vital contributions to understanding diseases and creating treatments for them, they almost always lack the immense resources required to test drugs or devices. Obtaining approval from the FDA takes many years and requires trials involving thousands of people and millions of dollars. That's where companies come in; they have the resources, financial and logistical, to carry out the testing that is as much a part of research as the original discovery is. So while it is in fashion to denounce the biggest breakthroughs of recent decades as the products of universities, scooped up and exploited by avaricious industry, these treatments would almost never have made it to the market—and thereby to patients—without the intervention of companies. We have seen a long history of benefit from interaction and collaboration between academia and industry, and by excluding or restricting this cooperation, universities and other scientific institutions are making it more difficult for new technologies and drugs to be created, tested, and eventually made available to those who will benefit from them.[17]

The creation of new drugs may enrich scientists and companies, but as many studies have borne out, "Many more patients have benefited from this partnership than have the pockets of doctors or members of industry."[18] Studies conducted by University of Chicago economists Kevin Murphy and Robert Topel estimate that from 1970 to 2000, increased longevity from new medicines and devices added approximately $3.2 trillion per year to national wealth, the equivalent of half of the average annual gross domestic product over the period. Half of these gains were due to progress against heart disease alone, with reduced mortality from heart disease increasing the value of life by about $1.5 trillion per year since 1970.[19]

The tabloid medicine crowd claims "[academic] medical research was every bit as productive before Bayh-Dole as it is now, despite the lack of patents," cleverly sidestepping the fact that it is not the productivity of medical research at universities that is at issue here but the translation of that study into available treatments. Former *New England Journal of Medicine* editor Marcia Angell once argued, "I'm reminded of Jonas Salk's response when asked whether he had patented the polio vaccine. He seemed amazed at the very notion. The vaccine, he explained, belonged to everybody. 'Could you patent the sun?' he asked."[20] But what she had forgotten is that he went on to establish the Salk Institute and pursued research funding from industry, collaborating with companies to move discoveries into development. This cooperation has produced in excess of 350 patents, over 250 license agreements, and 22 start-up firms.[21]

Critics of collaboration between scientists and industry also ignore the fact that many innovations come out of the United States precisely because it has provided fertile ground for developing, testing, and, yes, commercializing new discoveries. As other countries heed the siren song of cost-effectiveness, this is becoming truer than ever. In the United Kingdom, the National Institute for Health and Clinical Effectiveness (which goes by the oh-so-ironic acronym NICE) refuses coverage by the National Health System of medications deemed to cost too much. This creates a disincentive for companies to produce new medications that, after hundreds of millions have been spent to bring them to market, will not be covered by the NHS. In addition, several companies have already reduced the inclusion of British patients in trials because, due to NICE recommendations, "few patients in Britain are receiving 'gold standard' treatment, so there is too small a group against which to compare their experimental drugs."[22]

In 2007, drug and device companies in the United States spent $58.8 billion on research and development.[23] The National Institutes of Health added over $28 billion more.[24] Today, overall funding of research in the United States is more than twice what it was in 1994.[25] In total, the United States accounts for around 78 percent of spending on developing new biotechnology around the globe. The European share is only 16 percent, although the European Union is beginning to shift more emphasis—and money—toward drug research and development.[26] It is not surprising that one 2007 analysis said that the United States "has been the country of first launch for close to half of the oncology drugs brought to market in the last 11 years."[27]

Finally, while you probably would never know it from reading the press or trawling Google, some data indicate that the population would prefer greater "cooperation at the state and national level among funders and performers of health research." In 2005, Research! America found that 73 percent of people who participated in one of its surveys believed "government, universities, and the pharmaceutical industry do not work together to develop new treatments," and 95 percent advocated such collaboration. In addition, 69 percent held that doctors and other researchers should be allowed to make a monetary profit from the results of their work.[28]

FEWER DRUGS

Scandals like the one surrounding the withdrawal of Vioxx, and the greater scrutiny of drug safety they've engendered, have reduced the number of drugs that are approved and, in some cases, increased the time it takes to approve successful drugs. The FDA has repeatedly denied that its standards have become stricter, but there are many indications that it has certainly become more wary of new drugs that may have unknown side effects. This has led to denials for some medications and requirements for additional data or tests on others, stretching out the approval process and driving up the cost of development. This can mean higher prices for the consumer when the drug makes it to market—if it ever does.

Overall, drug approvals were only slightly down in the three years after Vioxx, as compared to the three prior years, going from ninety-five per year to eighty-nine. But for drugs that went through the Center for Drug Evaluation and Research (CDER), which evaluates all drugs other than biologics (drugs produced using DNA technology from living cells), the number of successful medications went from eighty-four down to sixty-seven. That's a difference of 20 percent.[29] This trend has actually increased as a result of subsequent panics over drugs; in 2004, the year Vioxx was pulled from the market, thirty-two new molecular entities (drug molecules that have never been previously marketed) were approved by CDER, but 2005 and 2006 each saw only nineteen reach the market. And this trend has remained steady. In 2007, there were fifteen new molecular entities approved; in 2008, twenty-one; and in 2009, nineteen.[30]

Yet a comparison of the number of clinical trials of new drugs to the number of approvals indicates that the decline isn't the product of dry pipelines at pharmaceutical companies, as many allege. Indeed, the number of trials continued to go up in the two years following the Vioxx scandal, even as fewer medications were getting through the FDA.[31] New drug applications (NDAs) did fall to 102 in 2004, the year of Vioxx, after rising from 74 in 1993 to 129 in 1999, according to the Government Accountability Office (GAO).[32] But this was only part of the picture; an analysis found that in 2007, the FDA approved 60 percent of the NDAs it received, versus 76 percent the previous year. Among new molecular entities, the percentage of approvals was down 18 percent, and approvals of biologics, which have made up an increasing part of the new applications, were also down considerably.[33]

In response to a more difficult climate for getting medications to market, companies are now using genetic tools called biomarkers to more precisely predict which potential drugs will deliver benefits without severe side effects. Increasingly, new drugs will be launched with a test kit that allows physicians and patients to determine whether the treatment is likely to offer benefits or not. In particular, physicians can now use such tests in tailoring and adjusting the care of people with cancer or AIDS. At the same time, however, even targeted therapies based on these more accurate assessments of risks and benefits are facing high hurdles, further increasing the percentage of products facing delays in approval or outright rejections. Rather than confront these challenges, companies will create fewer innovative medicines developed for niche markets. Drug development is simply too costly for companies to risk being unable to recoup the investment. This is exactly the opposite of the intent of the Critical Path but is precisely the objective of the tabloid medicine forces.

In general, drugs within types or classes where previous treatments have been accused of being too risky, however minor or spurious the danger actually was, have been especially scrutinized, and require increased evidence of safety. The FDA has become especially vigilant about watching drugs for indications that they contribute to heart or liver problems, since such side effects have been at the center of numerous recent conflicts over drug safety.[34]

In order to counter these trends, the FDA's vision has been to use genetic tools and encrypted medical data to monitor products once they are on the market, gathering valuable new data while also enhancing public health. For example, scientists within the FDA and academia are seeking to find ways to individualize the use of diabetes drugs such as Avandia by testing how well patients process the drug and how it affects cholesterol levels.

Yet tabloid medicine crusaders simply ignore the value of such tools or dismiss such science as merely the adoption of a weaker standard for approval. Instead, they insist on studies to respond to false fears they themselves create. GlaxoSmithKline is currently conducting an FDA-approved study to compare how Avandia and a similar drug called Actos affect the risk of stroke or heart attack in diabetic patients with heart disease. This trial was prompted by studies claiming that Actos is "safer." The studies were authored by two researchers we have already encountered in their roles as instigators of the

Vioxx scandal: Steve Nissen, a paid consultant to Actos, who was also responsible for the original claim that Avandia was a dangerous drug; and David Graham, who believes that Actos is safer despite the fact that a government-run study of the two drugs found no difference.[35]

Instead of investing in tools that could help predict patient response to Avandia, GlaxoSmithKline is spending hundreds of millions of dollars on a study that will be attacked—if it ever gets off the ground. And that is looking doubtful; because of vitriol against the FDA by politicians, anti-pharma activists, and instant experts, patients are afraid to enroll in the Avandia study. Already two of the trial's research locations have been closed down due to difficulties recruiting enough patients. In the meantime, the attacks on the study have gone global because it also includes a dozen research sites overseas, some in developing countries, including Colombia, India, Latvia, Mexico, and Pakistan, and that has some critics of the company uneasy. Dr. Sidney Wolfe of the consumer advocacy group Public Citizen told the *Wall Street Journal* that he was concerned that patients at some of these overseas sites might not be aware of the safety questions surrounding Avandia and has made clear he wants to see the study scrapped.[36]

More money spent on clinical trials that will not move toward predictive medicine means less support for personalized medicine tools. Distracting the FDA from its pursuit of more sophisticated methods for regulating medicines likely means more failures and fewer drugs. Dr. Raymond Woosley of the Critical Path Institute has worked with the FDA and companies to develop blood tests to screen for serious side effects of medicines before they happen. Woosley notes that there is "a shift in focus by pharmaceutical companies to the development of medication for the causes of diseases, rather than the symptoms, a process that is 'just much more complex.'"[37] This may produce a higher likelihood of failure as long as drug regulation fails to embrace the potential of new personalized medicine tools that use biomarkers and genetic information to anticipate which patients will be helped by a drug and which ones may be harmed.

NOTHING NEW?

One of the main contentions of tabloid medicine is that most drugs not only carry hidden dangers but are also merely variations on existing medications and little or no better than those already on the market. Search for information on the Internet and this is what you are likely to get, not only from the critics and their own websites but also from a seemingly endless succession of ordinary citizens who parrot pharma scolds' talking points. In her book *The Truth About Drug Companies*, Marcia Angell asserts that "there is little evidence to support the notion that if one drug doesn't work for a patient, a virtually identical one will. Or if one drug causes side effects, another one won't."[38]

This accusation is wrong for two reasons. First, even among similar drugs, there are variations in exactly how they work, producing differences in which patients they work for and the side effect risks they present. No drug works for 100 percent of patients, and patients frequently find that one drug of a particular type is more effective for them than another. In other cases, each drug in a given class may have different side effect profiles, whether in terms of the relative risks of a given side effect or in terms of which side effects are common.

This is particularly true of drugs for conditions such as depression and anxiety, leading patients to need to try multiple medications before they find one that is effective. The most dramatic example of this (though a big splash was not made) can be found in the results of the NIMH Sequenced Treatment Alternatives to Relieve Depression (STAR*D) study, in which nearly half of all patients with difficult-to-treat depression needed either to switch to another medicine or to combine their existing therapy—behavioral therapy, drugs, or a combination—with another treatment in order to get well.[39] Patients with a variety of chronic illnesses, including cancer, may also need to switch drugs periodically if they begin to tolerate the one they are taking and therefore derive less efficacy from it.

Second, incremental improvement nonetheless produces measurable benefits. The principle of gradually improving technology is unquestioningly accepted in other spheres of our lives. Just look at our electronics. Yet, in medicine, this is somehow indicative of malfeasance. Furthermore, as we accept the principle of competition tending to improve quality in the rest of the economy, why do we reject it in the case of drugs? There are many examples where the first drug in a class is just a shadow of the ones that come later as knowledge increases and the workings can be refined to improve the drug's safety and effectiveness. It should be noted, for example, that Prozac, the first SSRI, was once regarded as no more effective than first-generation antidepressants called tricyclics. Yet SSRIs became front-line therapy once psychiatrists found that people had fewer side effects and better responses after not doing well on tricyclics.

In *Money-Driven Medicine*, Maggie Mahar asserts that companies squander millions producing "me-too tumor-shrinking drugs that 'don't perform better than existing treatments.'"[40] Yet we know that not only are there several types of cancers, such as breast, ovarian, and colon, but also that one person's cancer can progress quite differently from another's. By understanding how these different so-called "me-too" cancer drugs work, we can identify which drug or combination of drugs works best for a given patient and can develop more accurate tests to detect cancer earlier than ever. Would Mahar suggest that her family members simply use the oldest cancer drug or forego the use of "me-too-tumor" drugs? Would she avoid the use of these new medications if she had to be treated for cancer?

To be sure, both in the past and today, companies will sometimes unjustifiably promote their products to the nation as a whole or overstate the number of patients who can benefit from them. (Though they will add disclaimers in sotto voce that "drug X is not for everyone.") Yet this isn't an excuse to stop the development of new drugs or block their way to market. As companies compete to perfect an approach to treating a disease, increasing efficacy, reducing side effects, or tailoring it to certain types of patients, drugs can become better and better, superseding one another, carving out niches, or even being used in combination. This can mean steadily improving treatment for patients.[41]

Similarly maligned are new indications for drugs, often dismissed as a sneaky way for drugmakers to keep sales high and increase revenue. Yet many new breakthroughs have been spawned by discoveries made after a drug was released onto the market, either in postapproval testing or through simple physician use, and drugs in this category are increasing. A case in point is the wet macular degeneration drug Lucentis, which is an extraordinarily rare 95 percent effective in either halting or reversing damage to patients' sight, saving them from blindness. In December 2006, the medication was declared one of the year's top breakthroughs by the American Association for the Advancement of Science.

But Lucentis began life as another novel drug: Avastin, which was developed to treat colorectal cancer and is now either approved for or being studied in half a dozen other types of cancer, including breast, lung, kidney, ovarian, prostate, and pancreatic. Yet rather than celebrate Lucentis as a spectacular advance, many observers prefer to debate about using small amounts of regular Avastin instead of the specially engineered version in Lucentis in order to save money.

Another drug to find a second life treating other conditions is Gleevac, an innovative cancer treatment, which has also shown promise at stopping the development of diabetes. Viread, an HIV medication, can also be used against hepatitis B. Rituxan first got FDA approval to treat cancer before being found to be effective against rheumatoid arthritis, while two one-time rheumatoid arthritis drugs, Enbrel and Remicade, went on to be approved for new uses: psoriasis and Crohn's disease respectively. Even a drug to treat hypertension gained a second (and famous) life in the form of Viagra. And in turn, Viagra is now used to treat pulmonary hypertension in newborns. Should we bar patients from taking effective drugs because they also treat another condition or because they started out being developed for a different purpose?

Finally, as noted earlier, scientific data have revealed the importance of these types of drugs in helping Americans have longer and better lives. People often underestimate the extent to which medical innovation impacts them, especially if they have never faced a major health crisis. After observing that people in Mississippi and Louisiana lived only 74.2 years, versus 81.3 years for those in Hawaii, and that there were similar divergences in the rates at which life expectancy was increasing, economist Frank Lichtenberg went looking for the reason. What he discovered was that "the most important factor was medical innovation." More than rates of obesity, HIV/AIDs, and smoking, "longevity increased the most in those states where access to newer drugs—measured by their 'vintage' or FDA approval year—in Medicaid and Medicare programs has increased the most."

Lichtenberg found that an estimated 63 percent of "potential increase in longevity," or the change in life expectancy that would be expected if other factors stayed stable, came from the introduction of new medications. The more recent the average approval of the available drugs, the better the life expectancy: two months longer per one year increase in vintage. Other researchers have likewise documented the role played by new drugs in extending life and improving its quality. A 2006 report by the National Bureau of Economic Research concluded that medical progress was the primary factor in the reduction of cardiovascular mortality by 55 percent from 1975 to 1995.[42] Cancer rates in the United States have been steadily declining for more than fifteen years, with five year survival rates passing 90 percent for some cancers, such as breast cancer, if found early.[43] Examples abound and are increasing every day.

Lichtenberg's study—like many others he has conducted in the past—also dealt a blow to a common truism about innovation: that it inevitably means an increase in medical costs. He estimated that the use of newer drugs and devices increased overall drug costs associated with treating a disease by $18—and reduced the total hospital and other nondrug costs by $129.[44] Lichtenberg also found that spending did not appear any higher in states with more recent average drug vintages, and that labor productivity went up approximately 1 percent annually, since patients with ongoing conditions were out of work less often.[45] New medications can also control or prevent chronic illnesses, creating potential savings in the long run. It isn't just true in the United States, either. A National Bureau of Economic Research study has estimated that, in Europe, for each euro devoted to creating new medications and treatments, countries could avoid up to €3.95 in costs down the line.[46]

Innovation is all around us as we learn more about the mechanisms behind disease, discover how drugs work, and make the connections that allow us to turn existing discoveries to new uses. This is especially true in the domain of cancer drugs, where we are simultaneously recognizing the variations within single types of cancers and the similarities among different types. Doesn't it make sense to pursue greater understanding of the dynamics and abilities of the drugs we have, as well as to look for new ones? The campaign to portray innovation as only uncovering new molecules or mechanisms is ultimately hypocritical and contradictory.

The critics write off new uses of old drugs and additions to existing drug classes as mere "me-too"s and revenue enhancers. Yet these old medicines were yesterday's breakthroughs in treating ulcers, arthritis, heart disease, mental illness, and cancer. If the critics had been successful ten to twenty years ago in raising the bar for innovation and undermining reliance on medicines, what would the effect have been on both the number and the impact of medical technologies? To survive, tabloid medicine must reject these advances in the same way that those who insisted the earth was flat maintained their beliefs: by remaining ignorant, by attempting to silence those who disagree, and by conducting research that does little more than reframe medical innovation as too risky.

THE "BEST" TREATMENT

Tabloid medicine has also made use of the idea that using large, randomized trials that pit treatments against one another allows us to determine which therapies are really the best. Then, theoretically, we will use only the winning treatment and have little or no need for the others. Such research goes by the name comparative effectiveness, and has in recent years gained a lot of interest in the political, and medical, debate because it is perceived as a way to hold down health costs, particularly if a cheap or generic drug can be shown to be more or less equal to a pricier one. Money for a comparative effectiveness institute was even included in the 2009 federal stimulus bill. It is not surprising that a large number of doctors and scientists, and many politicians and bureaucrats, have flocked to this approach, since it purports to use gold standard research to find proven, cost-effective treatments. As for the public, well, the idea sounds impossible to argue against, at least until it means that they don't get the medication they want.

Advocacy of comparative effectiveness research is often fueled by the same beliefs that drive complaints about the proliferation of "me-too" drugs, but it runs aground on the same realities: even drugs that have comparable effects in studies often don't work the same way or in the same patients. Part of the problem with comparative effectiveness research is the failure of such analyses to look at how individuals respond differently to different or even the same treatment. Many of these trials use carefully selected homogenous populations that are not representative of the people who actually have the given condition. Scientists running a trial want to have the best chance to see a real divergence between treatments, so they choose participants who do not have other differences that would complicate the picture. Thus, randomized controlled trials have inclusion criteria that select out "a trial population that often differs from the target population in demographics, clinical status, and underlying risk for both benefits and harms."[47]

Even in studies that include a wider range of patients, most fail to dissect the data to look for subgroups of people who may react differently to the treatment, whether in terms of harm or benefit. One survey of clinical trials used in comparative effectiveness research found that "benefit or harm of most treatments in clinical trials can be misleading and fail to reveal the potentially complex mixture of substantial benefits for some, little benefit for many, and harm for a few."[48] Comparative effectiveness studies also may use outcomes or markers that have little to do with actual practice or the concerns of the patients themselves. Finally, not all scientific questions lend themselves to the randomized controlled trials prevalent in comparative effectiveness research. Given the limitation of comparative effectiveness studies, it is unwise to institutionalize them as a regulatory tool for governments and insurance companies.

The outcome in the idealized populations used in such studies is then generalized to society at large. Yet those to whom a drug or intervention will be prescribed are highly heterogeneous, including people of different ages, genders, and ethnicities. Real patients also frequently have other conditions that impact the advisability and efficacy of a given treatment. The challenges of translating from trial population to real population is a problem common to many studies, not just those done for the purpose of comparative effectiveness research, and that's where the real-world experience of physicians comes into play. As doctors use drugs, they learn more about how nonideal patients respond to those drugs and how differences among patients predict variations in efficacy and safety.

But comparative effectiveness research and its advocates aren't very interested in on-the-ground physician expertise. Many of its proponents believe that the study results, in their objectivity and rationality, are the truth, untainted by individual views or experiences. This raises the potential to create "one size fits all" medication that not only does not take into account individual variation but also imposes a solution that actually suits few. Comparative effectiveness used in this manner becomes a straightjacket for physicians, handing down dictums on "good" and "bad" drugs and "right" and "wrong" answers to clinical problems. The patients a doctor will see in practice represent the wide range of variation and complexity that is excluded from medical studies but ubiquitous in the real world. To apply evidence blindly, giving them all the same drug, at the same dose, is to break the fundamental dictum to do no harm.

The shading of comparative effectiveness into cost effectiveness is a worrisome trend, and payers are already talking about using the results of comparative effectiveness studies to decide what they will cover and how much they will pay. Government and insurance companies, after all, have an incentive to find that older and/or cheaper treatments are just as efficacious as newer, pricier ones. We already have a case study of the dangers of rigid government decisions on comparative effectiveness and the dangers of integrating it with questions of cost: Britain's aforementioned NICE, which regularly rejects drugs that extend lives or improve their quality because they are deemed not to be cost-effective.

Patients in the United Kingdom do not have to wonder how much their lives are worth to the people who make these decisions. They know the answer: £30,000 (around $50,000) per quality adjusted life year. No more. Among the drugs rejected or restricted by NICE are four drugs for kidney cancer, Sutent, Nexavar, Torisel, and Avastin; several drugs for rheumatoid arthritis; Aricept for Alzheimer's; and Lucentis for macular degeneration. Such decisions have left many patients without effective treatments and, predictably, have provoked public outrage and, in some cases, reversals of the decision. Yet many proponents of comparative effectiveness believe that the United States needs an American version of NICE, and they argue in blogs and editorials, on forums and television shows, that cost-effectiveness is the cure to all those pernicious expensive pills that Americans are so devoted to popping and would be better off without.

The problems with comparative effectiveness research do not mean that we should abandon the objective of giving patients the best treatments, based on the best science. There is another way to achieve the valuable goals behind comparative effectiveness research. We can provide better, and potentially cheaper, health care by using new medical technologies in the fields of genetics and biometrics to produce individualized, personalized medicine that makes sure that each patient receives the most appropriate and most efficacious treatment.

BESPOKE MEDICINE

At the same time that tabloid medicine threatens both individual and public health by scaring people away from important and beneficial treatments and undermining trust in doctors and scientists, we are also making unparalleled progress in creating customized, targeted therapies for some of the most difficult diseases and most pressing medical problems. The new paradigm of personalized medicine is emerging in health care as advances in genomics, proteomics (the study of proteins), and other areas are driving the creation of highly targeted tests and therapies tailored to the specific characteristics of subpopulations and individual patients. At its core are the four rights: right treatment, right patient, right time, and right dose.

Personalized medicine draws on information from a range of sources, including individual genetic variation, differences in molecular-level and cellular-level disease processes, health states, behavioral and environmental determinants, and personal patient response to interventions, to tailor care strategies and treatments to the needs of individuals. These tools also facilitate the discovery and validation of health care products and interventions. Many build on advances in the understanding and use of genetic markers that can catch conditions earlier, help doctors determine if a patient will benefit from a given drug, and even fix genetic defects that create devastating diseases.

Advances in genetics are revealing the nature of patient subgroups at an increasing rate, and thus the extent to which genetic variation plays a role in patient responses to treatments and predispositions to side effects. For many medications, from cancer treatments to blood thinners, patients can be given a genetic test that will tell their doctor whether they should take a certain drug. These tests can now frequently tell us whether a medication will work for a given patient and can reveal susceptibility to complications. For patients who are more likely to experience adverse events, doctors can either chose another drug or put into place additional monitoring.

The movement toward personalized medicine has perhaps gone farthest for the diagnosis and treatment of cancer. Researchers have discovered that cancer is far from one disease and that even within each type of cancer, there are differences that determine whether a given treatment will work and what the most effective medical approach is. Many breakthrough cancer drugs can now target certain variants of cancer and be prescribed only to patients who are identified through the use of tests as likely to respond to them. Genetic tests can even in some cases indicate how much of the drug should be used.

One example is Herceptin, a targeted medication for human epithelial growth factor receptor-2 (HER2) positive breast cancer, a kind of cancer that makes up around 20 to 30 percent of breast cancer cases.[49] After a 2005 study found the drug halved the frequency with which this type of cancer returned after treatment, the prestigious *New England Journal of Medicine* said the trial "suggests a dramatic and perhaps permanent perturbation of the natural history of the disease, maybe even a cure." Later research proved the drug yet more efficacious than previously thought, showing reductions in deaths a mere two years into the trial.[50]

Another example is colorectal cancer. According to a 2009 study, the leading drugs for the condition, Erbitux and Vectibix, are not effective in people with a particular mutation. But there is a test for the genetic marker, and since a course of Erbitux costs $61,000 and the mutation is present in 35 to 46 percent of cases, the $452 test pays for itself many times over by saving insurance companies and government programs from spending money on a drug that will not work. The total savings could be $604 million annually. Meanwhile, patients can live longer, higher-quality lives by immediately getting the drug or other treatment most likely to work for them.[51]

These are just two examples. In the last decade, we have seen an explosion of innovative cancer drugs that use genetics to provide unparalleled results when the right regimen is matched with the right patient. New mutations linked to different cancers are being discovered every day, underlining both the need and the potential for carefully tailored treatment of each patient based on his or her individual genetic makeup.

But personalized medicine based on new discoveries in genetics isn't confined to cancer treatments. One of the poster children for personalized medicine, for both supporters and opponents, is the blood-thinning drug warfarin. Individual response to warfarin is unpredictable and idiosyncratic, and for decades, determining how much of the drug to prescribe to a given patient has been a matter of trial and error. It can require months of testing and monitoring to find the optimal dose. This may soon change. Recent research has shown that there are two genetic variants that impact how the body deals with warfarin, CYP2C9 and VKORC1, both of which increase the action of the drug and reduce the dose needed to be effective. Reportedly, these genetic differences are together responsible for 30 percent of patient response to the drug versus 15 to 20 percent for other factors such as age and weight.[52] Other research has put it as high as 60 percent for these two genes and 30 percent for other clinical considerations.[53]

About two million Americans take warfarin annually, yet it is estimated that twice as many could be helped by the drug. But dangerous side effects from improper doses of the drug lead to approximately forty-three thousand emergency hospital stays each year, the second most of any medication.[54] Researchers believe that about 10 to 20 percent of the white and African American populations have the variant CYP2C9, and 14 to 37 percent have the variant VKORC1. In the Asian American population, however, up to 89 percent have the variant of VKORC1 that affects warfarin dosing.[55] In 2007, the FDA approved a test for these genes and changed the drug's label to advise that "lower initiation doses should be considered for patients with certain genetic variations in CYP2C9 and VKORC1."[56]

Still, the use of the genetic test isn't yet widespread because some, including Medicare, claim it's too expensive, even though more accurate dosing could prevent costly complications, and the price of the test will go down as the genetic technology is refined and developed.[57] Indeed, Medicare's announcement that it would not pay for the test for all but a few patients has proved a serious challenge to the hopes of supporters of personalized medicine that incorporating genetic considerations could change the way warfarin is prescribed and dosed. A clinical trial using genetics is under way and may eventually change the government's mind.

Genetic discoveries are also helping us to understand who develops various diseases, making possible preventive measures to stop or slow the diseases' development, catch the symptoms early, and mitigate a condition when it appears. From the BRCA1 and BRCA2 genes tied to breast cancer and ovarian cancer to genes predisposing people to colon cancer, Alzheimer's disease, prostate cancer, and many more, we are identifying new markers all the time. For example, a recently discovered gene, STK39, raises carriers' risk of high blood pressure and attendant complications such as heart problems, stroke, and kidney disease, and it may be present in around 20 percent of the population. The head of the study, Yen-Pei Christy Chang, has explained, "What we hope is that by understanding STK39 we can use that information for personalized medicine, so we can actually predict which hypertensive patients should be on what class of medication and know that they will respond well and have minimal risk for side effects."[58]

Indeed, some one thousand genetic tests already exist, and while neither these tools nor our knowledge of the genetic components of disease are perfect, that doesn't negate how far we've come or that the foundation has been laid for future advances.[59] Thanks to genetics research, the United States now tests babies at birth for twenty-nine rare but very serious genetic diseases. Some of these diseases can be essentially stopped with special diets or lifestyle changes; others have treatments but not yet cures. But many can be fatal or cause severe permanent damage if they are not caught early. Thanks to the genetic tests, doctors now identify and treat these diseases quickly, and a number of states are adding testing for even more conditions.[60] As sequencing whole genomes becomes easier and cheaper, and as scientists continue to link genes to diseases, the number of genetic tests (and their availability) is likely to expand exponentially.

Genetics may be one of the biggest and most exciting mechanisms for customizing treatments, but it isn't the only one. Simply by studying subgroups in clinical trials, and by making trial populations more representative of society at large, we can gain valuable data about how both results and adverse events differ by gender, ethnicity, age, and other factors. And with this knowledge, better, more targeted decisions can be made both in future research and everyday prescribing. Bruce Chabner, the former director of the National Cancer Institute's Drug Development Program, argued:

> The characterization of subgroups of patients who are likely to have responses would reduce the needless cost of ineffective therapy and size of clinical trials, and it might even broaden the range of indications to include diseases with common molecular features but with dissimilar pathologic manifestations. Many specialties in medicine have become too accustomed to low response rates and have emphasized the search for new drugs without making a sufficient effort to define the markers of response.[61]

Furthermore, personalized medicine may have a salutary effect on costs, preventing expensive trial and error, reducing wasted time and money on ineffective therapies, and mitigating complications that are pricey to deal with and may require a hospital stay.

Finally, personalized medicine is allowing us to create advanced biologic drugs capable of prolonging or saving the lives of people afflicted with the rarest, often genetic, diseases, patients who even ten years ago had no hope and no treatments. Because they affect so few people, these ailments can be difficult to diagnose and are little known even among doctors. Novel treatments are being found and developed for a wide range of rare conditions, ranging from phenylke-tonuria, or PKU, in which patients lack an enzyme to process protein and which causes brain damage if not caught early; to molybdenum cofactor deficiency, a disease that typically kills babies born with it within a few months; to Batten's disease, a degenerative condition that destroys vision, motor skills, and cognitive abilities.[62]

Another example is Fabry disease, a rare genetic condition that inhibits the body's ability to produce a certain enzyme and can leave sufferers with a wide variety of serious complications, including kidney failure. But thanks to advanced scientific techniques and committed researchers, there is now a highly effective drug to replace the enzyme. As Fabry patient Jenny Dickinson said, "The treatment has given me back my normal life."[63] Similar is Pompe disease, a genetic enzyme disease like Fabry that atrophies muscles and often keeps patients in a wheelchair and on a respirator. Thanks to the extraordinary effort of one father, there is now a drug to treat the disease, Genzyme's Monozyme. New research has also revealed that Rituxan, a drug used to treat non-Hodgkin's lymphoma and rheumatoid arthritis, can help patients with a particular form of Pompe, who have limited response to the enzyme-replacement drug.[64]

These treatments are often made possible by the Orphan Drug Act, along with similar legislation in other countries. Drug development doesn't get any less expensive because the disease is rare, and finding treatments for these genetic conditions can take many years of single-minded work and many setbacks. But since the patient population is so small, recouping the costs by selling the final drug, if one ever makes it to market, is impossible. So the Orphan Drug Act gives companies creating drugs for rare diseases special tax incentives and seven years of exclusivity. Even then, the medications have to be extremely expensive, often hundreds of thousands of dollars a year, for the companies even to begin to cover the money spent on developing them.

The NIH's Office of Rare Diseases has also stepped up to try to find the causes of—and even put names to—ultra-rare and unknown diseases. Up to one hundred "undiagnosable" patients each year will get free medical treatment, accommodation, and transport to the agency headquarters. Not only may patients who have fruitlessly gone from doctor to doctor finally have answers, but the information and data gained by studying them will advance knowledge, help patients not just with these super rare ailments but with more common ones as well, and open the way to eventual treatments and cures.

The NIH also runs some fifteen hundred studies, with ten thousand patients, every year, many of them focused on rare diseases, and in 2009 it launched the Therapeutics for Rare and Neglected Diseases Program to help fund the development of potential treatments for rare diseases. This will help successful treatments make it to approval and availability and also keep track of ones that don't work to add to scientific knowledge. Already genetic research has helped offer a diagnosis, if not yet a treatment, to patients like Amanda Conyers, who has an extremely uncommon condition called IRAK4 deficiency. The disease affects her immune system, giving her a childhood history of life-threatening infections, including one that led to the amputation of her leg at age eight.[65]

Although rare diseases may individually have few sufferers, their collective impact is big: around twenty-five to thirty million Americans have one.[66] The science of rare illnesses is truly personalized medicine, drawn from these small groups of patients, designed to pinpoint the causes and mechanisms that create the diseases and their symptoms, and aimed at finding ways to improve and extend lives and, eventually, to prevent future patients from suffering from these illnesses. This research has already had some startling successes, despite the many and devastating failures that are unfortunately an integral part of expanding medical knowledge and developing new treatments. There are even signs that gene therapy capable of replacing the faulty genes may finally be becoming a reality after many years of setbacks.[67]

Americans overwhelmingly support the objectives of personalized medicine, but they don't hear very much about it from the media, at least compared to the coverage of medical risks. While the discovery of new genetic markers and the creation of novel tests may draw enough notice to receive a television news story or a blog entry, the scientific details are too esoteric and too dull to hold the attention of most Americans. With a few exceptions, such as BRCA1 and BRCA2, the odd names of the genes involved don't stick in many people's minds.

Meanwhile, though breakthroughs on rare diseases can produce heartstring-tugging human interest stories, perfect for linking and reproducing online, they tend to focus more on the plight of the patient than on the science, and all too often they give way to commentary on how the drugs cost far too much and drug companies should be ashamed of themselves.

Finally, the success of personalized medicine has produced its own challenges: all too many Americans believe that even the most complex diseases can be cured with some funding and a couple of years of research. To maximize the potential of personalized medicine, we must do a better job of educating Americans about the realities of scientific research and drug development, repurposing money spent on large studies to allay tabloid medicine–generated fears and using it instead to create easy-to-use tools for individualizing care.

LOOKING FORWARD

Tabloid medicine's proponents are aware that personalized medicine holds great promise for a new kind of medical future. That's why they fear it so much and oppose it so vehemently. At the core of the Precautionary Principle is an opposition to change, indeed a terror of new developments, in whatever form and for whatever purpose. They say they are fighting against not innovation, not progress, but risk. Yet the future will always come with risk, whether it is moving forward or trying to stand still. To pretend otherwise is to act like a child who believes that he can escape what he does not want to hear simply by holding his hands over his ears.

Medicine has plenty of problems and plenty of dangers, but it has allowed us lives of unparallel length and has turned diseases that were once death sentences into curable conditions or chronic illnesses. Personalized medicine offers the potential to identify diseases before they hit and to create treatments tailored to each patient and what will work most effectively and safely for his or her specific genetic makeup. Against this, tabloid medicine offers only one-size-fits-all solutions that actually fit almost no one. It also threatens to destroy an environment that has made possible immense progress in developing new drugs and tests and uncovering the mechanisms of disease. It will take all of us, scientists, doctors, universities, companies, government agencies, and regular Americans, to ensure that tabloid medicine does not triumph and that personalized medicine will be allowed to grow and flourish.

CHAPTER 9

Battling Tabloid Medicine: The Personalized Medicine Revolution

THE ROLE OF TABLOID medicine in shaping medical and public health decisions is growing and will continue to do so if left unchecked. The objective of this book has been to explain how the Web has not only made possible this expansion but also changed the way Americans gather and use medical information. I have argued that tabloid medicine seeks to promote fear about the risks of drugs and technologies because it believes that the commercialization of science is inherently immoral. To advance this goal, it helps to promote a culture of distrust about important medical innovations and a definition of risk shaped not by science but by moral and political choices. And I have described the defects of this movement and the largely hidden dangers of tabloid medicine.

If we are not careful, the progress biomedical researchers are making in understanding the mechanisms of disease and in discovering how to treat and prevent conditions such as heart disease and cancer will remain just information. Tabloid medicine is already using the Precautionary Principle to erect barriers and regulations in academia, government agencies, and journals and to convince the public that scientists and physicians are not to be trusted. This is also a way of silencing or stifling a more optimistic view of commercialization and increasing the influence of a more negative one.

Years ago, Nobel laureate Joshua Lederberg warned that if our political, legal, and scientific institutions were not reshaped to respond to the new science of genomics, then future medical progress would be made more difficult. He argued that if decisions about what is safe and effective are not guided by scientists and doctors but by politicians, lawyers, and "safety" groups, then nothing will ever be safe enough. It would seem that Lederberg was right to worry. Tabloid medicine has become a means to spread scare stories across the United States and around the world and to advance the interests and ideologies of instant experts.

Yet the influence of tabloid medicine can be minimized in many ways. Its apocalyptic claims depend upon individuals reacting to a new potential danger instead of thinking it through. The most effective way to neutralize the impact of tabloid medicine is, as Dr. Lederberg suggested, to introduce ways to individualize and predict the benefits and risks of medical technology. What is broadly called personalized medicine consists of using diagnostic tests, targeted therapies, and information sharing among patients to give us the ability to know in advance what treatments are most likely to help each of us as individuals.

Genetic differences among patients not only help determine who will develop a disease but also affect the activity of drugs in the body, impacting whether the medication works and the likelihood of adverse events. Establishing a strong association between these changes at a genetic level and improvement in other measures of health is making medicine more predictive. At the same time, online communities offer a wealth of data on real-world use of medications that will help us to understand who benefits, who doesn't, and why. Research into personalized medicine will let us answer questions of risk and benefit in advance and reduce uncertainty. And as we have seen, uncertainty is the mother of fear.

Personalized medicine will put tabloid medicine—those who profit from it—out of business. If we and our doctors can make decisions based on targeted, individualized information, then tabloid medicine's narrative of a corrupted conspiracy doing harm to the public health will fade away. That's why those who promote tabloid medicine are on a campaign to slow down the move toward personalized medicine by claiming it is simply a way to water down product approval standards on behalf of industry.

To prevent them from succeeding, the medical community, from drug companies, to government agencies, to practicing physicians, must take back and use the Web. The same qualities that make it the strongest weapon of tabloid medicine can also be wielded by doctors and scientists. Companies must stop avoiding the Internet because they fear running afoul of regulators. Science bloggers must continue to fight back against the spread of misinformation and untruth. And Americans must become more critical of the information they find online—and of those who dispense it.

THE MEDICINE OF THE FUTURE

The key to reducing concerns about the danger of drugs is to provide doctors and patients with better information about their relative risks and benefits. To this end, the FDA has pledged to support the development and advancement of personalized medicine designed to match patients with the right treatment in order to minimize risks and maximize efficacy. By tailoring treatments to individual patients, we can mitigate many of the safety concerns that currently plague drugs and improve our ability to heal. In an editorial, FDA commissioner Margaret Hamburg and principal deputy commissioner Joshua Sharfstein called personalized medicine an "emerging opportunity" and argued that "the agency should work with scientific leaders on novel approaches to treating illness."[1]

This view has already been reflected in the vision of the Critical Path Initiative, set up by the FDA in 2004. Its objective is to bring together the agency with researchers from both academia and industry to apply the same twenty-first-century scientific tools being used to discover new treatments to the process of product development. These include genetic tests and validated biomarkers—molecules that are proxies for how a disease is progressing or for response to a treatment—both of which can help determine earlier than ever before whether a drug or device will have serious side effects and which patients will be vulnerable to them. These tests can be used in combination with other measures of medical benefit to allow studies to target those who are most likely to benefit and to let companies and the FDA use clinical trial designs and statistical methods that zero in on the information we really need to improve health.

The FDA set up the Critical Path program because it realized that "without such tools there would be a continuing inability to achieve the benefits of molecular medicine and further delay in the personalized, predictive, and preemptive health care outcomes such medicine could bring."[2] Most importantly, it was developed to encourage and ultimately require companies to develop and market medicines based on information about how individuals process and respond to various treatments.

Janet Woodcock, MD, the director of the FDA's Center for Drug Evaluation and Research and the godmother of Critical Path, has noted:

> One size does not fit all when it comes to drugs. This means that people who don't benefit from therapy get harmed and then think that therapy should be taken off the market. And then people who needed that therapy but have no way to get it become very resentful. My theory for a number of years has been that we

have to use science to get out of this box. No drug is all bad or all good—it's about who's going to have a positive response to a drug and who will have a suboptimal response. Personalized medicine, in my view, is the key. But we need to find better predictive safety biomarkers and other ways of predicting adverse events. Also, and equally important, we need to have markers of positive response.[3]

So far the emergence of targeted treatments for cancer represent the first fruits of this new investment in personalized medicine. The now-classic example is the identification of a variation in a gene called HER2, which causes breast cancer. A drug was then developed to switch off the part of the gene influenced by the mutation and responsible for causing tumor development. Last, a test to see if patients carried the mutation was created to pinpoint good candidates for the medication. Richard Schilsky, president of the American Society of Clinical Oncology, believes that at the current pace of progress, personalized medicine will be standard in ten years.[4]

Increasingly, researchers have also identified genes that contribute to the sort of adverse drug events that fuel tabloid medicine. This has been a focus of the nonprofit Critical Path Institute, which brings together companies and researchers from the FDA and its European counterpart, the EMEA, to work on projects that involve linking genetic factors with drug response. Already one of these collaborations has resulted in the development of a test to screen for genes that cause medicines to have toxic side effects that lead to kidney damage and liver failure. Other tests to identify patients at increased risk of heart failure or arrhythmia are being developed.[5] The institute's founder and president, Dr. Raymond Woosley, has explained, "C-Path is neutral because it is not vested in the development of any medical products, so we will act as catalyst for bringing resources together to break new ground in science and then share it broadly to be used by different entities in product development."[6]

Companies are also independently testing existing drugs for differences in individual response and side effects, and there are currently two hundred such clinical trials looking for strong genetic links to outcomes or adverse drug events. One such study is seeking to "identify variations in differentially expressed genes that may be involved in the development of suicidal events and certain behaviors in youth exposed to antidepressant medications," and there is already evidence that mutations in genes regulating drug metabolism contribute to these differences.[7] Hopefully, such research will make dangerous controversies like the one over pediatric antidepressant use a thing of the past.

But the development of genetic tests to predict response and improve safety has been attacked by the advocates of tabloid medicine, who see them as a shortcut for industry to produce drugs that don't have any benefit. Century Foundation health care fellow Maggie Mahar, who has maintained that there are too many cancer drugs, asks, "How much faith should we be putting in biomarkers, i.e., genes, biochemical molecules that indicate the presence of a disease, but aren't the disease itself?" She then answers the question with reference not to scientific data or medical discoveries but to the amount of money that has been invested in developing such tools, implying that this invalidates their benefit.[8] Similarly, persistent industry opponent Merrill Goozner asserts that much biomarker research is just a way to avoid finding out that new drugs aren't that much better than old ones.

But for instant experts, the last straw was the creation of the Reagan-Udall Foundation, which was set up in 2007 to "identify unmet scientific needs in the development, manufacture, and evaluation of the safety and effectiveness of FDA-regulated products, including post-market evaluation, and establish scientific projects and programs to address those needs." The foundation is private, independent, and nonprofit, headed by a board made up of members from industry, academia, patient and consumer advocacy groups, and health care professionals, and four representatives at large with relevant expertise or experience.

Dr. Mark McClellan, the chairman of the Reagan-Udall Foundation and the head of the Engelberg Center for Health Care Reform at the Brooking Institution, has explained that these goals are so important because the "FDA today still has to rely on methods for demonstrating safety effectiveness, reliable manufacturing and effective use that are based on technologies from the 1970s that don't reflect new techniques, like genomics or predictive testing, or new statistical methods and the like."

The agency, along with other stakeholders, has made a list of Critical Path opportunities that includes seventy-six concrete examples of how new scientific discoveries in fields such as genomics and proteomics, imaging, and bioinformatics could be applied during medical product development to improve the accuracy of the tests used to predict the safety and efficacy of investigational medical products. There has, however, been insufficient investment in translating these ideas into treatments for patients. That's where the Reagan-Udall Foundation comes in; it links scientists from both the private and public spheres to make these opportunities realities.[9]

Yet the tabloid medicine crowd quickly jumped into action at the news of Reagan-Udall's creation. The Foundation for Integrity and Responsibility, the Union of Concerned Scientists, and the Center for Science in the Public Interest all immediately criticized what they claimed was "the potential for influence of industry over the direction of the Reagan-Udall Foundation."[10] Representative Rosa DeLauro from Connecticut, who chairs the House Appropriations Subcommittee that controls the FDA budget, enthusiastically took up these attacks and sent a letter to then–FDA commissioner Andrew von Eschenbach that reads as if it were taken straight from tabloid medicines talking points.

In addition to deliberately misstating the role of biomarkers and claiming that they are less accurate than traditional clinical trials in predicting safety problems and measuring efficacy, the letter all but accused the FDA of creating the Reagan-Udall Foundation to aid industry efforts to weaken regulation. DeLauro told von Eschenbach, "Although the mission of the foundation is intended to support research that encourages an expedited FDA approval process, I believe the Reagan-Udall Foundation has the potential of endorsing the approval of drugs and devices based on lower standards of safety and efficacy, and without appropriately designed clinical trials."[11]

The irony is that one of the cosponsors of the legislation that set up the Reagan-Udall Foundation was Senator Edward Kennedy, not most people's idea of someone who was too cozy with the drug industry. He said that the foundation "will make new research tools and techniques available to the entire research community, shortening the time it takes to develop new drugs and reducing costs for patients."[12] DeLauro has also been a strong critic of the Critical Path Initiative in general and has repeatedly impeded its work by slashing its budget.

The Critical Path is a crucial driver of personalized medicine that deserves to be protected and fostered rather than slandered. Without it, we risk foregoing the fruits of current research into the molecular and genetic factors that determine whether we will get sick, what medicines will work on us, and if we are in danger of having an adverse event while taking them. The FDA already has much more on its plate than its funding and staff can support, especially as its scope widens and its role in advancing the future of medicine becomes larger. Politicians should provide the agency with the money it needs to carry out the myriad responsibilities assigned to it and stop attacking the agency to score political points and up their bona fides on "safety." They should support the Critical Path Institute and the Reagan-Udall Foundation instead of decrying the fact that some of their members have ties to industry.

However, the FDA and supporters of the Critical Path can also do more to reach out to the public, which knows very little about the initiative but widely supports its purpose and objectives. Ask most Americans what the Critical Path is or to innumerate its goals and few could answer you. But explain to the public what it does to reduce uncertainty and risk at the individual level and almost all of them would resoundingly endorse the program. In 2008, the Center for Medicine in the Public Interest conducted a survey of 1,049 adults across the continental United States and found that 9 in 10 of them supported Critical Path.

Further, 78 percent said they were in favor of expanded use of biomarkers to match patients with the best drug, and 77 percent backed bringing together the FDA, industry, and academia to improve drug development and approval. When asked whether they would be in favor of a voluntary, confidential Web portal that allowed patients to share their experiences taking various medications, half the respondents said they would use the site and 87 percent said that it would boost their confidence in the safety of medications on the market.[13]

The unscientific attack on the use and development of genomics and biomarkers flows from the political and cultural beliefs of tabloid medicine's adherents and beneficiaries. The Critical Path reduces uncertainty by giving individual patients and their doctors the ability and the power to make accurate and personalized decisions about drugs, devices, and other treatments, but in so doing, it will weaken the ability of tabloid medicine elites to impose their views on society. It's no surprise, then, that they are fighting this future with everything they have.

TAPPING THE POTENTIAL OF THE INTERNET

Ensuring that personalized medicine thrives and is able to increase the freedom of doctors and patients to make individualized treatment decisions will require both recognizing and channeling the power of the Internet and other digital technologies. Medical scientists and pharmaceutical firms should use the Web to track the risks and benefits of products throughout the time a drug or device is on the market and must also realize the potential of these tools to address new risks and benefits with transparency and speed.

The pharmaceutical industry could learn something from Apple; companies and researchers should actively involve patients in the design or beta-testing of clinical trials and studies, keeping participants up-to-date with the status of research. And once products are approved, companies and the FDA should provide consumers with regularly updated information that can be used to improve the selection and use of medicines. Every drug ad has the same disclaimer: our drug is not for everybody. So why not find out who *will* benefit from it and help others find something else?

Too often the medical community reacts to the Web rather than using it. Yet digital technologies allow the creation of complex networks that make possible rapid adaptation to new information and lets challenges be shared, discussed, and addressed quickly. That is what makes it such a strong tool for advancing tabloid medicine and the Precautionary Principle. Now it is time for researchers and physicians to make use of this power and fight back against tabloid medicine, turning the weapons wielded against science and medicine back on the charlatans and ideologues. Ignorance is the midwife of fear and dependence, and the influence of those who back tabloid medicine relies on keeping people in the dark. It thrives only when scientists and innovators fail to act toward the public in ways that respect the wisdom and freedom of the people they ultimately serve.

If companies, doctors, and credible scientists do not use the Internet and other technologies to engage the public, preempt the purveyors of tabloid medicine, and put more pressure on traditional media outlets to report objectively and carefully about biomedical innovation, the war for trust and for control over what new medical technologies are available will be lost. The key to winning this war is to provide individuals with real-time and individualized information about adverse events. Drug companies and scientists must be proactive and go on the offensive to shape public perceptions before the forces of tabloid medicine can do so.

The pharmaceutical industry has already begun to seek to make use of the Web, setting up sites to provide information on their drugs and the conditions they treat. But the FDA's rules regarding online communication by industry are not always clear, and as technology develops far faster than bureaucracy can, drugmakers must often either forego the use of new communications tools, from blogs to Twitter, or risk ending up on the wrong side of the agency. Yet to do nothing is irresponsible.

As my colleague Peter Pitts, a former associate FDA commissioner, recently observed:

I know of one large pharmaceutical company whose policy is not to monitor social media sites because they don't want to unearth adverse events. Is this responsible? Is it even supportable? If this company received a call from a reporter and was asked if they purposely avoid social media so as not to find adverse experiences would the truth set them free? Legally they may be in compliance, but it wouldn't look good on Page One or sound very good in front of a congressional subcommittee.[14]

Pitts believes that companies cower in fear at their own peril because "[w]ithout the participation of regulated healthcare players, the social media field is left to snake-oil salesmen, Internet drug dealers, unscrupulous trial lawyers and others who operate without almost any constraints whatsoever. Nature abhors a vacuum. It is irresponsible not to correct healthcare information errors. And yet that is precisely the advice being regularly given by regulatory consultants."[15]

THE LIMITS OF TRANSPARENCY

Government agencies such as the FDA must likewise refuse to abandon the Internet to tabloid medicine and must launch and sustain concerted efforts to displace bad information with good. In general, they are already farther along this road than companies; many have already debuted new Internet sites and content targeted at the needs and wants of Googlers, and most are committed to continuing to make their inner workings more understandable to the American population. The FDA in particular has embraced greater openness by implementing several initiatives designed to make the analyses and evaluations of the agency more transparent and has also worked to raise and expand its Web presence.

While the FDA's online efforts have long centered on countering the sale of counterfeit drugs and fraudulent cures on websites and via emails and advertisements, it is now making available a wide range of information on how it operates.[16] The FDA has also become more proactive, no longer waiting for concerns about various treatments to reach a fever pitch but, rather, seeking to address them early and clearly using both on- and offline tools.

However, as the FDA has recently learned, more information for the public means more information for those who attack the agency, and going too far to placate opponents who will never be satisfied can produce dangerous effects. In order to try to quell public concerns quickly, the FDA has initiated the release of a document called an "Early Communication About an Ongoing Safety Review," to provide an interim analysis of data regarding a product's safety. The FDA is careful to note that an early report does not mean a product is unsafe or that doctors should stop prescribing it, but rather, simply that the agency is considering regulatory action. However, the agency is constrained by regulatory rules from saying more than that.

The result is that tabloid medicine adherents use these communications—and the fact that the FDA has yet to make a determination—to spread more fear. For these critics, it does not matter what the agency's eventual verdict is, either way the FDA and the drug company are considered guilty of malfeasance. If the FDA does later issue a warning about the drug, then it is accused of having allowed a dangerous product to remain on the market too long. The benighted medication soon appears on Public Citizen's "Worst Pill" list and starts popping up all over the Internet as disgruntled patients, lawyers, alternative medicine sites, and others jump on the bandwagon. If the agency determines that there is no new indication of danger, then it is accused of caving in to industry and letting a risky drug continue to be prescribed to patients.

Similarly, the FDA now makes reports of side effects from drugs available on its Adverse Event Reporting System. The agency does warn that "there is no certainty that the reported event was actually due to the product. FDA does not require that a causal relationship between a product and event be proven, and reports do not always contain enough detail to properly evaluate an event." But this disclaimer is easily overlooked by those who prefer to ignore it and by searchers angry or fearful because of what they find in the database.[17]

The fact that reports are not verified means that the system can be manipulated by those who erroneously blame the drugs and who deliberately submit claims of adverse events in order to advance the perception that it is unsafe. We have already seen this happen with the similar reporting system for potential vaccine adverse events, which has been repeatedly used by anti-vaccine groups to claim inflated rates of injuries and deaths from immunizations.

Thus, however good the intentions behind them, FDA initiatives designed to reassure scared patients and aggressive "safety" crusaders may actually do the opposite. In general, despite its valiant attempts to allay concerns about transparency and objectivity, the FDA's efforts are likely a losing proposition because critics will not rest until the agency adopts their overstringent standards of safety and all those who work with pharmaceutical companies are replaced with anti-industry activists. According to the canons of tabloid medicine, the

FDA can't be transparent enough. It must adopt the risk perception of the tabloid medicine crowd if it is to be deemed "pure."

It is an important lesson for not just the FDA but for other agencies, companies, and any other organization seeking to combat tabloid medicine. But it is also not an excuse to hold back or to abandon initiatives to use the Internet more effectively. Rather than bend over too far in a vain attempt to please critics, the FDA and the whole scientific and medical community must continually make clear that there is both benefit and potential for harm in every product, and they must oppose the belief that 100 percent safety exists. So long as we cling to the craving for perfect certainty and zero risk, our public debate will be stunted and our ability to innovate restricted.

FDA commissioner Dr. Margaret Hamburg and principal deputy commissioner Dr. Joshua Sharfstein wrote truly and insightfully when they said in their article in the *New England Journal of Medicine*:

> [O]ne of the greatest challenges facing any public health agency is that of risk communication. We all accept small risks in our daily lives, from the risk of falling in the shower and sustaining a head injury to the risk of having a car accident on the way to the grocery store. One reason we are rarely fearful of these risks is our perception that we have control over them. When it comes to food and drugs, even small risks can cause considerable fear and anxiety, especially when they seem to be out of our control. Yet all pharmaceuticals have some potential adverse effects.[18]

CHANGING THE ROLE OF PATIENTS IN RESEARCH

There is a lot more to using the Web than getting ahead of the curve on negative reports about products. We must also change how we make public the information on clinical research conducted both before and after a drug or device is available to patients. In 1998, in a *BMJ* editorial that still feels oddly current, Richard Sykes, chairman of then Glaxo Wellcome, wrote:

> What does it mean to be a modern pharmaceutical company? Rapid changes in society and advances in science and medicine mean that the pharmaceutical industry has several important roles today that would not have been apparent as recently as 10–15 years ago ... It has to harness scientific advances, particularly in genetics and information technology, and work in partnership with researchers, healthcare providers, and governments. One substantial outcome of these partnerships is a better understanding of the need for openness and transparency in clinical trials.[19]

We may still be working on most of Sykes's goals, but when it comes to clinical trials, we've come a long way. Already details on more than 85,000 studies, both government- and industry-sponsored, in 172 countries can be found on *www.clinicaltrials.gov*, a site created by the NIH in association with the FDA and other federal organizations.

Trials can now be searched by location, condition, sponsor, or drug being studied, and the listings include the status of the trial, how to join if it is recruiting, and links to available publications. The site also offers laypersons assistance in understanding clinical trials, including a glossary and an overview of how trials are set up and what participating in one would mean. According to the site, around sixty-five thousand people visit each day, accounting for over fifty million page views in a month.[20]

Many government agencies that fund or monitor clinical trials also have information on their websites for patients considering participating in a trial or Web users interested in what joining a study entails. Furthermore, many pharmaceutical companies have listings of trials on their websites, and the Pharmaceutical Research and

Manufacturers of America has a voluntary study database as well. Indeed, some pharmaceutical companies see being more transparent about the methodologies and results of clinical trials as necessary not only to combat a climate of ever-increasing public distrust of industry and its products but also to protect and expand their business. Access to all the research that has been done also helps scientists and funders avoid duplicating trials, isolate why a certain study produced different results, and identify new areas to explore. Last, bolstering openness on existing trials and their results aids government agencies in showing that nothing is being hidden and, it is hoped, improves public trust.

However, transparency in clinical trial reporting on its own is not enough. Just as they exploit preliminary information from the FDA, instant experts and industry critics spread fear by mining data from these studies and producing reports that claim drugs are dangerous or ineffective and that this information is being hidden. Thus unless companies get and stay in touch with doctors and patients, transparency will be just another tool for generating tabloid medicine. As one expert noted, "Just to say you want data available to hold people accountable and responsible on the surface sounds like a good thing ... But transparency just for the sake of transparency isn't. Just because data are out there, we are not necessarily better informed." The information available in databases and trial websites is not necessarily complete, and it lacks context that allows people to understand what the trial actually found and why the data showed what they did. The listing might also be written in terminology that is difficult for laypeople to understand. Studies can be flawed and a "negative study could be picked up ... and could inappropriately set public opinion that drug X is worthless."[21]

Research is also evolving in ways that require companies to collect information that goes far beyond that available from clinical trials. Getting a better, fuller picture of drugs from discovery to approval to real-world use requires industry to make patients a resource. This has the double benefit of also addressing patients' feeling of being shut out by researchers and pharmaceutical firms, and therefore their distrust of those who create and test drugs. Up to now, companies have done a horrible job of staying in touch with those who use their products—including both patients and their family members—to learn about their experiences with the drug or device and discuss risks and benefits. When firms have reached out, it has been kept quiet or confidential, as if patients' experiences were a trade secret. This approach is a mistake and a missed opportunity. Instead, we should use the Internet and the communities it has forged among patients to further our understanding of and research into diseases.

Particularly for patients with chronic conditions or life-threatening diseases such as cancer, the Web has become an increasingly important way of exchanging knowledge and providing support, and while there are risks to this uninhibited sharing of information, especially when personal experience is overstated or misinterpreted, there is also potential for greater understanding of disease and better treatment. More and more patients and families are using the Web to search not only for more information about medicines or other treatments but also for answers about whether or not those medicines and treatments work. Online patient groups allow individuals to share experiences and give them the ability to combine these stories to produce important data about whether a drug or regimen is making a difference.

Tabloid medicine has long targeted these patients, taking advantage of their influence and avid involvement in analyzing and disseminating information on diseases and treatments. But these patients also represent a vast, hitherto untapped resource for researchers, companies, and organizations committed to a future defined by personalized medicine and increased choice for patients and physicians, goals that are strongly supported by this group of patients. Not only do these sites and groups feature lists of hundreds or thousands of people with every disease imaginable, stretching around the globe, but many of these people are highly involved patients eager to take part in research.

And, increasingly, these patients are no longer content to sit on the sidelines of research but, rather, want to participate in it in new ways that make use of the ability of the Web to connect people all over the world. These online communities are using the Internet not only to bring together patients but also to collect thousands of pieces of data about symptoms, drugs, treatment responses, and more. Although many Americans remain concerned about confiding too much medical information to the Web, patients with chronic and potentially deadly diseases are often an exception, especially if doing so may help lead to cures or better treatments. Furthermore, the anonymity of the Internet allows patients to keep their real identities separate from the information they provide, a concern when it comes to determining whose advice to listen to, but less of a problem for collecting data that will be aggregated and analyzed.

One of the biggest such patient communities is PatientsLikeMe, with more than forty thousand people registered. A pioneer in gathering clinical data online, the site now makes the valuable information provided voluntarily by its members available to companies and organizations involved in health care. Another example is iGuard, a health care service that helps monitor the safety of medications (including prescription drugs, over-the-counter drugs, nutritional supplements, and herbal extracts). Its more than two million members worldwide routinely share their experiences with various regimens, helping researchers to learn how to treat diseases better and minimize medication side effects. In 2009, iGuard members participated in ninety-two clinical research trials studying new medications for multiple sclerosis, epilepsy, diabetes, and others.[22]

iGuard is able to detect potential problems or safety signals for newly marketed medicines months and years before the company can do so through conventional approaches. It is also able to identify potential reasons why certain people are reacting well or poorly to the therapy. This means that if drugmakers allied themselves with a community like iGuard, they could quickly investigate, or even anticipate, the isolated scary stories that tabloid medicine seizes on to spread fear.

Some e-patients are already using the Internet to carry out clinical research, whether or not companies are willing to participate. In 2008, a group of patients with ALS, intrigued by data suggesting that lithium could treat the condition, decided to create a quasi-clinical trial. They obtained and took the drug and discussed their results online.[23] The findings were a disappointment to patients—they refuted an earlier, much smaller study suggesting that lithium could alter the disease's rapid decline—but they also confirmed what many had already begun to suspect, and more importantly, they managed to come to this conclusion eighteen months earlier, and at far less cost, than research into lithium for ALS that used traditional methods.[24]

There are many problems with this approach, and it is not likely for the foreseeable future that Web-based trials will supersede existing methodologies. But this case does demonstrate the huge potential of such research when it comes to showing how medications work in the real world, with real patients. Dr. Mark Roberts of the University of Pittsburgh believes that such studies exemplify that "[t]he beauty of observational trials is that you can see how an intervention works in the real world."[25]

Even for companies and clinical investigators who aren't yet ready to embrace new types of studies, the Web has proved a boon for connecting researchers with patients interested in clinical trials. Indeed, some of the world's best research facilities have teamed up with online patient groups in order to promote and recruit for studies.[26] To exploit this potential, companies such as TrialX and Healogica now offer what amounts to an online matchmaking service. Both use a short list of questions to gather information about patients and then connect them to the studies that are the best fit. TrialX is even now using Twitter to make clinical trial connections. As cofounder Sharib Khan explains, "Patients send a tweet to @trialX, preceded by 'CT' describing the type of clinical trials they are seeking. If you say, 'I am 35 years old, have multiple sclerosis, and live in New York,' we can tweet you back a tiny link that brings you to a list of trials." For patients who want more information or who are seeking out clinical trials but prefer to stay anonymous, companies such as Private Access offer them the ability to share as much data as they want and with whomever they want without revealing their identity.[27]

The question is whether pharmaceutical and biotech companies are willing to integrate these new approaches into research about their products, both pre- and postapproval, especially if it means more patient control. There are important issues industry will have to address, in particular, concerns about privacy and control of the data. But whether or not industry decides to participate, the emergence of online patient communities and e-patients is shifting control of the clinical research process to patients and their needs and accelerating the development and adoption of personalized medicine. Researchers who fail to seize this opportunity not only risk becoming less competitive and innovative but also show themselves to be shortsighted.

USING THE INTERNET AGAINST TABLOID MEDICINE

Companies and government agencies are not the only ones who need to lend their voices to the Internet debate over medicine and health. To counterbalance the claims of tabloid medicine, researchers and physicians must offer online opposition to these spurious and scary claims. In fact, a growing number of doctors and scientists already have blogs and Web pages and have acquired devoted audiences of their own. A thriving science and medicine blogosphere has developed, drawing on researchers and scientists from just about every specialty and area. While some blogs cater to those with scientific or medical training and a deep interest in the topics covered, most are intended for the public, albeit a fairly educated and engaged segment of it.

One center of this trend is ScienceBlogs, an online blog collective whose members are specially invited to participate. Its founders explain on the site that they set up ScienceBlogs in January 2006 because "[s]cience is driving our conversation unlike ever before," and "[a]t a time when public interest in science is high but public understanding of science remains weak, we have set out to create innovative media ventures to improve science literacy and to advance global science culture."[28] The site now has more than eighty bloggers.

Another site, *www.getbetterhealth.com*, was established by Dr. Val Jones to "support and promote healthcare professional bloggers, provide insightful and trustworthy health commentary, and help to inform health policy makers about the provider point of view on healthcare reform, science, research, and care." Dr. Jones notes that all the Better Health bloggers respect scientific integrity in health care and strongly support evidence- and science-based practices. They also seek to provide their audience with evaluations about new technologies in terms of individual risk and benefit and often offer a valuable counterpoint to the "facts" spread far and wide by tabloid medicine—which are actually misunderstandings, urban legends, or outright lies.

Indeed, perhaps the most valuable effect such bloggers have is dismantling the so-called evidence marshaled by charlatans and ideologues. The Internet has made articles in scientific and medical journals far more available to everyone, but most of the public lacks the background and training to truly understand the statistics and analyses involved. So the unscrupulous often cite studies that do not support their contention or that misrepresent what the research found. Science and medical bloggers have proved capable of explaining in terms that even relative laypeople understand what the data actually show and how they are being misused.

As a result, some of the most effective opposition to the manifestations of tabloid medicine, from claims of alternative miracle cures to scaremongering about drugs, has come from scientists and doctors who are fighting to take back Internet territory from charlatans and quacks. This was especially apparent in the conflict over vaccines and autism, where a network of blogs and sites arguing against the connection, many of them created by scientists or doctors, slowly developed to counter the myriad anti-immunization sites that were broadcasting their message across the Web and imperiling vaccination rates.

In addition, scientists and physicians are not the only ones who have built Internet sites and blogs to spread good information and sound science. Medical facilities are embracing the Web, using online resources not only to inform patients but also to help themselves better understand what draws and satisfies patients. Some even offer virtual tours and videos featuring their physicians. In 2009, Dr. Richard Bedlack of Duke University brought together forty other leaders of facilities treating ALS patients to create a Twitter stream "where patients can ask questions about off-label therapies. A team of doctors then investigates each query and posts their medical opinion online."[29] Established health websites are likewise branching out into new, more interactive tools and features to tap into patients' interests and desires and to keep them coming back.

Even Google itself may be changing (again) how people get health information—this time for the better. Two-thirds of people begin looking for answers to medical questions on a search engine, one of the few numbers in the Pew Research Center Internet surveys that has moved little since the surveys started a decade ago.[30] What's more, multiple analyses have found that Google accounts for nearly three-quarters of searches.[31] That means that changing Google and its fellows might do more to improve the information Americans find online than even altering Internet users' behavior.

In August 2009, to not very much notice, Google Health added a search feature that picks Web pages not by how popular they are—the traditional method for search engines and a serious pitfall when it comes to finding accurate information—but by taking into account the reliability of the source. Now, theoretically at least, WebMD will score higher than sites belonging to safety groups or the blogs of ordinary citizens.

Roni Zeiger of Google Health told Pew's Susannah Fox, "For this health search feature we decided to offer users one source each from a governmental health agency, a medical institution, and a commercial site. We'll study how users like these choices and continue to iterate. None of these sites is paying any money to Google to be included in the feature."[32]

And finally, thanks to the increasing mobility of Internet access, the Web itself is evolving in ways that have enormous meaning for everyone involved in health care, from industry to government, from instant experts to researchers to physicians. One of the top observers of these trends is Jay Bryne, CEO of v-Fluence, a company that works with industry, patient groups, and regulators to manage and monitor online medical information. The company is at the forefront of efforts to evaluate the potential impact of technologies such as the iPhone and the Web apps that are now available for multiple devices. V-Fluence has discovered that the percentage of the public who turn to mobile devices to find medical information has expanded enormously in a very short time. Indeed, iTunes reports their health and fitness and medical apps have been downloaded by more than one million users.

Byrne has also found that 80 percent of physicians rely more on searches conducted using a Smartphone than on journal articles when making a diagnosis or deciding what medicine to prescribe.[33] Meanwhile, 37 percent of all Americans now access the Internet through mobile devices, and 25 percent get their news information this way. All told, more than ten million Americans have searched for answers on health or medical questions using such devices.[34]

These developments offer both the potential for tabloid medicine to expand far beyond its current bounds and a strong promise for advancing personalized medicine. Over the years to come, more and more information will be collected, captured, and exchanged through Twitter and Facebook, Smartphones, PDAs, and iPads. On one hand, this could strengthen the power of patient communities and pro-science blogs and expand the ability of companies, government agencies, and physicians to reach patients. Unfortunately, on the other hand, all of the current tactics of tabloid medicine could also be enhanced and improved by these technologies. If we allow it, the reach of its misinformation will soon expand farther and faster. That's why it is so critical that science and medicine fight back on all the fronts where pseudoscience and ideology have advanced so far.

The ultimate lesson is that patients will continue using the Internet as their go-to source for health information and medical answers, and if the scientific and medical community shuns the Web, it will only get worse. Rather, doctors, researchers, scientists, government officials, and, yes, patients can push back by getting involved in disseminating the correct information, disputing the half truths and untruths, and understanding and engaging what the public is finding online. Physicians and scientists should continue to become involved members of the online debate, lending their knowledge and expertise to helping Web users understand what information to trust and what to avoid, what is true and what is not, what is overhyped and what risks are going unstated. To this end, you are welcome to submit your own examples of tabloid medicine to this book's website, *www. tabloidmedicine.com*.

SKEPTICAL SEARCHERS

Ultimately, the battle against tabloid medicine can never be won unless Americans become less trusting about the information they find online. The great British mathematician and philosopher Alfred North Whitehead once observed, "The aim of science is to seek the simplest explanation of complex facts ... Seek simplicity and distrust it." This advice should guide our searches for medical information on the Web. Tabloid medicine is all about simplicity, the vivid image or example of danger repeated and widely distributed for immediate and easy consumption. At the same time, then, our search should be shaped by three important questions when we are faced with sensational findings or claims: Do I know this information is accurate? Where did it come from? And, finally, how does it fit in with other the research on the subject? In fact, if there is only one rule of thumb to follow, it would be the one provided by the blog Respectful Insolence: "*Of course* first attempts to answer a clinical question often produce incorrect or exaggerated results! It is the totality of evidence that has to be examined, and until it is, new findings should be treated with care and skepticism."[35]

Care and skepticism can be found in some Web sources and not others. As we discussed in chapter 3, websites offering medical information can be grouped into seven basic types: (1) official government or pharmaceutical websites, (2) reputable medical and professional organizations, (3) impartial news/database sites, (4) forums or blogs, (5) anti-pharmaceutical activist sites, (6) alternative treatment sites, and (7) class action/litigation sites.

Many organizations and government agencies are now beginning to get involved in sorting out the sites that make unreliable claims from those that don't. The World Health Organization, the FDA, and the CDC are now beginning to address the fact that, while they have jurisdiction over claims by regulated industries, tabloid medicine is beyond their control and asserts that certain treatments are unsafe and deadly without having to validate such statements with good science. Therefore, they are starting to step up to arm consumers of health information, both online and from other sources, with the tools they need to judge and use what they find safely and responsibly.

One of the earliest and most widely agreed upon standards for a good health or medical website comes from the Health on the Net Foundation, an international NGO based in Switzerland that, since 1995, has made its mission to fight online misinformation related to human health. Its goal "is to guide the growing community of health care consumers and providers on the World Wide Web to sound, reliable medical information and expertise."[36] They also created the HONcode to designate trustworthy websites, and thousands of sites bear its symbol. In order to meet the code, websites must conform to eight principles:

1. Authoritative: Indicate the qualifications of the authors ...

2. Complementarity: Information should support, not replace, the doctor-patient relationship ...

3. Privacy: Respect the privacy and confidentiality of personal data submitted to the site by the visitor ...

4. Attribution: Cite the source(s) of published information ...

5. Justifiability: Site must back up claims relating to benefits and performance ...

6. Transparency: Accessible presentation, accurate email contact ...

7. Financial disclosure: Identify funding sources ...

8. Advertising policy: Clearly distinguish advertising from editorial content.[37]

These are excellent guidelines for anyone evaluating Internet information on not just health or medicine but on any topic, and users should keep them in mind when reading content on websites. At the very least, everyone searching online for medical information should take a few moments to look for indications of who created the content, when it was updated, who else the site might be affiliated with, and where the money to run the page comes from. This often isn't easy; many websites do not display all or even any of this information. But there are usually clues. If there is an "About Us" section, this is a prime place to check for indications of the site's agenda and affiliations.

If a site has links to other sites offering products or advertisements that provide a "natural" alternative to the treatment or a 1-800-SUE-DRUG number, this is a sure sign that the information you are reading should at least be verified, if not simply dismissed as untrustworthy.

These elements indicate that the site is endorsing or working with people who have ideological and/or monetary motives for offering inaccurate health information, and these people may provide at least some of the funds that keep the site running.

Watch out for sites that want to sell you something, especially if they claim to be news sites, since their news is probably actually just advertising copy to make you buy their product. If someone is trying to scare you away from one treatment and selling services, goods, or products that profit from that fear, then they probably have a motive other than preserving your health and aren't to be trusted. The FDA advises Web users to "remember the adage 'If it sounds too good to be true, it probably is,'" and to beware of promises of immediate, spectacular effects.[38]

Other evidence that a site is producing tabloid medicine can be found by checking whether and when information about a particular illness or treatment has been updated. Most commonly, sites will show this information either in the header or at the bottom of the page. If the site does not tell you when the content was created or last changed, check the text and any citations to see if any years are referenced. But proceed cautiously if there is no indication of a date at all.

Searchers should also look out for who created the content and what their credentials are. Be aware that many websites reprint information or content from other sites, and sometimes the same text is posted and reposted on many sites to try to draw more readers and create a large Web presence. Some companies do nothing but aggregate and redistribute the same scary material to deliver content to many different sites. If the content comes from somewhere else, the source should be clearly noted and the citation(s) sufficiently comprehensive to make it easy to find the original. The source of statistics or data should be clearly identified. Forums or chat sites should say whether they are moderated, who the moderators are (at least by user name), and whom to contact if inaccurate or inappropriate material is being posted. Since there is no way to know who anyone posting on these sites actually is, the information they provide should be verified by a reputable source and taken with several grains of salt.

Unfortunately, almost all websites lack at least some of this information. In 2006, the Office of Disease Prevention and Health Promotion at the Department of Health and Human Services carried out a study on two samples, each of approximately fifty websites, drawn from two categories: "all health websites" and "frequently visited websites." The researchers evaluated the sites based on six criteria: "identity," "purpose," "content," "privacy," "user feedback," and "content updating." None of the Web pages studied met all six criteria, and only 0.3 percent of general sites and 3.9 percent of the most popular sites conformed to five criteria. In general, the most visited sites met more criteria than sites drawn from the rest of the Internet. Sites were least likely to comply with the "content" and "updating" criteria. This means that some of the most critical element for evaluating pages' reliability, such as information on the author, details on who reviews the site and how, and the date the site was last updated or checked for accuracy, were missing.[39]

Even when sites appear credible, it is always best to look at many different sources and more than one point of view. Because instant experts and true believers frequently succeed in overwhelming and outshouting their opponents, it can take some searching to find an alternate perspective. So it isn't any surprise that since most Americans looking online never get beyond the second page of results, they often believe that there is a consensus on the topic and take at face view the prevalent version of the situation and the evidence. Finding an opposing point of view may require deliberately looking for it, but failing to do so can have big consequences for the health of the user and his or her family—and for our public health.

Finally, when reading in the media about a new scare or a medical breakthrough, it pays to see if the source of the story was found on the Web, since the press increasingly fishes for new topics using the Internet. Also, the press is often instinctively sympathetic to the anti-pharma bias and to assertions that most new technologies are as unimportant and ineffective as they are unaffordable. And while they are quick to note the funding sources of researchers, many are allergic to examining the biases and viewpoints that inform the renegades or self-styled advocates. News stories are also likely to assign as much or more weight to studies conducted by advocacy groups as they do to the findings of well-designed clinical trials, usually in the name of balance. There are certainly good science and medical journalists who offer sound research, well-founded conclusions, and important insights, but they are, unfortunately, outnumbered by the credulous and the sensationalistic.

The other element information seekers should think about is the reliability of the research that underlies stories about health, both in the press and online. Dr. Alicia White of Bazian, a British organization promoting evidence-based medicine, recommends that when reading health headlines (and this goes just as much for the titles of blog posts, Web articles, and other online sources), people should ask a few fundamental questions. First, is there actual scientific study behind the thesis of the piece? If the article cannot cite any trials showing that a risk is real or a treatment is effective, "then treat [the article] with caution. A lot of caution, like balling the article up and throwing it in the (recycling) bin." But even if the research was published in a top journal, that doesn't automatically make it true. Take nothing on faith.[40]

John Ioannidis, an epidemiologist and expert in clinical trial design, has other warning signs to look for. Ionnidis says, "The probability that a research finding is indeed true depends on the prior probability of it being true (before doing the study), the statistical power of the study, and the level of statistical significance." Web users should watch out for small trials, because the fewer participants involved, the more likely there will appear to be a difference between the groups and the larger that difference will seem. They should also beware of methodologies and definitions that are ambiguous, flexible, or subject to interpretation, since, as we discussed in the context of SSRIs, this makes it easier both for the results to be deliberately manipulated and for bias to slip in unintentionally. Furthermore, "[t]he hotter a scientific field (with more scientific teams involved), the less likely the research findings are to be true," since researchers may be eager to produce controversial or sensational results or may be racing to be the first to publish on a topic.[41]

Finally, all risk is relative and absolute. Remember that numbers are used to shape the way you evaluate risk absent any other information. Be wary of statistics, and think carefully about what the numbers and percentages cited actually mean—it's rarely what it first appears. A 60 percent increase in the chance of something happening sounds scary, but then again, think about how many lottery tickets you would need to buy to increase your chances of winning by 60 percent. Even a 200 percent risk is pretty insignificant if it makes the chance of developing a disease or a complication 0.02 percent rather than 0.01 percent. Numbers are often used to scare and stick, not to inform.

Last, and most importantly, Internet users should share the information they find on the Web with their doctor or other health professional and never make medical decisions without the knowledge of their physician. Many doctors don't have the time to go through piles of Web printouts with patients in the short duration of an average doctor's visit, but they certainly would rather do so than have a patient make health decisions without consulting them. Several surveys show that patients whose doctors discuss and evaluate online information with them are more satisfied with the office visit and have more confidence in their physician. These patients also ask more questions, are more likely to follow their doctor's advice, and make more lifestyle changes to improve their health.[42]

FORWARD OR BACKWARD?

Tabloid medicine has a vision of the future. It is a world where a single, small study should be taken as the basis for a massive change in behavior when it comes to your health and that of your family. Where a rare risk should be avoided at all costs to the exclusion of other considerations and issues. Where the only source of conflict is money from the medical industry. Where no one should have access to new medicines or technologies until the critics are satisfied. And where new technologies from corporations are required to be proven safe in response to any theory about potential harms. It is a future with less innovation and medical progress, indeed, with fewer treatments than we have now.

Combating a largely imaginary threat of unsafe drugs, vaccines, and medical devices by eliminating each and every possible danger has been, and will continue to be, extremely costly, scientifically unsound, technologically impossible, and ultimately damaging to human prospects for longer life and prosperity. The goal of medical innovation is to reduce death, suffering, and risk, which it has done on a grand scale for the past one hundred years. There have been problems, mistakes, and cases of misconduct, but just as medicine without risk is impossible, so, too, is unblemished purity and perfection.

The cult of safety existed before the advent of the Internet, but enshrined in the Precautionary Principle, it has found in the Web a haven and an effective means of disseminating its point of view. Many of the fundamental failings of the human mind when it comes to evaluating and avoiding risks are heightened by the Internet, which extends personalization and the reach of information about new and rare dangers far beyond their previous limits and produces an illusion of control and agency. As Americans have increasingly turned to the Web as their default first opinion on medicine and health, online charlatans and instant experts, whether opportunistic or ignorant, have seen burgeoning influence. They are aided and abetted by a population hungry for information and empowerment but too trusting of those who offer it and insufficiently critical of the content they find.

Not taking chances with possible risks and heading off dangers before they are certain may seem sensible, but it brings its own threats to our health, individual and collective. When the FDA acted precipitously to warn against prescribing SSRI antidepressants to children and teens, the result was an uptick in the suicide rate. When the panic over vaccines drove down immunization rates, it led to outbreaks of diseases that had all but vanished in the first world and impeded research into the real causes of autism. When drugs such as Avandia, Crestor, and even Vioxx were attacked with hyperbole rather than rational analysis, patients were denied treatments that helped them or were turned away from medications from which they would have benefited.

Both the Precautionary Principle and tabloid medicine are the products of a shared belief that technology causes harm. Why do its proponents fear the smallest risks of medical innovation while others (like me) believe that the risks are not only worth taking but that they should be taken? Both views reflect choices about the kind of society we want and deeply held beliefs about the role technology can play in our lives. Tabloid medicine insists on not only having greater control over determining when innovations are safe but also controlling what research is conducted and how doctors practice medicine. Its proponents hold that without such limits, the dangers of medical innovation will overwhelm us.

In this book, I have tried to show that the tabloid medicine agenda has costs along with its supposed benefits. In their arrogance, its proponents glide over this fact and seek to silence those who object, but the risks of pursuing their course remain. Cass Sunstein observed on the subject of global warming that "if we take steps to reduce risks, we will always create fresh hazards. No choice is risk-free. For environmental and other problems, we need to decide which risks to combat—not comfort ourselves with the pretense that there is such a thing as a 'safe' choice."[43] The same is true of tabloid medicine.

Not only is it impossible to anticipate all risks, but relying on the claim that there is a "safe" choice creates a false sense of security and leaves us unable to cope with problems or dangers that were not supposed to happen. While everyone was focusing on finding a connection between autism and vaccines, no one paid attention to the fact people were not getting immunized. Vioxx was taken off the market, and now other painkillers of its class seem scary, too. But pain persists and more people either suffer or go on narcotics-based medicines, where overdose and addiction have become problems. Fears about the dangers of antibiotics have led to a decline in new product development, even as bacterial infections become harder and harder to treat. Academic detailers prescribe medicines according to their ideological bent, restricting the use of new drugs and demanding the use of old ones, and patients exposed to this experiment stop taking medicines altogether because of fear of side effects.

I am encouraged by personalized medicine, particularly the development and use of biomarkers, because it will allow people and institutions to manage the risks of disease (and treatment) in a dynamic fashion. Use of molecular and genetic markers allows patients to choose the right drug for them and helps society identify risks more quickly and adapt to them faster. The movement toward patient-centered clinical research should be encouraged, and the potential of Internet communities to capture personal experiences and variations in response to treatment should be employed to create data we can use to answer fundamental questions about how medications work and whom they may put at risk. Through encouraging—not prohibiting or censoring—collaboration between government, industry, and academia, these new methods can flourish and grow, producing treatments tailored to the patient and designed to offer unparalleled efficacy and safety.

But tabloid medicine has proved an inveterate enemy of personalized medicine, determined to cosset us in a world where progress is viewed with suspicion and is impeded unless it can offer the impossible.

Its proponents are tireless, because their beliefs are the source of their power, and they are loath to lose their ability to manipulate millions. To counter the expansion of their influence, much needs to be done. We should acknowledge that we have been used as pawns in tabloid medicine's game and make use of simple defenses: skepticism about websites and careful scrutiny of online information, ideally in collaboration with our physicians.

If we do nothing, we will become captives of an ideology that leaves little room for individual freedom and medical progress and of the impulse to restrict and control, if only for our own good and salvation. As Lionel Trilling wrote in *The Liberal Imagination*, "We must be aware of the dangers that lie in our most generous wishes. Some paradox of our nature leads us, when once we have made our fellow men the object of our enlightened interest, to go on to make them the objects of our pity, then of our wisdom, and ultimately of our coercion."[44] Would you rather live in a world where government allows one or two types of treatment to the exclusion of all others because of fear of side effects and the belief that all medicines are the same—or in a world where we have access to a diversity of medical technologies? We have the ability to overcome tabloid medicine and the sooner we start exercising it, the better. The future is already being written and it is up to us, to me and to you, to decide what it will look like. Choose wisely.

NOTES

INTRODUCTION

1. Nancy D. Berkman et al., "Management of Eating Disorders," Agency for Healthcare Research and Quality, U.S. Department of Health and Human Services, *Evidence Report/Technology Assessment* 135, April 2006, www.ahrq. gov/downloads/pub/evidence/pdf/eatingdisorders/eatdis.pdf.

2. Michael Shermer, "When Ideas Have Sex: How Free Exchange Between People Increases Prosperity and Trust," *Scientific American*, June 2010, www. scientificamerican.com/sciammag/?contents=2010-06.

CHAPTER 1—PROSPECT THEORY: THE RISKS WE CHOOSE TO LIVE WITH AND WHY

1. Paul Slovic, Baruch Fischhoff, and Sarah Lichtenstein, "Why Study Risk Perception?" *Risk Analysis* 2, no. 2 (1982): 83–93.

2. Valerie Reyna, "A Theory of Medical Decision Making and Health: Fuzzy Trace Theory," *Medical Decision Making* 28, no. 6 (2008): 850–65.

3. Ibid.

4. Angela Fagerlin, Brian J. Zikmund-Fisher, and Peter A. Ubel, "How Making a Risk Estimate Can Change the Feel of That Risk: Shifting Attitudes Towards Breast Cancer Risk in a General Public Survey," *Patient Education and Counseling* 57, no. 3 (June 2005): 294–99.

5. Angela Fagerlin et al., "Women's Decisions Regarding Tamoxifen for Breast Cancer Prevention: Responses to a Tailored Decision Aid," *Breast Cancer Research and Treatment* 119, no. 3 (February 2010): 613–20.

6. Reyna, "A Theory of Medical Decision Making and Health."

7. Scott Plous, *The Psychology of Judgment and Decision Making* (New York: McGraw-Hill, 1993), 178.

8. Craig R. Fox, "The Impact of Extreme Events in Decisions Under Uncertainty: A Cognitive Perspective," Fuqua School of Business Duke University, 2002, available at www.ldeo.columbia.edu/chrr/documents/meetings/roundtable/pdf/notes/fox_craig_note.pdf.

9. Steven Johnson, *Mind Wide Open: Your Brain and The Neuroscience of Everyday Life* (New York: Scribner's, 2004), 48, 50–51.

10. Daniel Gilbert, "If Only Gay Sex Caused Global Warming," *Los Angeles Times*, July 2, 2006.

11. Michael Schrage, "Daniel Kahneman: The Thought Leader Interview," *Strategy + Business*, 33 (Winter 2003), available at www.strategy-business.com/media/file/03409.pdf.

12. Leora Swartzman, "SARS Anxiety: The Psychology of Risk Perception," *Western News*, May 8, 2003, available at www.communications.uwo.ca/com/western_news/opinions/sars_anxiety_the_psychology_of_risk_perception_20030508436313.

13. Fox, "The Impact of Extreme Events in Decisions Under Uncertainty," 4–5.

14. Michael L. Rothschild, "Terrorism and You: The Real Odds," *Washington Post*, November 25, 2001, reprinted at www.aei.org/article/101141.

15. Gerd Gigerenzer and Wolfgang Gaissmaier, "Fear in the Wake of Terror," *MaxPlanckResearch* 3 (2007), available at www.mpg.de/english/illustrationsDocumentation/multimedia/mpResearch/2007/heft03/009/index.html.

16. Wenbo Wang, Hean Tat Keh, and Lisa E. Bolton, "Lay Theories of Medicine and a Healthy Lifestyle," *Journal of Consumer Research* (June 2010), available at www.personal.psu.edu/leb14/Docs/Bolton12%20HealthRemedies.pdf.

17. Centers for Disease Control, "Questions and Answers Regarding Estimating Deaths from Seasonal Influenza in the United States," September 4, 2009, available at www.cdc.gov/flu/about/disease/us_flu-related_deaths.htm.

18. The full email can be found at www.hoax-slayer.com/swine-flu-fear-mongering.shtml and, minus the opening comments, at www.snopes.com/medical/swineflu/asia.asp, along with a thorough debunking of the content.

19. Heather Whipps, "Urban Legends: How They Start and How They Persist," *Live Science*, August 26, 2006, available at www.livescience.com/strangenews/060827_urban_legends.html.

20. Chat with Jan Harold Brunvand, *CNN.com Book Chat*, September 22, 1999, accessed at www.edition.cnn.com/COMMUNITY/transcripts/jan.harold.brunvand.html.

21. Scott Reinardy, Jensen Moore, and Wayne Wanta, "How Do Newspaper Journalists Use the Internet in News Gathering?" Paper presented at the annual meeting of the International Communication Association, San Francisco, Calif., May 23, 2007.

22. Kayo Tomono, "Health, Risk and News: The MMR Vaccine and the Media," Reuters Institute for the Study of Journalism, March 3, 2008.

23. Ibid.; Tammy Boyce, *Health, Risk and News: The MMR Vaccine and the Media* (Oxford: Peter Lang Publishing, Inc., 2007), 46–47, 191.

24. Richard B. Philipp, *Herbal-Drug Interactions and Adverse Effects: An Evidence-Based Quick Reference Guide* (New York: McGraw Hill Companies, 2004).

25. M. Cirgliano, "Bioidentical Hormone Therapy: A Review of the Evidence," *Journal of Women's Health* 16, no. 5 (June 2007): 600–631.

26. Amos Tversky and Daniel Kahneman, "The Framing of Decisions and the Psychology of Choice," *Science* 211 (1981): 453–58.

27. Mary Douglas and Aaron Wildavsky, *Risk and Culture: An Essay on the Selection of Technological and Environmental Dangers* (Berkeley and Los Angeles: University of California Press, 1982), 10.

CHAPTER 2—THE PRECAUTIONARY PRINCIPLE: THE POLITICS OF PSEUDOCERTAINTY

1. Rebecca Ruiz, "Industrial Chemicals Lurking in Your Bloodstream," *Forbes*, January 21, 2010.

2. Jill Neimark, "The Dirty Truth About Plastic," *Discover*, July 2008, available at www.discovermagazine.com/2008/may.

3. U.S. Food and Drug Administration, "Draft Assessment of Bisphenol-A for Use in Food Contact Applications," August 2008, available at www.fda.gov/ohrms/dockets/AC/08/briefing/2008-0038b1_01_02_FDA%20BPA%20Draft%20Assessment.pdf.

4. E. Diamanti-Kandarakis et al., "Endocrine-Disrupting Chemicals: An Endocrine Society Scientific Statement," *Endocrine Reviews* 30, no. 4 (2009): 293–342.

5. U.S. Food and Drug Administration, "Update on Bisphenol-A for Use in Food Contact Applications," January 2010, available at www.fda.gov/downloads/NewsEvents/PublicHealthFocus/UCM197778.pdf.

6. Denise Grady, "FDA Concerned About Substance in Food Packaging," *New York Times*, January 15, 2010.

7. Stephanie Wood, "Eating Green," *Parenting*, March 1, 2008, reproduced at www.ewg.org/node/26097.

8. Courtney Perkes, "Laptops and Sperm Count," *Los Angeles Times*, October 5, 2009, available at www.latimes.com/sns-health-laptops-sperm-count,0,1576522.story.

9. Quoted in Cass R. Sunstein, "The Paralyzing Principle," *Regulation* (Winter 2002–03): 33.

10. "Wingspread Statement on the Precautionary Principle," drafted and signed by attendees of the Wingspread Conference on the Precautionary Principle, at the Wingspread Conference Center, Racine, Wisconsin, January 23–25, 1998, reproduced at www.gdrc.org/u-gov/precaution-3.html.

11. European Commission, "Communication from the commission on the precautionary principle," European Union, February 2, 2002.

12. "Wingspread Statement on the Precautionary Principle."

13. Ronald Bailey, "Precautionary Tale," *Reason*, April 1999, available at www.reason.com/archives/1999/04/01/precautionary-tale.

14. Daniel Gardner, *The Science of Fear: Why We Fear the Things We Shouldn't— and Put Ourselves in Greater Danger* (New York: Dutton Adult, 2008), 82.

15. From John Weingart, *Waste Is a Terrible Thing to Mind: Risk, Radiation, and Distrust of Government* (New Brunswick, N.J.: Rutgers University Press, 2007), quoted in Gardner, *The Science of Fear*, 107.

16. Paul Slovic, Baruch Fischhoff, and Sarah Lichtenstein, "Facts and Fears: Understanding Perceived Risk," in Richard C. Schwing and Walter A. Albers, Jr., eds., *Societal Risk Assessment: How Safe Is Safe Enough?* Proceedings of the General Motors Symposium on Societal Risk Assessment, Warren, Michigan, October 7–9, 1979 (New York: Plenum Press, 1980), 181–212.

17. Ali Siddiq Alhakami and Paul Slovic, "A Psychological Study of the Inverse Relationship Between Perceived Risk and Perceived Benefit," *Risk Analysis* 14, no. 6 (1994): 1,085–96.

18. Bruce Schneier, *Beyond Fear: Thinking Sensibly About Security in an Uncertain World* (New York: Copernicus Books, 2003), 23–24.

19. Melissa L. Finucane et al., "The Affect Heuristic in Judgment of Risks and Benefits," *Journal of Behavioral Decision Making* 13, no. 1 (Jan./Mar. 2000): 1–17.

20. Paul Slovic, "If Hormesis Exists . . . : Implications for Risk Perception and Communication," *Human and Experimental Toxicology* 17 (1998): 439–40.

21. Gardner, *The Science of Fear*, 228.

22. Winston Williams, "Polishing the Apple's Image," *New York Times*, May 25, 1986.

23. Timothy Egan, "Apple Growers Bruised and Bitter After Alar Scare," *New York Times*, July 9, 1991.

24. This discussion of Alar is based on Williams, "Polishing the Apple's Image"; Egan, "Apple Growers Bruised and Bitter"; Cynthia Crossen, *Tainted Truth: The Manipulation of Fact in America* (New York: Touchstone, 1996), 53–57; Steven J. Milloy, *Junk Science Judo: Self-Defense Against Health Scares and Scams* (Washington, D.C.: The Cato Institute, 2001), 18–19; and Elizabeth M. Whelan, *Toxic Terror: The Truth Behind the Cancer Scares*, 2nd edition (Amherst, NY: Prometheus Books, 1993), 187–198.

25. Sandy Starr, "Science, Risk and the Price of Precaution," Spiked-online.com, May 1, 2003, available at www.spiked-online.com/articles/00000006DD7A.htm.

26. Bailey, "Precautionary Tale."

27. Poul Harremoës, Professor of Environmental Science and Engineering at the Technical University of Denmark, quoted in European Environment Agency news release, "EEA Draws Key Lessons from History on Using Precaution in Policy-making," January 10, 2002, available at www.biotech-info.net/EEA_news.html.

28. Helen Guldberg, "Challenging the Precautionary Principle," Spiked-online.com, July 1, 2003, available at www.spiked-online.com/articles/00000006DE2F.htm.

29. Bailey, "Precautionary Tale."

30. Ronald Brunton, "The Perils of the Precautionary Principle," *Australasian Biotechnology* 5, no. 4 (August 1995): 236–38.

31. Trent Stephen and Rock Brynne, *Dark Remedy: The Impact of Thalidomide and Its Revival as a Vital Medicine* (Cambridge, Mass.: Perseus Publishing, 2001), 17.

32. This section is based on Stefan Timmermans and Marc Berg, *The Gold Standard: The Challenge of Evidence-Based Medicine and Standardization in Health Care* (Philadelphia, Pa.: Temple University Press, 2003), 170–73; Joe Schwarcz, MD, *The Genie in the Bottle: 67 All-New Commentaries on the Fascinating Chemistry of Everyday Life* (New York: Henry Holt and Company, 2002), 26–27; and Trent Stephen and Rock Brynne, *Dark Remedy: The Impact of Thalidomide and Its Revival as a Vital Medicine* (Cambridge, Mass.: Perseus Publishing, 2001).

33. Paul A. Offit, MD, *The Cutter Incident: How America's First Polio Vaccine Led to the Growing Vaccine Crisis* (New Haven, Conn.: Yale University Press, 2005), 179–81.

34. For more on DTP see Offit, *The Cutter Incident*, 179–84, 255–56; and Arthur Allen, *Vaccine: The Controversial Story of Medicine's Greatest Lifesaver* (New York: W.W. Norton and Company, 2007), 251–56.

35. "Helen Keller Quotes" in World of Quotes, available at www.worldofquotes.com/author/Helen-Keller/1/index.html (accessed January 26, 2010).

36. James M. Taylor, "Liberal Academic Shoots Down Precautionary Principle," *Environment and Climate News*, The Heartland Institute (July 2002), available at www.heartland.org/policybot/results/902/Liberal_academic_shoots_down_Precautionary_Principle.html.

CHAPTER 3—INSTA-AMERICANS: THE RISE OF ONLINE SELF-DIAGNOSIS

1. Susannah Fox and Sydney Jones, "The Social Life of Health Information," Pew Research Center Internet and American Life Project, June 2009, available at www.pewInternet.org/~/media//Files/Reports/2009/PIP_Health_2009.pdf, 2.

2. Susannah Fox, "Online Health Search 2006," Pew Research Center Internet and American Life Project, Oct. 2006, available at www.pewInternet.org/~/media//Files/Reports/2006/PIP_Online_Health_2006.pdf.pdf, 3.

3. "How Many U.S. Adults Have Searched for Health Information Online in the Past Year?" *iHealthBeat*, Nov. 5, 2008, available at www.ihealthbeat.org/Data-Points/2008/How-Many-US-Adults-Have-Searched-for-Health-Information-Online-in-the-Past-Year.aspx; Bill Tancer, "Bing: Rising Success (rate)," blog post, Hitwise Intelligence blog, Jan. 14, 2010, available at www.weblogs.hitwise.com/bill-tancer/2010/01/bing_rising_success_rate.html.

4. John Markoff, "Microsoft Examines Causes of 'Cyberchondria,'" *New York Times*, Nov. 25, 2008, available at www.nytimes.com/2008/11/25/technology/Internet/25symptoms.html.

5. Fox and Jones, "The Social Life of Health Information," 9.

6. Jennifer Huget, "No One Way to Hold Sway: Women Drive Online Health Traffic, but Use Varies," *Washington Post*, Oct. 2, 2007, available at www.washingtonpost.com/wp-dyn/content/article/2007/09/28/AR2007092801718.html.

7. Fox and Jones, "The Social Life of Health Information," 9.

8. Fox, "Online Health Search 2006," 3; Fox and Jones, "The Social Life of Health Information," 2.

9. Fox and Jones, "The Social Life of Health Information," 3.

10. Ibid., 11.

11. "How Many U.S. Adults Have Searched for Health Information Online in the Past Year?" *iHealthBeat*, November 5, 2008, available at www.ihealthbeat. org/data-points/2008/how-many-us-adults-have-searched-for-health-information-online-in-the-past-year.aspx.

12. Fox and Jones, "The Social Life of Health Information," 18–19.

13. "75 Percent of Consumers Say Internet Is Their First-Choice Resource for Drug Treatment Information, according to Prospectiv Survey," BusinessWire.com, July 24, 2007, available at www.businesswire.com/portal/site/home/permalink/?ndmViewId=news_view&newsId=200707 24005070&newsLang=en.

14. Fox, "Online Health Search 2006," 4.

15. Fox and Jones, "The Social Life of Health Information," 20.

16. Sarah Bauerle Bass et al., "Relationship of Internet Health Information Use with Patient Behavior and Self-Efficacy: Experiences of Newly Diagnosed Cancer Patients Who Contact the National Cancer Institute's Cancer Information Service," *Journal of Health Communication* 11, no. 2 (March 2006): 219–36.

17. See for example, S. L. Ayers and J. J. Kronenfeld, "Chronic Illness and Health-seeking Information on the Internet," *Health* 11, no. 3 (July 2007): 327–47; Susannah Fox, "E-patients with a Disability or Chronic Disease," Pew Research Center Internet and American Life Project, Oct. 8, 2007, available at www.pewInternet.org/~/media//Files/Reports/2007/EPatients_Chronic_Conditions_2007.pdf.pdf.

18. Susannah Fox, "The Engaged e-Patient Population," Pew Research Center Internet and American Life Project, Aug. 26, 2008, available at www.pewInternet.org/pdfs/PIP_Health_Aug08.pdf.

19. "Many Young Adults Struggle to Manage Multiple Chronic Conditions," California HealthCare Foundation, March 18, 2009, available at www.chcf.org/press/view.cfm?itemID=133897.

20. Mike Benigeri and Pierre Pluye, "Shortcomings of Health Information on the Internet," *Health Promotion International* 18, no. 4 (Dec. 2003): 381–86.

21. Ryen W. White and Eric Horvitz, "Cyberchondria: Studies of the Escalation of Medical Concerns in Web Search," Microsoft Research, Dec. 2008, available at www.research.microsoft.com/apps/pubs/default.aspx?id=76529, 7.

22. Markoff, "Microsoft Examines Causes of 'Cyberchondria.'"

23. White and Horvitz, "Cyberchondria," 26.

24. Marisa Osario Colon, "Medical Web Advice," *Star News Online*, Sept. 4, 2007, available at www.starnewsonline.com/article/FP/20070904/HEALTHMATTERS/70904005/-1/health.

25. Shirley S. Wang, "Drug-Safety Data: Too Much Information?" *Wall Street Journal*, Dec. 9, 2008.

26. R.J.W. Cline and K. M. Haynes, "Consumer Health Information Seeking on the Internet: The State of the Art," *Health Education Research* 16, no. 6 (Dec. 2001): 671–92.

27. W. M. Silberg et al., "Assessing, Controlling, and Assuring the Quality of Medical Information on the Internet: *Caveat lector et viewor*—Let the Reader and Viewer Beware," *Journal of the American Medical Association* 277 (1997): 1,244–45, quoted in Cline and Haynes, "Consumer Health Information Seeking on the Internet."

28. Fox, "Online Health Search 2006," 18–19.

29. "Search users 'stop at page three,'" *BBC News*, April 12, 2006, available at www.news.bbc.co.uk/2/hi/technology/4900742.stm; Deborah Fallows, "Search Engine Users," Pew Research Center Internet and American Life Project, Jan. 2005, available at www.pewInternet.org/pdfs/PIP_Searchengine_users.pdf, 1.

30. Enid Burns, "U.S. Search Engine Ranking," SearchEngineWatch.com, April 2007, available at www.searchenginewatch.com/showPage.html?page=3626021; "How Many U.S. Adults Have Searched for Health Information Online in the Past Year?"

31. "How Many U.S. Adults Have Searched for Health Information Online in the Past Year?" The percentages add up to more than 100 percent because some searchers used multiple sites.

32. A. M. Minino, M. P. Heron, and B. L. Smith, "Preliminary Data for 2004 National Vital Statistics Reports," National Center for Health Statistics (Hyattsville, Md.), vol. 54, no. 19 (2006).

33. "Heart Disease and Stroke Statistics," American Heart Association, 2007, available at www.americanheart.org/downloadable/heart/1166712318459HS_StatsInsideText.pdf, 9; "State Specific Cholesterol Screening Trends," *CDC Morbidity and Mortality Weekly* 49, no. 33 (Aug. 25, 2000), available at www.cdc.gov/mmwr/preview/mmwrhtml/mm4933a2.htm.

34. Based on data from the "Third Report of the Expert Panel on Detection, Evaluation, and Treatment of High Blood Cholesterol in Adults," *Journal of the American Medical Association* 106, no. 25 (Dec. 2002): 2,486–97.

35. See "Interview with Dr. Sidney Wolfe," *CNN in the Money*, July 17, 2004, available at www.transcripts.cnn.com/TRANSCRIPTS/0407/17/cnnitm.00.html and "Statement of Sidney Wolfe, MD, regarding the FDA's decision to leave Crestor on the market (HRG Publication no. 1730)," Public Citizen, March 14, 2005; see www.citizen.org/publications/release.cfm?ID=7371, for examples.

36. "Rosuvastatin Calcium (marketed as Crestor) Information," U.S. Food and Drug Administration, March 14, 2005, available at www.fda.gov/cder/drug/infopage/rosuvastatin/default.htm.

37. Steven K. Galson, "Letter from FDA in Response to Citizen Petition," Department of Health and Human Services, March, 11, 2005.

38. Matthew Herper and Robert Langreth, "A New Age of Statins?" *Forbes*, Nov. 11, 2008.

39. "FDA Panel Backs Crestor for Heart Attack, Stroke Prevention," *USA Today*, Dec. 15, 2009.

40. "AstraZeneca gets OK for Expanded Crestor Use," *USA Today*, Feb. 8, 2010.

41. Andrew C. von Eschenbach, "Statement of Andrew C. von Eschenbach, M.D., Commissioner of Food and Drugs," Department of Health and Human Services, June 6, 2007, available at www.oversight.house.gov/documents/20070606105302.pdf, 2.

42. "Type 2 Diabetes," American Diabetes Association, available at www.diabetes.org/type-2-diabetes.jsp.

43. "Direct and Indirect Costs of Diabetes in America," American Diabetes Association, www.diabetes.org/diabetes-statistics/cost-of-diabetes-in-us.jsp.

44. Robin Pagnamenta, "Avandia Flop Forces Glaxo Rethink," *Times Online*, Aug. 13, 2007, available at www.business.timesonline.co.uk/tol/business/industry_sectors/health/article2249837.ece; Stephanie Saul, "V.A. Limits Glaxo Drug Widely Used for Diabetes," *New York Times*, Aug. 18, 2007, available at www.query.nytimes.com/gst/fullpage.html?res=9C0CE4DF103EF93BA25753C1A9619C8B63.

45. von Eschenbach, "Statement of Andrew C. von Eschenbach, M.D."

46. Private survey of endocrinologists conducted for Lazard, Inc., June 18, 2007.

47. See "Age-Adjusted Percentage of Adults with Diabetes Using Diabetes Medication, by Type of Medication, United States, 1997-2008," Centers for Disease Control and Prevention, updated Feburary 9, 2010, available at www.cdc.gov/diabetes/statistics/meduse/fig2.htm; "Crude and Age-Adjusted Percentage of Adults with Diabetes Using Any Diabetes Medication, United States, 1997-2008," Centers for Disease Control and Prevention, updated Feburary 9, 2010, available at www.cdc.gov/diabetes/statistics/meduse/fig3.htm; "Crude and Age-Adjusted Incidence of Diagnosed Diabetes per 1,000 Population Aged 18-79 Years, United States, 1980-2008," Centers for Disease Control and Prevention, updated June 25, 2010, available at www.cdc.gov/diabetes/statistics/incidence/fig2.htm.

48. Gardiner Harris, "A Face-Off on the Safety of a Drug for Diabetes," *New York Times*, February 22, 2010, available at www.nytimes.com/2010/02/23/health/23niss.html.

49. Gardiner Harris, "Diabetes Drug Maker Hid Test Data, Files Indicate," *New York Times*, July 12, 2010, available at www.nytimes.com/2010/07/13/health/policy/13avandia.html.

50. David J. Graham et al., "Risk of Acute Myocardial Infarction, Stroke, Heart Failure, and Death in Elderly Medicare Patients Treated With Rosiglitazone or Pioglitazone," *JAMA* 304, no. 4 (2010), available at http://jama.ama-assn.org/cgi/content/full/jama.2010.920; Steven E. Nissen and Kathy Wolski, "Rosiglitazone Revisited: An Updated Meta-analysis of Risk for Myocardial Infarction and Cardiovascular Mortality," *Archives of Internal Medicine* 170, no. 14 (2010), available at http://archinte.ama-assn.org/cgi/content/abstract/2010.207.

51. Emily Walker and Dan Childs, "Au Revoir, Avandia? FDA Reviewers Urge Agency to Pull Drug," ABC News, February 23, 2010; January W. Payne, "6 Things You Should Know About Avandia," *U.S. News & World Report*, Feb. 25, 2010.

52. M. C. Lunik, "What's There for Me? The Internet for Pharmacists," *Pharmacy Practice Management Quarterly* 17, no. 4 (1998): 37–47, quoted in Cline and Haynes, "Consumer Health Information Seeking on the Internet."

53. B. Richards et al., "The Current and Future Role of the Internet in Patient Education," *International Journal of Medical Informatics* 50 (1998): 279–85, quoted in Cline and Haynes, "Consumer Health Information Seeking on the Internet."

54. M. Tascilar, F. A. de Jong, J. Verweij, and R. H. Mathijssen, "Complementary and Alternative Medicine During Cancer Treatment: Beyond Innocence," *The Oncologist* 11, no. 7 (Jul.–Aug. 2006): 732–41.

55. Huget, "No One Way to Hold Sway."

56. Benigeri and Pluye, "Shortcomings of Health Information on the Internet."

57. Gretchen K. Berland et al., "Health Information on the Internet: Accessibility, Quality, and Readability in English and Spanish," *Journal of the American Medical Association* 285, no. 20 (May 23, 2001): 2,612–21.

58. Bernie Monegain, ed. "Online Info Has Patients Doubting Doctors, Survey Finds," *Healthcare IT News*, July 30, 2008, available at www.healthcareitnews.com/news/online-info-has-patients-doubting-doctors-survey-finds.

59. Fox, "The Engaged e-Patient Population."

60. Tom Ferguson, MD, and the e-Patient Scholars Working Group, "E-Patients: How They Can Help Us Heal Health Care," e-Patients, March 2007, chapter 1, available at www.acor.org/epatientswiki/index.php/Main_Page.

61. Rahul K. Parikh, "Not My Best Day Doctoring," blog post, "sWell," on Salon.com, Dec. 15, 2008, available at www.open.salon.com/content.php?cid=61914.

62. Michelle Slatalla, "Visits to Doctors Who Are Not in, Ever," *New York Times*, May 24, 2007, available at www.nytimes.com/2007/05/24/fashion/24Cyber. html; Susannah Fox, "Recruit Doctors: Let e-Patients Lead. Go Mobile," remarks at Health 2.0 Conference, March 4, 2009, available at www. pewInternet.org/pdfs/Fox_Health_March_2008.pdf.

63. Humphrey Taylor and Robert Leitman, eds., "4-Country Survey Finds Most Cyberchondriacs Believe Online Health Care Information Is Trustworthy, Easy to Find and Understand," *Harris International Health Care News* 2, no. 12 (2002), available at www.harrisinteractive.com/news/newsletters/ healthnews/HI_HealthCareNews2002Vol2_Iss12.pdf.

64. Monegain, ed., "Online Info Has Patients Doubting Doctors, Survey Finds."

65. Sam Vaknin, PhD, "The Demise of the Expert and the Ascendance of the Layman," Global Politician.com, available at www.globalpolitician.com/print. asp?id=3920.

CHAPTER 4—A DAMAGING PRECEDENT: THE SIDE EFFECTS OF THE VIOXX PANIC

1. Raja Mishra and Jeffrey Krasner, "Pulling of MS Drug Calls FDA Actions into Question," *The Boston Globe*, March 6, 2005, available at www.boston. com/news/globe/health_science/articles/2005/03/06/pulling_of_ms_drug_ calls_fda_actions_into_question; Jeffrey Krasner, "Biogen Calls Halt to Its MS Drug," *The Boston Globe*, March 1, 2005, available at www.acceleratedcure. org/news/bcp/20050301-bostonglobe.php.

2. David Henderson and Charles Hooper, "Clear Thinking About Vioxx: The Risk Is Not What You Think," *Reason*, Jan. 3 2005, available at www.reason. com/news/show/36510.html.

3. Robert Burton, "How Merck Stacked the Vioxx Deck," Salon.com, March 31, 2005, available at www.salon.com/news/feature/2005/03/31/vioxx/print. htm.

4. Jenkins, "Good Drugs, Bad Customers."

5. Duncan Emerson, "Will FDA's Axe Fall on COX-2s," *Data Monitor*, Jan. 8, 2005, available at www.countrydoctor.co.uk/precis/precis%20-%20Cox2s%20 and%20Datamonitor.htm.

6. Mary Anne Crandall, *The World Market for Pain Management Drugs and Devices*, 2nd edition (Rockville, MD: Kalorama Information, MarketResearch, 2004).

7. Burton, "How Merck Stacked the Vioxx Deck."

8. G. A. FitzGerald, Y. Cheng, and S. Austin, "COX-2 Inhibitors and the Cardio-vascular System," *Clinical Experimental Rheumatology* 19, no. 6, suppl. 5 (Nov.–Dec. 2001): S31–36; G. A. FitzGerald, "Cardiovascular Pharmacology of Nonselective Nonsteroidal Anti-Inflammatory Drugs and Coxibs: Clinical Considerations," *American Journal of Cardiology* 89, no. 6A (March 21, 2002): 26–32; G. A. FitzGerald, "Prostaglandins: Modulators of Inflammation and Cardiovascular Risk," *Journal of Clinical Rheumatology* 10, suppl. 3 (June 2004): S12–17.

9. Frederick Wolfe et al., "Increase in Lifetime Adverse Drug Reactions, Service Utilization, and Disease Severity Among Patients Who Will Start COX-2 specific Inhibitors: Quantitative Assessment of Channeling Bias and Confounding by Indication in 6689 Patients with Rheumatoid Arthritis and Osteoarthritis," *The Journal of Rheumatology* 29, no. 5 (2002): 1,015–22.

10. Frederick Wolfe, Sean Zhao, and Dan Pettitt, "Blood Pressure Destabilization and Edema Among 8538 Users of Celecoxib, Rofecoxib, and Nonselective Nonsteroidal Anti-inflammatory Drugs (NSAIDs) and Non-users of NSAID Receiving Ordinary Clinical Care," *The Journal of Rheumatology* 31, no. 6 (2004): 1,143–51; S. Z. Zhao et al., "Comparison of the Baseline Cardiovascular Risk Profile Among Hypertensive Patients Prescribed COX-2-specific Inhibitors or Nonspecific NSAIDs: Data from Real-life Practice," *American Journal of Managed Care* 8, suppl. 15 (Oct. 2002): S392–400.

11. See figure 3 in Peter Jüni et al., "Risk of Cardiovascular Events and Rofecoxib: Cumulative Meta-analysis," *The Lancet* 364 (Dec. 4, 2004): 2,021–29.

12. Jüni et al., "Risk of Cardiovascular Events and Rofecoxib."

13. C. Bombardier et al., "Comparison of Upper Gastrointestinal Toxicity of Rofecoxib and Naproxen in Patients with Rheumatoid Arthritis," *New England Journal of Medicine* 343, no. 21 (Nov. 23, 2000): 1,520–28.

14. Ibid.

15. Statement of Sandra Kweder, MD, deputy director, Office of New Drugs, U.S. Food and Drug Administration, before the Committee on Finance, U.S. Senate, Nov. 18, 2004, available at www.fda.gov/ola/2004/vioxx1118.html.

16. Sid Kirchheimer, "Painkiller Vioxx Often Taken at Too High Dose," WebMD.com, July 14, 2004, available at www.webmd.com/content/Article/90/100801.htm?pagenumber=1; Statement of Sandra Kweder, before the Committee on Finance.

17. Jüni et al., "Risk of Cardiovascular Events and Rofecoxib."

18. Alex Berenson, Gardiner Harris, Barry Meier, and Andrew Pollack, "Despite Warnings, Drug Giant Took Long Path to Vioxx Recall," *New York Times*, Nov. 14, 2004.

19. See table 1 and figure 3 of Jüni et al., "Risk of Cardiovascular Events and Rofe-coxib." Because of lack of labeling, it is difficult to match all of the numbers in figure 3 to table 1, but the dichotomy of early and late trials is striking and, to the extent that the points can be matched to trials, highly correlated with the use of naproxen or another NSAID. Ironically, the authors of the article used this data to argue that Vioxx should have been withdrawn several years earlier.

20. Marvin A. Konstam et al., "Cardiovascular Thrombotic Events in Con-trolled Clinical Trials of Rofecoxib," *Circulation* 104, no. 19 (Nov. 6, 2001): 2,280–88.

21. FitzGerald, Cheng, and Austin, "COX-2 Inhibitors and the Cardiovascular System"; FitzGerald, "Cardiovascular Pharmacology of Nonselective Nonste-roidal Anti-Inflammatory Drugs and Coxibs"; FitzGerald, "Prostaglandins: Modulators of Inflammation and Cardiovascular Risk."

22. Jüni et al., "Risk of Cardiovascular Events and Rofecoxib."

23. Debabrata Mukherjee, Steven E. Nissen, and Eric J. Topol, "Risk of Cardio-vascular Events Associated with Selective COX-2 Inhibitors," *Journal of the American Medical Association* 286, no. 8 (2001): 954–59.

24. Susan Ferraro, "Easing Arthritis: Are Controversial New Drugs Worth the Risk?" *New York Daily News*, Oct. 15, 2001.

25. Mukherjee, Nissen, and Topol, "Risk of Cardiovascular Events Associated with Selective COX-2 Inhibitors."

26. Interview with Steve Nissen by Patricia O'Connell, "Early Twinges over Vioxx," *Business Week*, Oct. 1, 2004, available at www.businessweek.com/bwdaily/dnflash/oct2004/nf20041011_4033_db008.htm.

27. Henderson and Hooper, "Clear Thinking About Vioxx."

28. Berenson, Harris, Meier, and Pollack, "Despite Warnings, Drug Giant Took Long Path to Vioxx Recall."

29. Robert S. Bresalier et al., "Cardiovascular Events Associated with Rofecoxib in a Colorectal Adenoma Chemoprevention Trial," *New England Journal of Medicine* 352, no. 11 (March 17, 2005): 1,092–102.

30. For one look at patient medication patterns in the wake of the Vioxx with-drawal see, M. P. Sukel et al., "Large-scale Stopping and Switching Treatment with COX-2 Inhibitors After the Rofecoxib Withdrawal," *Pharmacoepidemio-logical Drug Safety* 17, no. 1 (Jan. 2008): 9–19.

31. Rita Rubin, "How Did Vioxx Debacle Happen?" *USA Today*, Oct. 11, 2004, available at www.usatoday.com/life/lifestyle/2004-10-11-vioxx-main_x.htm.

32. Burton, "How Merck Stacked the Vioxx Deck."

33. James Doran, "US Officials 'Knew of Vioxx Threat,'" *Times*, Oct. 9, 2004, available at www.timesonline.co.uk/tol/news/uk/article492326.ece?print=yes&r andnum=1235769983951.

34. "Pazdur's Revenge," editorial, *Wall Street Journal*, Dec. 20, 2004.

35. Henderson and Hooper, "Clear Thinking About Vioxx."

36. Sukel et al., "Large-scale Stopping and Switching Treatment with COX-2 Inhibitors After the Rofecoxib Withdrawal."

37. Heather Won Tesoriero, "Patients Weigh Pain vs. Risk: Some Former Vioxx Takers Say Alternatives Fall Short or Carry Other Dangers," *Wall Street Journal*, Dec. 21, 2004.

38. "Vioxx: How Safe Is FDA Approval?" *Wired*, March 10, 2004.

39. Testimony of David Graham before the Committee on Finance, Nov. 18, 2004, reprinted at www.consumersunion.org/pub/campaignprescription forchange/001651.html.

40. Susan Dentzer, "Drug Failure," *NewsHour*, PBS.org, Nov. 18, 2004, available at www.pbs.org/newshour/bb/health/july-dec04/vioxx_11-18.html.

41. Rubin, "How Did Vioxx Debacle Happen?"

42. Ibid.

43. See table 3 and figure 4 of Jüni et al., "Risk of Cardiovascular Events and Rofecoxib."

44. Fadia T. Shaya et al., "Selective Cyclooxygenase-2 Inhibition and Cardiovascular Effects," *Archives of Internal Medicine* 165, no. 2 (Jan. 24, 2005): 181–86.

45. Rubin, "How Did Vioxx Debacle Happen?"

46. Rebecca Leung, "FDA: Harsh Criticism from Within," CBS News, Feb. 16, 2005, available at www.cbsnews.com/stories/2005/02/15/60II/main674293.shtml.

47. Statement of Sandra Kweder, before the Committee on Finance, Nov. 18, 2004.

48. Leung, "FDA: Harsh Criticism from Within."

49. Statement of Sandra Kweder, before the Committee on Finance, Nov. 18, 2004.

50. Leung, "FDA: Harsh Criticism from Within."

51. Doran, "US Officials 'Knew of Vioxx Threat.'"

52. Rubin, "How Did Vioxx Debacle Happen?"

53. Leung, "FDA: Harsh Criticism from Within."

54. Mary Duenwald, Anahad O'Connor, and Gardiner Harris, "For Pain Management, Doctors Prescribe Caution," *New York Times*, Feb. 20, 2005.

55. Ibid.

56. Matthew Herper and Robert Langreth, "Merck's High-Stakes Mistake," *Forbes*, Dec. 9, 2005, available at www.forbes.com/2005/12/09/vioxx-merck-nejm-cx_mh_rl_1209merckscience.html.

57. Stephanie Saul, "Pfizer to Finance $100 Million Safety Study of Celebrex," *New York Times*, Dec. 14, 2005, available at www.nytimes.com/2005/12/14/business/14drugs.html.

58. Amy Barrett, with John Carey, "Big Pharma's Favorite Gadfly," *BusinessWeek*, Dec. 19, 2005, available at www.businessweek.com/magazine/content/05_51/b3964073.htm.

59. Ibid.

60. Saul, "Pfizer to Finance $100 Million Safety Study of Celebrex."

61. Matthew Herper, "Saving A Potential Heart Breakthrough," *Forbes*, Sept. 27, 2004, available at www.forbes.com/2004/09/27/cx_mh_0927agix.html.

62. Peggy Peck, "Valdecoxib Meta-Analysis Suggests Increased Cardiovascular Risk," American Heart Association 2004 Scientific Sessions: Russell Ross Memorial Lectureship in Vascular Biology: Inflammatory Processes in Atherosclerosis, delivered Nov. 9, 2004, available at www.medscape.com/viewarticle/493612.

63. Gurkirpal Singh, Shweta Vadhavkar, Alka Mithal, and George Triadafilopoulos, "A New Safety Warning: Decreased Gastroprotection Is Associated with an Increase of Serious Ulcer Complications in Elderly Users of NSAIDs," American College of Rheumatology Annual Scientific Meeting, presentation 668, Nov. 8, 2007.

64. Christopher Maggos, "Blunt Instrument," *BioCentury: The Bernstein Report on BioBusiness* 13, no. 4 (Jan. 17, 2005).

65. "Pazdur's Revenge."

CHAPTER 5—WEB OF FEAR: VACCINES, AUTISM, AND THE EMERGENCE OF "INSTANT EXPERTS"

1. A. J. Wakefield et al., "Ileal-lymphoid-nodule Hyperplasia, Non-specific Colitis, and Pervasive Developmental Disorder in Children," *The Lancet* 351, no. 9103 (Feb. 1998): 637–41.

2. Arthur Allen, "A Recipe for Disaster," Salon.com, August 2, 2000, available at www.archive.salon.com/health/feature/2000/08/02/autism.html.

3. Paul A. Offit, *Autism's False Prophets: Bad Science, Risky Medicine, and the Search for a Cure* (New York: Columbia University Press, 2008), 44.

4. Allen, "A Recipe for Disaster."

5. Offit, *Autism's False Prophets*, 19.

6. V. Uhlmann et al., "Potential Viral Pathogenic Mechanism for New Variant Inflammatory Bowel Disease," *Molecular Pathology* 55, no. 2 (April 2002): 84–90.

7. O. Shiels et al., "Development of an 'Allelic Discrimination' Type Assay to Differentiate Between the Strain Origins of Measles Virus Detected in Intestinal Tissue of Children with Ileocolonic Lymphonodular Hyperplasia and Concomitant Developmental Disorder," abstract no. 20, presented at Pathological Society of Great Britain and Ireland (2002).

8. Offit, *Autism's False Prophets*, 64–65.

9. Gary L. Freed et al., "Policy Reaction to Thimerosal in Vaccines: A Comparative Study of the United States and Selected European Countries," Program for Appropriate Technology in Health (PATH), July 2001, available at www.path.org/vaccineresources/files/thimerosal_decision.pdf.

10. For details on how methyl and ethyl mercury differ in the body and why the use of methyl mercury guidelines may not be accurate, see Michael E. Pichichero et al., "Mercury Levels in Newborns and Infants After Receipt of Thimerosal-containing Vaccines," *Pediatrics* 121, no. 2 (Feb. 2008): e208–14.

11. Karin B. Nelson and Margaret L. Bauman, "Thimerosal and Autism," *Pediatrics* 111, no. 3 (March 3, 2003): 674–79.

12. Michael Pollack, "Doctors Fighting Backlash Over Vaccines," *New York Times*, April 27, 1999, available at www.query.nytimes.com/gst/fullpage.html?res=9E01E0D71E3AF934A15757C0A96F958260.

13. When a *New York Times* article supporting the connection between thimerosal and autism portrayed Halsey in what he believed was a misleading manner, he fired back to set the record straight and criticize the vaccine-autism hypothesis. See the *New York Times* article at www.query.nytimes.com/gst/fullpage.html?res=9B03EFD7153EF933A25752C1A9649C8B63, and Halsey's response at www.vaccinesafety.edu/NYT-LttE.htm. The author of the article, Arthur Allen, would turn his back on the thimerosal theory and become an influential opponent in his book *Vaccine: The Controversial Story of Medicine's Greatest Lifesaver* (New York: W.W. Norton, 2007).

14. Mark R. Geier and David A. Geier, "Neurodevelopmental Disorders after Thimerosal-Containing Vaccines: A Brief Communication," *Experimental Biology and Medicine* 228 (2003): 660–64.

15. Mark R. Geier and David A. Geier, "Thimerosal in Childhood Vaccines: Neurodevelopmental Disorders and Heart Disease in the United States," *Journal of American Physicians and Surgeons* 8, no. 1 (Spring 2003): 6–11; J. Bradstreet et al., "A Case-Control Study of Mercury Burden in Children with Autistic Spectrum Disorders," *Journal of American Physicians and Surgeons* 8, no. 3 (Summer 2003): 76–79.

16. A. S. Holmes, M. F. Blaxill, B. E. Haley, "Reduced Levels of Mercury in First Baby Haircuts of Autistic Children," *International Journal of Toxicology* 22, no. 4 (July–Aug. 2003): 277–85.

17. M. Waly et al., "Activation of Methionine Synthase by Insulin-Like Growth Factor-1 and Dopamine: A Target for Neurodevelopmental Toxins and Thimerosal," *Molecular Psychiatry* 9, no. 4 (2004): 358–70.

18. R. F. Berman et al., "Low-level Neonatal Thimerosal Exposure: Further Evaluation of Altered Neurotoxic Potential in SJL Mice," *Toxicology Science* 101, no. 2 (Feb. 2008): 358–70.

19. Rosalynn Carter and Betty Bumpers, "Some Parents Fall for Vaccination Scare Stories, with Deadly Results," Immunization Action Coalition, January 3, 2001, available at www.immunize.org/reports/report038.asp.

20. Annamari Patja et al., "Serious Adverse Events After Measles-Mumps-Rubella Vaccination During a Fourteen-Year Prospective Follow-Up," *Pediatric Infectious Disease Journal* 19, no. 12 (2000): 1,127–34.

21. Kreesten Madsen, Anders Hviid, et al. "A Population-based Study of Measles, Mumps, and Rubella Vaccination and Autism," *New England Journal of Medicine* 347, no. 19 (Nov. 7, 2002): 1,477–82.

22. P. Stehr Green et al., "Autism and Thimerosal-Containing Vaccines: Lack of Consistent Evidence for Association," *American Journal of Preventive Medicine* 25, no. 2 (August 2003): 101–6.

23. K. M. Madsen et al., "Thimerosal and the Occurrence Of Autism: Negative Ecological Evidence from Danish Population-Based Data," *Pediatrics* 112, no. 3, part 1 (Sept. 2003): 604–6.

24. A. Hviid et al., "Association Between Thimerosal-Containing Vaccine and Autism," *Journal of the American Medical Association* 290, no. 13 (October 2003): 1,763–66.

25. Immunization Safety Committee, "Immunization Safety Review," Institute of Medicine, May 17, 2004, available at www.nap.edu/catalog.php?record_id=10997#toc.

26. Daniel J. DeNoon, "Debate over Autism-Vaccine Link Intensifies," Fox News, July 13, 2005, available at www.foxnews.com/printer_friendly_story/0,3566,162314,00.html.

27. Shinnar et al., "Language Regression in Childhood," *Pediatric Neurology* 24, no. 3 (March 2001): 182–89, referenced in "What Do Parents Attribute Regression To?" blog post, Natural Variation, autism blog, Dec 27, 2006, available at www.autismnaturalvariation.blogspot.com/2006/12/what-do-parents-attribute-regression.html.

28. Julie Osterling and Geraldine Dawson, "Early Recognition of Children with Autism: A Study of First Birthday Home Videotapes," *Journal of Autism and Developmental Disorders* 24, no. 3 (1994): 247–57.

29. Arthur Allen, "Inoculated into oblivion," Salon.com, April 13, 2000, available at www.archive.salon.com/health/feature/2000/04/13/shot/index.html.

30. Offit, *Autism's False Prophets*, 121.

31. Arthur Allen, "Thimerosal on Trial," Slate.com, March 28, 2007. The Geiers would later begin to use a yet stronger prostate cancer drug, Androcur, which carries serious risks and is not FDA approved.

32. James R. Laidler, "Chelation and Autism," originally on Autism Watch, reproduced at www.neurodiversity.com/weblog/article/14.

33. Catherine Elsworth, "Autism Boy Dies After Alternative Therapy," *Telegraph*, Aug. 27, 2005, available at www.telegraph.co.uk/news/uknews/1496949/Autism-boy-dies-after-alternative-therapy.html.

34. Joanne Lauclus, "Research Gives Hope to Autistic Kids," *The Leader Post*, CanWest News Service, Dec. 7, 2007.

35. John Stossel, Kristina Kendall, and Patrick McMenamin, "Should Parents Worry About Vaccinating Their Children? Fears of Vaccinations Rise, Diseases Reemerge," ABC News, Feb. 22, 2007.

36. Mitzi Waltz and Paul Shattock, "Autistic Disorder in Nineteenth-century London," *Autism* 8, no. 1 (2004): 13, 15.

37. Dr. J. Landon Down, who would be credited with identifying Down syndrome, wrote in 1887 about both what we now call late-onset, or regressive, autism and "early-onset" autism in "mentally retarded" patients. (See "Abstract of the Lettsomian Lectures on Some of the Mental Affection of Childhood and Youth," Lecture II, delivered by J. Langdon Down, published in *The Lancet* [Jan. 22, 1887]: 256–59.) In 1908, Theodor Heller wrote about six children who regressed at age three or four, acquiring autistic behaviors. Once called dementia infantilism, today this is known as childhood disintegrative disorder (CDD), or Heller syndrome, and is on the autistic spectrum. (See Leo Kanner, "Childhood Psychosis: A Historical Overview," *Journal of Autism and Childhood Schizophrenia* 1, no. 1 [1971]: 16; and Marco T. Mercadante, Rutger J. Van der Gaag, and Jose S. Schwartzman, "Rett's Syndrome, Childhood Disintegrative Disorder and Pervasive Developmental Disorder Not Otherwise Specified," *Revista Brasileira de Psiquiatria* 28, suppl. 1 [2006]: 14, available at www.scielo.br/pdf/rbp/v28s1/en_a03v28s1.pdf.) Then, in 1926, a Russian scientist named G. E. Ssucharewa described six boys with what she called "schizoid personality," more or less identical to what is now called Asperger's syndrome. (See G. E. Ssucharewa, "Die schizoiden Psychopathien im Kindesalter," *Monatsschrift für Psychiatrie und Neurologie* 60 [1926]: 235–261. A translation is available as S. Wolff, "The First

Account of the Syndrome Asperger Described?" *European Child & Adolescent Psychiatry* 5, no. 3, [1996]: 119–132). In many cases, early researchers placed these cases under the heading of "infantile schizophrenia," a condition with which autism would remain identified, both by Kanner himself and by other doctors, until the 1970s. Indeed the term *autism* itself was coined in 1911, by Eugen Bleuler, to describe schizophrenia, although its meaning was somewhat changed by Asperger and Kanner.

38. Hans Asperger, "Die 'autistischen psychopathen' im kindesalter [The 'Autistic Psychopath' in Childhood]," *Archiv fur Psychiatrie und Nervenkrankheiten* 117 (1944): 128. An English translation can be found in Uta Frith, ed., *Autism and Asperger Syndrome* (Cambridge, UK: Cambridge University Press, 1991). Asperger actually first spoke about autism in 1938 to the Vienna Medical School (reprinted in *Wiener klinische Wochenschrift*), therefore predating Kanner. All translations from the German are by Caroline Patton.

39. Asperger, 134–35. The unnamed patient was highly academically accomplished; in addition to his PhD dissertation, he wrote a *Habilitationsschrift*, a second dissertation or thesis required in German-speaking countries to be qualified to be a professor. Unfortunately, because Asperger's records were destroyed when his clinic was bombed at the end of World War II, we do not know more about this patient or the others seen by Asperger and their identities have been lost. Excerpt from Roy Richard Grinker, *Unstrange Minds: Remapping the World of Autism* (New York: Basic Books, 2007), available at www.unstrange.com/unstrangeintro.html.

40. One such case is "Autism Misdiagnosis 'Ruined a Life,'" BBC News, June 27, 2000, available at www.news.bbc.co.uk/1/hi/health/787526.stm.

41. "Autism Misdiagnosis 'Ruined a Life,'" BBC News, June 27, 2000, available at www.news.bbc.co.uk/1/hi/health/787526.stm.

42. Meri Svoboda, "Forum School at Waldwick Offers 'Attic Children' Hope," *New York Times*, June 2, 1972.

43. Brita Schirmer, "Autismus und NS-Rassengesetze in Österreich 1938: Han Aspergers Verteidigung der 'autistischen Psychopathen' gegen die NS-Eugenik [Autism and NS Race Law in Austria 1938: Hans Asperger's Defense of the 'Autistic Psychopaths' Against NS Eugenics]," available at www.beltz.de/neusonderschule/s_02_04.htm. There unfortunately does not appear to be an English translation available.

44. For example, in the United Kingdom, the number of adults diagnosed increased from 4,220 in 1997/1998 to 9,170 in 2005, an increase of 217 percent, compared to a 199 percent increase in diagnoses for children under age sixteen. (Nic Fleming and Pat Hagan, "Pesticides Blamed as Autism Rate Soars," *Daily Telegraph*, March 25, 2006.)

45. The Committee on Nomenclature and Statistics of the American Psychiatric Association, *Diagnostic and Statistical Manual: Mental Disorders*, 2nd ed. (Washington, D.C.: American Psychiatric Association Mental Hospital Service, 1968), available at www.psychiatryonline.com/DSMPDF/dsm-ii.pdf, and the Committee on Nomenclature and Statistics of the American Psychiatric Association, *Diagnostic and Statistical Manual: Mental Disorders* (Washington, D.C.: American Psychiatric Association Mental Hospital Service, 1952), available at www.psychiatryonline.com/DSMPDF/dsm-i.pdf.

46. American Psychiatric Association, *Diagnostic and Statistical Manual of Mental Disorders*, 3rd ed. (Washington, D.C.: American Psychiatric Association, 1980).

47. Claudia Wallis, "Is the Autism Epidemic a Myth?" *Time*, Jan. 12, 2007.

48. John Stossel, Kristina Kendall, and Patrick McMenamin, "Should Parents Worry About Vaccinating Their Children?" ABC News, Feb. 22, 2007, available at www.abcnews.go.com/2020/Health/story?id=2892683&page=1.

49. Lidia Wasowicz, "Ped Med: Confounding Autism Counts," UPI, Oct. 18, 2006.

50. Allen, "Inoculated into Oblivion."

51. Wallis, "Is the Autism Epidemic a Myth?"

52. Arthur Allen, "Sticking up for Thimerosal," Slate.com, Aug. 2, 2005.

53. Offit, *Autism's False Prophets*, 237.

54. L. K. Ball, R. Ball, and R. D. Pratt, "An Assessment of Thimerosal Use in Childhood Vaccines," *Pediatrics* 107, no. 5 (2001): 1,147–54.

55. The introduction is reprinted on Kirby's website at www.evidenceofharm.com/introduction.htm.

56. The following blog post explains thoroughly and clearly the problems with such a study: "'Let's Put on a Study!'" blog post, A Photon in the Darkness, November 3, 2008, available at www.photoninthedarkness.com/?p=154.

57. Robert F. Kennedy, Jr., "Deadly Immunity," Salon.com, June 16, 2005, available at www.dir.salon.com/story/news/feature/2005/06/16/thimerosal.

58. Verstraeten et al., "Safety of Thimerosal-Containing Vaccines: A Two-Phase Study of Computerized Health Maintenance Organization Databases," *Pediatrics* 112, no. 5 (Nov. 2003): 1,039–48.

59. To see how the quotes were parsed in order to produce a false impression, see "Lies, Damn Lies, and Quote Mining," blog post, Skeptico.com, June 29, 2005, available at www.skeptico.blogs.com/skeptico/2005/06/lies_damn_lies_.html.

60. Darshak Sanghavi, "The Secret Truth," *Boston Globe*, Dec. 4, 2005, reprinted at www.darshaksanghavi.com/columns/secrettruth.htm.

61. Sanghavi, "The Secret Truth"; Offit, *Autism's False Prophets*, 47–48.

62. For details on the problems with the biopsy samples, please see Dr. Nicholas Chadwick's testimony to the court of the National Immunization Compensation Program, U.S. Court of Federal Claims, docket 98–916V, June 22, 2007, 2284-229-0.

63. "Journal Repents Over Vaccine-Autism Link," *The Sydney Morning Herald*, Feb. 23, 2004, available at www.smh.com.au/articles/2004/02/22/1077384637563. html.

64. Glenn Frankel, "Charismatic Doctor at Vortex of Vaccine Dispute," *Washington Post*, July 11, 2004, available at www.washington-post.com/wp-dyn/articles/A41450-2004Jul10.html.

65. Michael Fitzpatrick, "'The MMR-Autism Theory? There's Nothing in It,'" Spiked.com, July 4, 2007, available at www.spiked-online.com/index.php?/site/article/3562.

66. Offit, *Autism's False Prophets*, 48–49.

67. Gardiner Harris and Anahad O'Connor, "On Autism's Cause, It's Parent vs. Research," *New York Times*, June 25, 2005, available at www.nytimes. com/2005/06/25/science/25autism.html.

68. H. Honda et al., "No Effect of MMR Withdrawal on the Incidence of Autism: A Total Population Study," *Journal of Child Psychology and Psychiatry* 46, no. 6 (2005): 572–79.

69. Eric Fombonne et al., "Pervasive Developmental Disorders in Montreal, Quebec, Canada: Prevalence and Links with Immunizations," *Pediatrics* 118, no. 1 (July 2006): e139–50.

70. William W. Thompson et al., "Early Thimerosal Exposure and Neuropsychological Outcomes at 7 to 10 Years," *New England Journal of Medicine* 357, no. 13 (Sept. 27, 2007): 1,281–92.

71. Offit, *Autism's False Prophets*, xi.

72. Virginia Hughes, "Mercury Rising," *Nature Medicine* 13 (Aug. 1, 2007): 896–97.

73. Dan Childs, "Death Threats, Hate Mail: Autism Debate Turns Ugly: Vaccine Researchers, Autism Community React to Account of Death Threats," ABC News, Oct. 31, 2008, available at www.abcnews.go.com/print?id=6150482.

74. Mady Hornig et al., "Lack of Association Between Measles Virus Vaccine and Autism with Enteropathy: A Case Control Study," *PLoS ONE* 3, no. 9 (2008): e3,140.

75. Alberto Eugenio Tozzi et al., "Neuropsychological Performance 10 Years After Immunization in Infancy with Thimerosal-Containing Vaccines," *Pediatrics* 123, no. 2 (Feb. 2, 2009): 475–82.

76. Virginia Hughes, "Unraveling Mitochondria's Mysterious Link To Autism," Simmons Foundation Autism Research Initiative, March 24, 2008, available at www.sfari.org/news/unraveling-mitochondria-s-mysterious-link-to-autism.

77. Donald G. McNeil, Jr., "Court Says Vaccines Not to Blame for Autism," *New York Times*, Feb. 12, 2009, available at www.nytimes.com/2009/02/13/health/13vaccine.html?_r=1; U.S. Court of Federal Claims, Office of Special Masters, no. 98-916V, decision by George L. Hastings, Jr., in *Cedillo v. U.S. Department of Health and Human Services*, Feb. 12, 2009, pp. 2, 173, available at www.neurodiversity.com/court/cedillo_v_hhs_docket.html.

78. U.S. Court of Federal Claims, Office of Special Masters, no. 01-162V, decision by Denise K. Vowell in case of *Snyder v. U.S. Department of Health and Human Services*, Feb. 12, 2009, p. 278, available at www.uscfc.uscourts.gov/sites/default/files/vaccine_files/Vowell.Snyder.pdf.

79. Steven Salzberg, "Vaccine Court Ruling: Thimerosal Does Not Cause Autism," blog entry, The Science Business, *Forbes*, March 15, 2010, available at www.blogs.forbes.com/sciencebiz/2010/03/vaccine-court-ruling-thimerosal-does-not-cause-autism.

80. Centers for Disease Control, "National, State, and Local Area Vaccination Among Children 19–35 Months: United States, 2007," *MMWR Weekly* 57, no. 35 (Sept. 5, 2008), available at www.cdc.gov/mmwr/preview/mmwrhtml/mm5735a1.htm.

81. "Measles Returns," editorial, *New York Times*, Aug. 24, 2008.

82. "Fears of Measles Epidemic as Cases Soar to 13-year High in Wake of MMR Scare," *Daily Mail*, Dec. 3, 2008, available at www.dailymail.co.uk/health/article-1090149/Fears-measles-epidemic-cases-soar-13-year-high-wake-MMR-scare.html.

83. "Whooping cough makes a comeback," ABC News, Dec. 26, 2008, available at www.abclocal.go.com/wtvd/story?section=news/health&id=6573439; Laura Unger, "Whooping Cough Rates Rise," *Detroit Free Press*, Dec. 24, 2008, available at www.freep.com/article/20081224/FEATURES08/812240397; Riki Markowitz, "Pertussis Outbreak in Austin and Travis County," *Examiner*, Feb. 23, 2010, available at www.examiner.com/x-38309-Austin-Allergy-Examiner~y2010m2d23-Pertussis-outbreak-in-Austin-and-Travis-County; Alicia Gallegos, "South Bend Couple Loses Baby to Pertussis," *South Bend Tribune*, Feb. 28, 2010, available at www.southbendtribune.com/article/20100228/News01/2280367/1129/News.

84. K. Henry et al., "Mumps Outbreak at a Summer Camp—New York, 2005," *MMWR*, Feb. 24, 2006, available www.immunize.org/reports/report083.asp; Liz Szabo, "Missed Vaccines Weaken 'Herd Immunity' in Children," *USA Today*, Jan. 6, 2010.

85. Szabo, "Missed Vaccines Weaken 'Herd Immunity' in Children."

86. Brian Deer, "Hidden Records Show MMR Truth," *Sunday Times*, Feb. 8, 2009, available at www.timesonline.co.uk/tol/life_and_style/health/article5683643.ece.

87. General Medical Council, "Fitness to Practise Panel Hearings," Jan. 28, 2010, available at www.scribd.com/doc/25983372/FACTS-WWSM-280110-Final-Complete-Corrected.

88. Nick Triggle, "Lancet Accepts MMR Study 'False,'" BBC, Feb. 2, 2010, available at www.news.bbc.co.uk/2/hi/health/8493753.stm; Associated Press, "Vaccine-Autism Study Is Retracted," *New York Times*, Feb. 2, 2010, available at www.nytimes.com/aponline/2010/02/02/health/AP-EU-Britain-Medical-Journal.html?_r=1&em.

89. While the article—Laura Hewitson et al., "Delayed Acquisition of Neonatal Reflexes in Newborn Primates Receiving a Thimerosal-containing Hepatitis B Vaccine: Influence of Gestational Age and Birth Weight," electronic publication only, *Neurotoxicology* (2009)—is still available online (as of Feb. 21, 2010), it is clearly marked as withdrawn and contains a note on the decision and a link to the journal's policy on the decision.

90. Sam Lister, "Disgraced MMR-scare Doctor Andrew Wakefield Quits U.S. Clinic He Founded," (London) *Times*, Feb. 19, 2010, available at www.timesonline.co.uk/tol/life_and_style/health/article7032762.ece.

91. Amy Wallace, "An Epidemic of Fear: How Panicked Parents Skipping Shots Endangers Us All," Wired.com, Oct. 19, 2009, available at www.wired.com/magazine/2009/10/ff_waronscience.

CHAPTER 6—THE SUICIDE CRISIS: SOWING FEAR ABOUT ANTIDEPRESSANTS

1. Kevin Roy, "Too Young to Die," special segment on ABC-7 News, March 31, 2008, available at http://abclocal.go.com/wls/story?section=news/special_segments&id=6051243.

2. Walter A. Brown, "Understanding and Using the Placebo Effect," *Psychiatric Times* 23, no. 11 (Oct. 1, 2006).

3. Jeffrey A. Bridge et al., "Placebo Response in Randomized Controlled Trials of Antidepressants for Pediatric Major Depressive Disorder," *American Journal of Psychiatry* 166 (2009): 42–49.

4. Treatment for Adolescents with Depression Study (TADS) Team, "Fluoxetine, Cognitive-Behavioral Therapy, and Their Combination for Adolescents with Depression," *JAMA* 292 (2004).

5. Graham J. Emslie et al., "A Double-blind, Randomized, Placebo-Controlled Trial of Fluoxetine in Children and Adolescents with Depression," *Archives of General Psychiatry* 54, no. 11 (1997).

6. Ibid.

7. A few examples are: Daniel A. Geller et al., "Fluoxetine Treatment for Obsessive-Compulsive Disorder in Children and Adolescents: A Placebo-Controlled Clinical Trial," *Journal of the American Academy of Child and Adolescent Psychiatry* 40, no. 7 (July 2001); Michael R. Liebowitz et al., "Fluoxetine in Children and Adolescents with OCD: A Placebo Controlled Trial," *Journal of the American Academy of Child and Adolescent Psychiatry* 41, no. 12 (Dec. 2002); Boris Birmaher et al., "Fluoxetine for the Treatment of Childhood Anxiety Disorders," *Journal of the American Academy of Child and Adolescent Psychiatry* 42, no. 4 (April 2003).

8. Quoted in Erica Goode, "Researchers Find Zoloft, a Popular Antidepressant, to Be Effective in Treating Children," *New York Times*, Aug. 27, 2003; Karen Dineen Wagner et al., "Efficacy of Sertraline in the Treatment of Children and Adolescents with Major Depressive Disorder: Two Randomized Controlled Trials," *JAMA* 290, no. 8 (2003).

9. J. John Mann et al., "ACNP Task Force Report on SSRIs and Suicidal Behavior in Youth," *Neuropsychopharmacology* 31 (2006).

10. Jeffrey A. Bridge, PhD et al., "Clinical Response and Risk for Reported Suicidal Ideation and Suicide Attempts in Pediatric Antidepressant Treatment," *JAMA* 297, no. 15 (April 18, 2007).

11. Sarah Boseley, "GPs Accused of Not Reporting Seroxat Suicides," *The Guardian*, May 9, 2003.

12. Erica Goode, "Once Again, Prozac Takes Center Stage, in Furor," *New York Times*, July 18, 2000.

13. M. H. Teicher, C. Glod, and J. O. Cole, "Emergence of Intense Suicidal Preoccupation During Fluoxetine treatment," *American Journal of Psychiatry* 147 (1990): 207–10.

14. Goode, "Once Again, Prozac Takes Center Stage, in Furor."

15. Donald F. Klein, "The Flawed Basis for FDA Post-Marketing Safety Decisions: The Example of SSRIs and Children," *Neuropsychopharmacology* 31 (2006): 689–99.

16. M. B. Keller et al., "Efficacy of Paroxetine in the Treatment of Adolescent Major Depression: A Randomized Controlled Trial," *Journal of the American Academy of Child and Adolescent Psychiatry* 40 (2001): 762–72.

17. Jim Rosack, "Data Fail to Answer Key Questions About SSRIs," *Psychiatry News* 39, no. 6 (2004): 2.

18. Ibid.

19. Goode, "Once Again, Prozac Takes Center Stage, in Furor."; Lauren Neegard, "FDA Cites Possible Suicide Risk in Paxil," Associated Press, June 19, 2003.

20. Gardiner Harris, "Britain Says Use of Paxil By Children Is Dangerous," *New York Times*, June 11, 2003.

21. Gardiner Harris, "Antidepressants Restudied for Relation to Child Suicide," *New York Times*, June 20, 2004.

22. Tarek A. Hammad, Thomas Laughren, and Judith Racoosin, "Suicidality in Pediatric Patients Treated with Antidepressant Drugs," *Archives of General Psychiatry* 63, no. 3 (March 2006); Wayne K. Goodman, Tanya K. Murphy, and Eric A. Storch, "Risk of Adverse Behavioral Effects with Pediatric Use of Antidepressants," *Psychopharmacology* 191 (2007), 89; Susan J. Landers, "Panel: SSRIs Don't Increase Teen Suicide Risk," *American Medical News*, Feb. 9, 2004, available at www.ama-assn.org/amednews/2004/02/09/hlsb0209.htm.

23. Robert D. Gibbons et al., "The Relationship Between Antidepressant Medication Use and Rate of Suicide," *Archives of General Psychiatry* 62 (2005): 165–72.

24. M. Olfson et al., "Relationship Between Antidepressant Medication Treatment and Suicide in Adolescents," *Archives of General Psychiatry* 60 (2003): 978–82.

25. Statistic quoted from Dr. Rudorfer in Gardiner Harris, "F.D.A. Panel Urges Stronger Warning on Antidepressants," *New York Times*, Sept. 15, 2004, available at www.nytimes.com/2004/09/15/health/15depress.html.

26. Elaine Schmidt, "New UCLA Study Disputes Antidepressant/Suicide Link; Scientists Fear Rise in Deaths from Untreated Depression," news release, UCLA, Feb. 2, 2005, available at www.newsroom.ucla.edu/portal/ucla/New-UCLA-Study-Disputes-Antidepressant-5880.aspx?RelNum=5880.

27. One example of a combination is the aforementioned study by the TADS Team, "Fluoxetine, Cognitive-Behavioral Therapy, and Their Combination for Adolescents with Depression."

28. Quoted in Daniel DeNoon, "Link Between Teen Suicides, Antidepressants Question," Fox News, Dec. 15, 2004, available at www.foxnews.com/story/0,2933,141607,00.html.

29. Quoted in Chris Catizone, "Focus on Your Health: Antidepressants," *The Next Generation* 2, no. 1 available at www.nextgenmd.org/vol2-1/antidepressantsv2i1.html.

30. Hiroko Akagi and T. Manoj Kumar, "Akathisia: Overlooked at a Cost," *British Medical Journal* 324 (June 22, 2002); "Teen Suicide and Antidepressants: Harvard Psychiatrists Review Black Box Warning," press release, Harvard Medical School, Dec. 5, 2005, available at www.hms.harvard.edu/news/pressreleases/cha/1105teensuicide.html.

31. Shankar Vedantam, "FDA Links Antidepressants, Youth Suicide Risk," *Washington Post*, Feb. 3, 2004.

32. Ian R. Sharp and Jason E. Chapman, "Antidepressants and Increased Suicidality: The Media Portrayal of Controversy," *The Scientific Review of Mental Health Practice* 3, no. 1 (Summer 2004), available at www.srmhp.org/0301/media-watch.html.

33. Wayne Kondro and Barbara Sibbald, "Drug Company Experts Advised Staff to Withhold Information About SSRI Use in Children," *Canadian Medical Association Journal* 170, no. 5 (March 2, 2004), available at www.cmaj.ca/cgi/content/full/170/5/783.

34. Martin B. Keller et al., "Efficacy of Paroxetine in the Treatment of Adolescent Major Depression: A Randomized, Controlled Trial," *Journal of the American Academy of Child & Adolescent Psychiatry* 40, no. 7 (2001); SmithKline Beecham (which would become GlaxoSmithKline), "A Multi-center, Double-blind, Placebo Controlled Study of Paroxetine and Imipramine in Adolescents with Unipolar Major Depression-Acute Phase: 329," Nov. 24, 1998, available at www.gsk.com/media/paroxetine/Depression_329_full.pdf.

35. SmithKline Beecham, "A Double-blind, Multicentre Placebo Controlled Study of Paroxetine in Adolescents with Unipolar Major Depression: 377," Nov. 19, 1998, available at www.gsk.com/media/paroxetine/Depression_377_full.pdf.

36. Kondro and Sibbald, "Drug Company Experts Advised Staff to Withhold Information About SSRI Use in Children."

37. All these studies can be found at www.gsk.com/media/paroxetine.htm.

38. "GlaxoSmithKline CEO: 'We Had to Absorb a Number of Hits,'" Alliance for Human Research Protection, Feb. 16, 2004, available at www.ahrp.org/infomail/04/02/16.php.

39. Julie Wilson, "Seroxat/Paxil Adolescent Depression: Position Paper on the Phase III Clinical Studies," internal document, October 1998 and accompanying cover letter by Jackie Westaway, Oct. 14, 1998. Both available at www.ahrp.org/risks/SSRI0204/GSKpaxil/index.php.

40. Benedict Carey, "U.S. Panel Recommends Extending Suicide Warnings on Antidepressants," *New York Times*, Dec. 14, 2006.

41. Quoted in "FDA Tones Down Warning: Shyra Kallas an SSRI Suicide Victim," Alliance for Human Research Protection, March 4, 2005, available at www.ahrp.org/infomail/05/03/04a.php.

42. Jay M. Pomerantz, "After the Black Box Warning: Treating Children and Adolescents Who Have Depression," Medscape, Aug. 24, 2005, available at www.medscape.com/viewarticle/504164.

43. Ann M. Libby et al., "Decline in Treatment of Pediatric Depression After FDA Advisory on Risk of Suicidality with SSRIs," *American Journal of Psychiatry*

164, no. 6, (2007): 883–91; Gibbons et al., "The Relationship Between Anti-depressant Medication Use and Rate of Suicide."

44. Libby et al., "Decline in Treatment of Pediatric Depression."

45. "Suicide Trends Among Youths and Young Adults Aged 10–24 Years: United States 1990–2004," *MMWR* 56, no. 35 (2007), available at www.cdc.gov/mmwr/preview/mmwrhtml/mm5635a2.htm.

46. John L. McIntosh, PhD, "U.S.A. Suicide 2006: Official Final Data," American Association for Suicidology, April 19, 2009; data for 2006 and 2007 from Centers for Disease Control's Web-based Injury Statistics Query and Reporting System (WISQARS), accessed June 4, 2010.

47. Quoted in Daniel J. DeNoon, "Did FDA Teen Suicide Warning Backfire?" WebMD, Sept. 13, 2007, available at www.children.webmd.com/news/20070913/did-fda-teen-suicide-warning-backfire.

48. Libby et al., "Decline in Treatment of Pediatric Depression."

49. Michael Johnsen, "Doctors May Remain Loyal to SSRIs Despite Well-Publicized Teen Suicides," Drug Store News, March 22, 2004, reprinted at http://findarticles.com/p/articles/mi_m3374/is_4_26/ai_114742881/; Owen Dyer, "Did We Get It All Wrong About SSRIs and Youth Suicide?: New Data Shows Suicide Spike After Warning. Kids Undertreated," *National Review of Medicine* 4, no. 16 (2007).

50. Statistics quoted by Dr. David Fassler in Johnsen, "Doctors may remain loyal to SSRIs."

51. Anne M. Libby, Heather D. Orton, and Robert J. Valuck, "Persisting Decline in Depression Treatment after FDA Warnings," *Archives of General Psychiatry* 66, no. 6 (2009).

52. Joseph Mercola, "How Could Drug Companies Be So Evil?" May 15, 2004, available at www.mercola.com/2004/may/15/drug_companies_evil.htm.

53. Libby et al., "Decline in Treatment of Pediatric Depression"; Gibbons et al., "The Relationship Between Antidepressant Medication Use and Rate of Suicide."

54. Benji T. Kurian et al., "Effect of Regulatory Warnings on Antidepressant Prescribing for Children and Adolescents," *Archives of Pediatrics and Adolescent Medicine* 161, no. 7 (2007).

55. Benedict W. Wheeler et al., "The Population Impact on Incidence of Suicide and Non-Fatal Self-Harm of Regulatory Action Against the Use of Selective Serotonin Reuptake Inhibitors in Under 18s in the United Kingdom: Ecological Study," *British Medical Journal* 336 (March 8, 2008).

56. Gibbons et al., "The Relationship Between Antidepressant Medication Use and Rate of Suicide."

57. Amy Cheung, MD et al., "Pediatric Prescribing Practices and the FDA Black Box Warning on Antidepressants," *Journal of Developmental and Behavioral Pediatrics* 29, no. 3 (2008).

58. Laurence Y. Katz et al., "Effect of Regulatory Warnings on Antidepressant Prescription Rates, Use of Health Services and Outcomes Among Children, Adolescents, and Young Adults," *Canadian Medical Association Journal* 178, no. 8 (2008).

59. Ibid. Statistics on suicides in children age five to nineteen between 2000 and 2005 are drawn from Statistics Canada, accessed Nov. 27, 2009.

60. Quoted in Andrea Gordon, "Unintended Consequences: Teen Suicides Rise as Antidepressant Use Falls," Health Zone, April 9, 2008, available at www.healthzone.ca/health/mind%20amp;%20mood/article/412587-teen-suicides-rise-as-antidepressant-use-falls.

61. Quoted in Tony Dokoupil, "Trouble in a 'Black Box': Did an Effort to Reduce Teen Suicides Backfire?" *Newsweek*, July 16, 2007.

62. Gibbons et al., "The Relationship Between Antidepressant Medication Use and Rate of Suicide"; Benedict Carey, "U.S. Panel Recommends Extending Suicide Warnings on Antidepressants," *New York Times*, Dec. 14, 2006.

63. Silvia Paddock et al., "Association of GRIK4 with Outcome of Antidepressant Treatment in the STAR*D Cohort," *American Journal of Psychiatry* 164 (Aug. 2007). Other research indicates that genetic tests may allow psychiatrists to choose the drug that is the best and the most likely to work for their patients and to anticipate whether adverse effects are likely. Richard A. Friedman, MD, "On the Horizon, Personalized Depression Drugs," *New York Times*, June 19, 2007; Zhe-Yu Chen et al., "Genetic Variant BDNF (Val66Met) Polymorphism Alters Anxiety-Related Behavior," *Science* 314, no. 5,796 (2006).

CHAPTER 7—ASSAULT ON SCIENTISTS: THE CONFLICT-OF-INTEREST CANARD

1. David Willman, "Stealth Merger: Drug Companies and Government Medical Research," *Los Angeles Times*, Dec. 7, 2003, available at www.articles.latimes.com/2003/dec/07/nation/na-nih7.

2. Editorial, "Double Dipping at NIH: 'The Gaming Must End,'" *Washington Post*, July 6, 2004.

3. Rick Weiss, "NIH Ban Collaboration with Outside Companies," *Washington Post*, Sept. 24, 2004; Rick Weiss, "NIH Clears Most Researchers in Conflict-of-Interest Probe," *Washington Post*, Feb. 23, 2005; Jocelyn Kaiser, "Feeling the Heat, NIH Tightens Conflict-of-Interest Rules," *Science* 305, no. 5,680 (2004);

Bette-Jane Crigger, "The Curious Saga of Congress, the NIH, and Conflict of Interest," *Hastings Center Report* 35, no. 2, (March–April 2005): 13–4.

4. Marcia Angell, "Drug Companies & Doctors: A Story of Corruption," *The New York Review of Books*, January 15, 2009.

5. Vannevar Bush, "Science: The Endless Frontier," Washington, D.C.: U.S. Government Printing Office, 1945, available at www.nsf.gov/od/lpa/nsf50/vbush1945.htm#summary.

6. Susan Hockfield, "The Next Step in Stimulus: Long-Term Economic Growth," *Boston Globe*, Feb. 13, 2009.

7. U.S. Food and Drug, "The History of Drug Regulation in the United States," available at www.fda.gov/AboutFDA/WhatWeDo/History/FOrgsHistory/CDER/CenterforDrugEvaluationandResearchBrochureandChronology/ucm114470.htm.

8. Cari Tuna, "When Combined Data Reveal the Flaw of Averages," *Wall Street Journal*, Dec. 9, 2009, available at www.wsj.com/article/SB125970744553071829.html.

9. Tammy J. Clifford, Nicholas J. Barrowman, and David Moher, "Funding Source, Trial Outcome and Reporting Quality: Are They Related? Results of a Pilot Study," *BMC Health Services Research* 2 (2002): 18.

10. Daniele Fanelli, "Do Pressures to Publish Increase Scientists' Bias?: An Empirical Support from U.S. States Data," *PLoS One* 5, no. 4 (2010): e10,271.

11. Bodil Als-Nielsen et al., "Association of Funding and Conclusions in Randomized Drug Trials: A Reflection of Treatment Effect or Adverse Events?" *JAMA* 290 (2003): 921–28.

12. Joel Lexchin et al., "Pharmaceutical Industry Sponsorship and Research Outcome and Quality: Systematic Review," *British Medical Journal* 326 (2003).

13. See for instance Benjamin Djubegovic et al., "The Uncertainty Principle and Industry-Sponsored Research," *Lancet* 356, (2000): 635–638, Lise L. Kjaergard et al., "Association between Competing Interests and Authors' Conclusions: Epidemiological Study of Randomised Clinical Trials Published in the BMJ," *BMJ* 325, (2000): 249–53, and Jennifer J. Anderson et al., "Secular Changes in Published Clinical Trials of Second-Line Agents in Rheumatoid Arthritis," *Arthritis & Rheumatism* 34 (1991): 1,304–9.

14. David Conen, Jose Torres, Paul M. Ridker, "Differential citation rates of major cardiovascular clinical trials according to source of funding: a survey from 2000 to 2005," *Circulation*, vol. 118, no. 13 (2008): 1,321–1,327.

15. Henry Thomas Stelfox et al., "Conflict of Interest in the Debate over Calcium-Channel Antagonists," *New England Journal of Medicine* 338, no. 2 (Jan. 8, 1998).

16. Neal S. Young, John P. A. Ioannidis, and Omar Al-Ubaydli, "Why Current Publication Practices May Distort Science," *PLoS Medicine* 5, no. 10 (2008): e201.

17. Anthony N. DeMaria, "Your Soul for a Pen?" *Journal of the American College of Cardiology* 49, no. 11 (2007).

18. "About Academic Detailing," RxFacts, available at www.rxfacts.org/detailing. php.

19. One example is Randall S. Stafford et al., "Impact of the ALLHAT/JNC7 Dissemination Project on Thiazide-type Diuretic Use," *Archives of Internal Medicine* 170 (2010): 851–58.

20. S. Van McCrary et al., "A National Survey of Policies on Disclosure of Conflicts of Interest in Biomedical Research," *New England Journal of Medicine* 343, no. 22 (Nov. 30, 2000).

21. James Robert Brown, "Funding, Objectivity and the Socialization of Medical Research," *Science and Engineering Ethics* 8, no. 3 (2002).

22. John McKenzie, "Medical Journal Changes Independent Policy," ABC News, June 12, 2002, www.abcnews.go.com/WNT/story?id=130296&page=1.

23. Niteesh K. Choudhry, Henry Thomas Stelfox, and Allan S. Detsky, "Relationships Between Authors of Clinical Practice Guidelines and the Pharmaceutical Industry," *JAMA* 287, no. 5 (Feb. 6, 2002).

24. Lynn A. Jansen and Daniel P. Sulmasy, "Bioethics, Conflicts of Interest, and the Limits of Transparency," *Hastings Center Report* 33, no. 4, (2003).

25. Kenneth J. Rothman, "Conflict of Interest: The New McCarthyism in Science," *JAMA* 269, vol. 21, (1993): 2,782–84.

26. Martin J. Tobin, "Conflicts of Interest and AJRCCM: Restating Policy and a New Form to Upload," *American Journal of Respiratory and Critical Care Medicine* 167 (2003).

27. Jansen and Sulmasy, "Bioethics, Conflicts of Interest, and the Limits of Transparency."

28. The best source for a comprehensive look at the controversy is Daniel J. Kevles, *The Baltimore Case: A Trial of Politics, Science, and Character* (New York: W.W. Norton and Company, Inc., 1998). A good understanding of the evolution of the scandal and its depiction in the press can be found by looking at the *New York Times* coverage, of which selected articles include: "A Scientific Watergate," *New York Times*, March 26, 1991; Associated Press, "Scientist Accused of Faking Data Call the Scandal a 'Witch Hunt,'" *New York Times*, May 17, 1991; Philip J. Hilts, "Science and the Stain of Scandal," *New York Times*, Dec. 4, 1991; Philip J. Hilts, "Inquiry Finds a Researcher Faked Work," *New York Times*, Nov. 27, 1994; "Noted Finding of Scientific Fraud Is Overturned by a Federal Panel," *New York Times*, June 22, 1996; Gina Kolata,

"Inquiry Lacking Due Process," *New York Times*, June 25, 1996. The final verdict of the Research Integrity Adjudication Panel dismissing the charges is available at the Department of Health and Human Services, Departmental Appeals Board, Research Integrity Adjudication Panel, "Thereza Imanishi-Kari, Ph.D., DAB No. 1582 (1996)," June 21, 1996, available at www.hhs.gov/dab/decisions/dab1582.html.

29. Leon Jaroff, "Crisis in the Labs," *Time*, June 24, 2001, available at www.time.com/time/magazine/article/0,9171,157723,00.html.

30. Hamilton Moses III et al., "Financial Anatomy of Biomedical Research," *JAMA* 294, no. 11 (Sept. 21, 2005); Bekelman, Li, and Gross, "Scope and Impact of Financial Conflicts of Interest in Biomedical Research."

31. For more information on NIH appropriation, see the appropriations chart at www.nih.gov/about/almanac/appropriations/index.htm. Note that you must use the tabs for both section 1 and section 2 in order to see all of the funding.

32. Joseph B. Martin and Thomas P. Reynolds, "Academic-Industrial Relationships: Opportunities and Pitfalls," *Science and Engineering Ethics* 8, no. 3 (2002).

33. Moses et al., "Financial Anatomy of Biomedical Research"; Brandon Keim, "When Is a Conflict of Interest a Conflict?" *Wired Science*, Oct. 3, 2007, available at www.blog.wired.com/wiredscience/2007/10/when-is-a-confl.html.

34. James N. Weinstein, "Conflict of Interest: Art of Science? The Hippocratic Solution," *Spine* 27, no. 1 (2002).

35. Paul J. Friedman, "The Impact of Conflict of Interest on Trust in Science," *Science and Engineering Ethics* 8, no. 3 (2002).

36. Linda Brookes, "ALLHAT—Criticisms and Contradictions: An Expert Interview with Michael A. Weber, MD," Medscape Cardiology, Feb. 21, 2003, available at www.medscape.com/viewarticle/449606.

37. Remarks reproduced in "ALLHAT and CATIE Reconsidered: Reflections on Big Studies and Evidence Based Medicine as the Measure of Comparative Effectiveness," Center for Medicine in the Public Interest, available at www.cmpi.org/about-us/events/allhat-and-catie-reconsidered.

38. Ibid.

39. Norman G. Levinsky, "Nonfinancial Conflicts of Interest in Research," *New England Journal of Medicine* 347, no. 10 (Sept. 5, 2002).

40. Martin J. Tobin, "Conflicts of Interest and AJRCCM: Restating Policy and a New Form to Upload," *American Journal of Respiratory and Critical Care Medicine* 167 (2003).

41. Eliot Marshall, "When Does Intellectual Passion Become Conflict of Interest?" *Science* 257 (July 31, 1992).

42. Ibid.

43. Robert M. Goldberg and Peter Pitts, "Plaque Problem," The Washington Times, June 5, 2007. www.washingtontimes.com/news/2007/jun/5/2007 0605-092646-4828r.

44. Michael Tremblay, "Who to Trust?" Comment on Thomas P. Stossel, "Head to Head: Has the Hunt for Conflicts of Interest Gone too Far? Yes," British Medical Journal 336, no. 476 (March 1, 2008); and Kirby Lee, "Head to Head: Has the Hunt for Conflicts of Interest Gone too Far? No," British Medical Journal 336, no. 477 (March 1, 2008), posted March 1, 2008, available at www. bmj.com/cgi/eletters/336/7642/476#191338.

45. Keim, "When Is a Conflict of Interest a Conflict?"

CHAPTER 8—TABLOID MEDICINE'S VICTIMS: PUBLIC HEALTH AND MEDICAL PROGRESS

1. Tara Parker-Pope, The Hormone Decision (New York: Pocket Books, 2008).

2. JoAnn E. Manson et al., "Estrogen Therapy and Coronary-Artery Calcification," New England Journal of Medicine 356, no. 25 (June 21, 2007): 2,591–602.

3. National Heart, Lung, and Blood Institute, "Press Conference Remarks by Jacques Rossouw, M.D.: Release of the Results of the Estrogen Plus Progestin Trial of the Women's Health Initiative: Findings and Implications," press release, July 9, 2002, available at www.nhlbi.nih.gov/health/women/rossouw. htm.

4. Judith L. Turgeon et al., "Hormone Therapy: Physiological Complexity Belies Therapeutic Simplicity," Science 304, no. 5,675 (May 28, 2004): 1,269–73; Parker-Pope, The Hormone Decision.

5. Col et al., "Short-term Menopausal Hormone Therapy for Symptom Relief," Archives of Internal Medicine 164 (2004): 1,634–40.

6. David E. Gumpert, "Hormone Battle: Big Pharma vs. Small Biz," Business-Week, April 13, 2006.

7. Parker-Pope, The Hormone Decision.

8. Jenny Hope, "One Million Women 'Have Needlessly Abandoned HRT,'" Daily Mail, Oct. 9, 2007, available at www.dailymail.co.uk/pages/live/articles/ health/healthmain.html?in_article_id=486662&in_page_id=1774.

9. "Bad News About Hormone Replacement Therapy," Healthlink, Medical College of Wisconsin, available at www.healthlink.mcw.edu/article/1025191125. html.

10. Andrea Rinaldi, "Hormone Therapy for the Ageing," *European Molecular Biology Organization Report* 5, no. 10 (Oct. 2004): 938–41.

11. Rebecca Voelker, "Hormone Confusion Creates 'Credibility Gap,'" *JAMA* 284 (2000): 424–28.

12. John Stossel, Kristina Kendall, and Patrick McMenamin, "The Surprising Risks of Playing It Safe," ABC News, Feb. 22, 2007, available at www.abcnews. go.com/2020/story?id=2893122&page=1.

13. Siegel, "Polarized Pills."

14. Joanne Silberner, "FDA Works to Put Old Struggles Behind It," NPR, Jan. 8, 2010, available at www.npr.org/templates/story/story.php?storyId=122350772#.

15. "Appropriations Bill Bans Funds for Reagan-Udall Foundation," *FDA News* 4, no. 249 (Dec. 21, 2007).

16. Nils Hasselmo, "Individual and Institutional Conflict of Interest: Policy Review by Research Universities in the United States," Science and Engineering Ethics 8, no. 3 (2002): 421–27.

17. David Korn and Susan H. Ehringhaus, "NIH Conflict Rules Are Not Right for Universities," Nature 433, no. 7,035 (April 14, 2005): 821; Annetine G. Gelijns and Samuel O. Thier, "Medical Innovation and Institutional Interdependence: Rethinking University-Industry Connections," *JAMA* 287, no. 1 (Jan. 2, 2002): 72–77; Thomas P. Stossel, "Regulating Academic-Industrial Research Relationships—Solving Problems or Stifling Progress?" *New England Journal of Medicine* 353, no. 10 (2005): 1,060–65.

18. Robert James Cerfolio, "Politely Refuse the Pen and Note Pad: Gifts from Industry to Physicians Harm Patients: Con," *Ethics in Cardiothoracic Surgery* 84 (2007): 1,077–84.

19. Kevin M. Murphy and Robert H. Topel, "The Value of Health and Longevity," *Journal of Political Economy* 114, no. 4 (2006): 871–904.

20. Marcia Angell, "Big Pharma, Bad Medicine," *Boston Review* (May/June 2010), available at www.bostonreview.net/BR35.3/angell.php.

21. Salk Institute for Biological Studies, "Office of Technology Management and Development," available at www.salk.edu/faculty/technology_transfer.html.

22. Andrew Jack, "Big Drugs Companies Shift Trials from UK," *Financial Times*, June 26, 2008.

23. Pharmaceutical Research and Manufacturers of America, "R&D Spending by U.S. Biopharmaceutical Companies Reaches Record $58.8 Billion in 2007," press release, FierceBiotech, March 24, 2008, available at www.fiercebiotech. com/press-releases/r-d-spending-u-s-biopharmaceutical-companies-reaches-record-58-8-billion-2007-0.

24. "NIH budget," National Institute of Health, last reviewed June 11, 2009, available at www.nih.gov/about/budget.htm.

25. Tyler Cowen, "Poor U.S. Scores in Health Care Don't Measure Nobels and Innovation," *New York Times*, Oct. 5, 2006.

26. Rory Watson, "Europe's Research Council Calls for Spending to Be Doubled to 0.25% of GDP," *BMJ* 335 (Dec. 15, 2007); Daniele Capezzone, "Sicko Europe," *Wall Street Journal*, Aug. 3, 2007, available at www.online.wsj.com/article/SB118610945461187080.html.

27. Paul Howard, "A Story Michael Moore Didn't Tell," *Washington Post*, July 17, 2007.

28. Stossel, "Regulating Academic-Industrial Research Relationships."

29. Brian Lawler, "Scrutinizing FDA Drug Approvals," The Motley Fool, November 16, 2007, available at www.fool.com/investing/high-growth/2007/11/16/exploring-fda-drug-approvals.aspx.

30. Data from Drugs@FDA, available at www.accessdata.fda.gov/scripts/cder/drugsatfda/index.cfm.

31. Lawler, "Scrutinizing FDA Drug Approvals."

32. John Calfee, "The Golden Age of Medical Innovation," *The American*, March 1, 2007.

33. Aaron Smith, "Federal Drug Approvals Plunge," *CNN Money*, Nov. 15, 2007, available at www.money.cnn.com/2007/11/15/news/companies/fda/index.htm.

34. Linda A. Johnson, "FDA Takes Caution on Approving New Drugs," *Washington Post*, Aug. 17, 2007.

35. Information on the trial is available at www.clinicaltrials.gov/ct2/show/study/NCT00879970?term=avandia+TIDE&rank=1&show_locs=Y.

36. Alan M. Wolf, "2 Sites Pull Out of Trials for GSK's Avandia," *The News and Observer*, May 21, 2010, available at www.newsobserver.com/2010/05/21/492683/2-sites-pull-out-of-trials-for.html; Alicia Mundy, "Recruiting Lags for Avandia Drug Trial," *Washington Post*, May 20, 2010, available at www.online.wsj.com/article/SB10001424052748704691304575254613696899620.html.

37. "FDA Approved Only 19 New Medications in 2007, Analyst Reports," *Medical News Today*, Jan. 11, 2008, available at www.medicalnewstoday.com/articles/93690.php.

38. Marcia Angell, *The Truth About Drug Companies: How They Deceive Us and What to Do About It* (New York: Random House, 2005), 90.

39. National Institute of Mental Health, "Questions and Answers about the NIMH Sequenced Treatment Alternatives to Relieve Depression (STAR*D)

Study: All Medication Levels," Nov. 2006, available at www.nimh.nih.gov/trials/practical/stard/allmedicationlevels.shtml.

40. Maggie Mahar, *Money-Driven Medicine: The Real Reason Health Care Costs So Much* (New York: Collins, 2006), 54.

41. Calfee, "The Golden Age of Medical Innovation."

42. Ibid.

43. Howard, "A Story Michael Moore Didn't Tell."

44. Frank Lichtenberg, "Benefits and Costs of Newer Drugs: An Update," *Managerial and Decision Economics* 28, no. 4–5 (2007): 485–90.

45. Frank R. Lichtenberg, "Yes, New Drugs Save Lives," *Washington Post*, July 11, 2007, available at www.washingtonpost.com/wp-dyn/content/article/2007/07/10 /AR2007071001468.html.

46. Capezzone, "Sicko Europe."

47. David Atkins, "Creating and Synthesizing Evidence with Decision Makers in Mind: Integrating Evidence from Clinical Trials and Other Study Designs," *Medical Care* 45, no. 11, suppl. 2 (Oct. 2007): S16–S22.

48. Richard L. Kravitz, N. H. Duan, and J. Braslow, "Evidence-based Medicine, Heterogeneity of Treatment Effects, and the Trouble with Averages," *Milbank Quarterly* 82, no. 4 (2004): 661–87.

49. "Fact Sheet: Herceptin," National Cancer Institute, reviewed June 13, 2006, available at www.cancer.gov/cancertopics/factsheet/therapy/herceptin.

50. Calfee, "The Golden Age of Medical Innovation."

51. Liz Szabo, "Genetic Testing Boosts Efficacy in Cancer Care," *USA Today*, Jan. 14, 2009, available at www.usatoday.com/news/health/2009-01-13-cancer-cost-genetic_N.htm.

52. Dan Jones, "Steps on the Road to Personalized Medicine," *Nature Reviews Drug Discovery* 6, no. 10 (Oct. 2007): 770–71, available at www.nature.com/nrd/journal/v6/n10/full/nrd2434.html.

53. Allan E. Rettie and Guoying Tai, "The Pharmacogenomics of Warfarin," *Molecular Interventions* 6 (2006): 223–27.

54. Jones, "Steps on the Road to Personalized Medicine."

55. Rhonda Cooper-DeHoff, "Geno-type Guided Warfarin Dosing Now a Reality," *Cardiology Today*, Feb. 1, 2008, available at www.cardiologytoday.com/view.aspx?rid=29668.

56. Jones, "Steps on the Road to Personalized Medicine."

57. M. H. Eckman et al., "Cost-effectiveness of Using Pharmacogenetic Information in Warfarin Dosing for Patients with Nonvalvular Atrial Fibrillation," *Annuals of Internal Medicine* 150, no. 2 (Jan. 20, 2009).

58. Will Durham, "Key Gene Linked to High Blood Pressure Identified," Yahoo! Health, Dec. 29, 2008, available at www.health.yahoo.com/news/reuters/us_heart_gene.html.

59. Peter McKnight, "To Know Thyself—Genetically Speaking," *Vancouver Sun*, Dec. 19, 2009, available at www.vancouversun.com/health/know+thyself+genetically+speaking/2361457/story.html.

60. Associated Press, "Hunting Newborn Tests for Super-Rare Genetic Diseases," *New York Times*, Jan. 4, 2010, available at www.nytimes.com/aponline/2010/01/04/health/AP-US-MED-HealthBeat-Newborn-Screening.html.

61. Thomas G. Roberts, Jr., and Bruce A. Chabner, "Beyond Fast Track for Drug Approvals," *New England Journal of Medicine* 351, no. 5 (2004): 501–5.

62. Carolyn Johnson, "Doctors Develop Treatment For Rare Disease," ABC-7 News, May 9, 2008; "'World First' as Miracle Drug Saves Life of Baby with Rare Disease," *The Telegraph*, Nov. 5, 2009; "Family's Perseverance Helps Kids with Rare Diseases," *6 News*, Nov. 10, 2008.

63. Christine Doyle, "Too Rare for Them to Care?" *The Telegraph*, Oct. 5, 2005.

64. "New Therapy Helps US Boy with Rare Disease," Reuters, Jan. 8, 2009.

65. *USA Today* Staff, "Diagnosing the Undiagnosible," *USA Today*, May 19, 2008, available at www.blogs.usatoday.

66. "New Institute Will Study Rare Diseases," Reuters, May 21, 2009, available at www.in.reuters.com/article/healthNewsMolt/idINTRE54J7F220090520.

67. Joe Palca, "Rare Disease Treated Using Gene Therapy," NPR, Nov. 5, 2009, available at www.npr.org/templates/story/story.php?storyId=120118988; Robert Langreth, "Will Gene Therapy Finally Work?" *Forbes*, April 27, 2008, available at www.forbes.com/2008/04/27/eye-trial-gene-biz-healthcare-cx_rl_0427genetherapy.html.

CHAPTER 9—BATTLING TABLOID MEDICINE: THE PERSONALIZED MEDICINE REVOLUTION

1. Margaret A. Hamburg and Joshua M. Sharfstein, "The FDA as a Public Health Agency," *New England Journal of Medicine* 360, no. 24 (June 11, 2009): 2,493–95.

2. www.fda.gov/oc/oms/ofm/budget/2007/HTML/4CPPO.

3. "Interview with Dr. Janet Woodcock," U.S. Food and Drug Administration, March 2007, available at www.ageofpersonalizedmedicine.org/experts/government_policymakers/janet_woodcock.asp.

4. Elizabeth Whittington, "Cancer Treatment Gets Personal," *Cure Magazine*, ASCO EDITION 2009, available at www.media.curetoday.com/htmlemail/CURExtra/ASCO2009.html.

5. Information from C-path website at www.cpath.org.

6. Food and Drug Administration, "FDA Announced Partnership with Critical Path Institute to Conduct Essential Research to Spur Medical Innovation," press release, Dec. 16, 2005, available at www.fda.gov/NewsEvents/Newsroom/PressAnnouncements/2005/ucm108532.htm.

7. "Pharmacogenomics of Antidepressant Response in Children and Adolescents (PARCA)," last updated April 6, 2009, available at www.clinicaltrials.gov/ct2/show/NCT00516932.

8. Maggie Mahar, "The Prostate as Crystal Ball," Health Beat blog, Jan. 25, 2008, available at www.healthbeatblog.com/2008/01/the-prostate-as.html.

9. Center for Medicine in the Public Interest, "The Patient Centric Health Leadership Forum: Towards a Critical Path for Patient-Centered Medicine," Aug. 2008, available at www.cmpi.org/uploads/File/cmpi7-25.pdf.

10. Joel Finkelstein, "Members of New FDA Board Tied to Industry," *Journal of the National Cancer Institute* 100, no. 5 (2008): 296–97.

11. "Calls on FDA to Cease Activities Creating Reagan-Udall Foundation," press release, Office of Representative Rosa DeLauro, Nov. 1, 2007, available at www.delauro.house.gov/text_release.cfm?id=839.

12. Matthew Perrone, "New FDA Research Center Rife with Risks," Associated Press, Oct. 14, 2007.

13. "New CMPI Survey Shows Overwhelming Support for FDA Initiative," Center for Medicine in the Public Interest, Feb. 1, 2008, available at www.cmpi.org/PDFs/Reports/CMPIReportOnCriticalPathInitiativePRUpdated07RS.pdf.

14. Peter Pitts, "Friday the 13th—Day 2," Drugwonks blog, Nov. 14, 2009, available at www.drugwonks.com/blog_post/show/7055.

15. Peter Pitts, "Speaking up," Communiqué Live, April 7, 2010, available at www.communiquelive.com/features.

16. "NIH and Wikipedia Collaborate to Improve Online Health Information," press release, *NIH News*, July 14, 2009, available at www.nih.gov/news/health/jul2009/od-14.htm.

17. "Adverse Event Reporting System (AERS)," U.S. Food and Drug Administration, accessed Feb. 9, 2010, at www.fda.gov/Drugs/GuidanceComplianceRegulatoryInformation/Surveillance/AdverseDrugEffects/default.htm.

18. Hamburg and Sharfstein, "The FDA as a Public Health Agency."

19. Richard Sykes, "Being a Modern Pharmaceutical Company," *BMJ* 317, no. 7,167 (Oct. 31, 1998): 1,172–80.

20. "About ClinicalTrials.gov," U.S. National Institutes of Health, last updated April 2, 2008, available at www.clinicaltrials.gov/ct2/info/about.

21. Steve Benowitz, "Clinical Trial Transparency: Registries, Databases Raise Questions, Stir Debates," *Journal of the National Cancer Institute* 97, no. 22 (Nov. 16, 2005): 1,640–41.

22. "iGuard.org Drug Safety System Registers Two Million Users," press release, iGuard, Dec. 22, 2009, available at www.iguard.org/help/about-us/press-releases.html.

23. Thomas Goetz, "Practicing Patients," *New York Times*, March 23, 2008, available at www.nytimes.com/2008/03/23/magazine/23patients-t.html?_r=1&pagewanted=1.

24. Karen Felzer and Humberto Macedo, "The Lithium ALS Worldwide Study: Six Month Update," Nov. 16, 2008, available at www.its.caltech.edu/~kfelzer/SixMonthUpdate.pdf.

25. Emily Singer, "Patients' Social Network Predicts Drug Outcomes," *Technology Review*, May 11, 2010, available at www.technologyreview.com/biomedicine/25276/?a=f.

26. Jacob Goldstein, "In a Switch, Online Patient Groups Inform Research," blog post, *Wall Street Journal Health Blog*, June 13, 2007, available at www.blogs.wsj.com/health/2007/06/13/in-a-switch-online-patient-groups-inform-researchers.

27. Malory Allison, "Can Web 2.0 Reboot Clinical Trials?" *Nature Biotechnology* 27 (2009): 895–902.

28. "About ScienceBlogs," ScienceBlogs, available at www.scienceblogs.com/channel/about.php.

29. Bonnie Rochman, "When Patients Share Medical Data Online," TIME, February 8, 2010, available at www.time.com/time/magazine/article/0,9171,1957460,00.html.

30. Susannah Fox, "Online Health Search 2006," Pew Research Center Internet and American Life Project, Oct. 2006, www.pewInternet.org/~/media//Files/Reports/2006/PIP_Online_Health_2006.pdf.pdf.

31. "How Many U.S. Adults Have Searched for Health Information Online in the Past Year?" iHealthBeat, Nov. 5, 2008, www.ihealthbeat.org/Data-Points/2008/How-Many-US-Adults-Have-Searched-for-Health-Information-Online-in-the-Past-Year.aspx.

32. Susannah Fox, "Health Sites: Some Are More Equal Than Others," e-patients.net blog, January 21, 2010, available at www.e-patients.net/archives/2010/01/health-sites-some-are-more-equal-than-others.html.

33. Jay Byrne, "Healthcare "Apps" Exploding in Mobile, Are You Ready?" v-Fluence blog, March 5, 2010, available at www.v-fluence.com/blog/459/healthcare-apps-exploding-in-mobile-are-you-ready.

34. Jay Byrne, "v-Fluence Study Shows Healthcare Applications For Mobile Devices Exploding," WebWire, March 8, 2010, available at www.webwire. com/ViewPressRel.asp?aId=113803.

35. Orac, "The Cranks Pile On John Ioannidis' Work on the Reliability Of Science"; blog post, "Respectful Insolence," Sept. 24, 2007, available at www.scienceblogs.com/insolence/2007/09/the_cranks_pile_on_john_ ioannidis_work_o.php.

36. "About HON: Our Mission," Health on the Net Foundation, last modified April 11, 2006, available at www.hon.ch/Global/HON_mission.html.

37. "The HONcode in Brief," Health on the Net Foundation, last modified Oct. 22, 2008, available at www.hon.ch/HONcode/Patients/Conduct.html.

38. "How to Evaluate Health Information on the Internet," Food and Drug Administration, Dec. 2005, www.fda.gov/Drugs/EmergencyPreparedness/ BioterrorismandDrugPreparedness/ucm134620.htm.

39. Office of Disease Prevention and Health Promotion, "Report on Objective 11-4: Estimating the Proportion of Health Related Websites Disclosing Information That Can Be Used to Assess Their Quality," Department of Health and Human Services, May 30, 2006, available at www.health.gov/ communication/healthypeople/obj1104.

40. Alicia White, "How to Read Articles About Health and Healthcare," Bazian, 2008, available at www.bazian.com/pdfs/HowToReadANewsStory_ vers03_26Nov08.pdf.

41. John P. A. Ioannidis, "Why Most Published Research Findings Are False," *PLoS Medicine* 2, no. 8 (2005): e124.

42. S. A. Iverson, K. B. Howard, and B. K. Penney, "Impact of Internet Use on Health-Related Behaviors and the Patient-Physician Relationship: A Survey-Based Study and Review," *Journal of the American Osteopathic Association* 108, no. 12 (2008): 699–711.

43. Cass R. Sunstein, "Throwing Precaution to the Wind," *The Boston Globe*, July 13, 2008, available at www.boston.com/bostonglobe/ideas/articles/2008/07/13/ throwing_precaution_to_the_wind.

44. Lionel Trilling, *The Liberal Imagination* (New York: New York Review of Books Classics, 2008), 221.

INDEX

Index

University of Bristol
(United Kingdom), 120
University of British Columbia, 1
University of California–Los Angeles,
7, 213
University of California–San Diego, 204
University of Chicago, 219
"University of Google," 128, 144, 169
University of Kentucky, 118
University of Miami, 127
University of Michigan, 5
University of Missouri, 26
University of Pennsylvania, 136
University of Pittsburgh, 158, 165, 260
University of Toronto, Centre for
Addiction and Mental Health
(CAMH), 150
University of Wales, 14
University of Wisconsin, 10
U.S. Congress committees, 73–74, 98–101,
113, 218
U.S. Department of Agriculture, 38
U.S. Department of Health and Human
Services, 199–200, 269

V

vaccination, anti- — movement, 20, 41,
48–50, 110–144, 273, 274. *See also*
specific vaccinations
Vaccine Adverse Event Reporting System
(VAERS), 117–118
Vaccine Injury Compensation Program.
See National Vaccine Injury
Compensation Program
VAERS. *See* Vaccine Adverse Event
Reporting System
Vanderbilt University, 99, 137
Vectibix, 234
verbatim, 4–5, 8
Verstraeten, Thomas, 132
v-Fluence, 264
Viagra, 227
VICP. *See* National Vaccine Injury
Compensation Program
VIGOR trial. *See* Vioxx GI Outcomes
Research trial
Vioxx GI Outcomes Research (VIGOR)
trial, 88–91, 98, 102
Vioxx, 84–109, 185, 215–218, 222, 273, 274
Vired, 227
VKORC1, 235–236

vom Saal, Frederick, 26
von Eschenbach, Andrew C., 73,
248–249
von Koop, Carina, 79
Vorsorgungsprinzip, 30

W

Wakefield, Andrew, 111–113, 117, 133–134,
135, 139, 142–143, 150, 195
Wallace, Amy, 144
Wall Street Journal, 97, 224
Walther, Leonard, 119
Walther, Mary Catherine, 119
Walther, Suzanne, 119
warfarin, 235–236
Washington Post, 158–159, 174–175
water, drinking, 12, 42
Web. *See* Internet
Weber, Michael A., 105, 205
WebMD, 55, 263–264
Websites, types of, 67–69, 266
Weingart, John, 32
Western Psychiatric Institute and
Clinic, 158
WHI. *See* Women's Health Initiative
White, Alicia, 270
Whitehead, Alfred North, 265
whooping cough vaccine, 48–50, 142
Wildavsky, Aaron, vii, 23, 24
Winfrey, Oprah, 20, 129
Wingspread Statement, 30, 31
Wired magazine, 144
Wolfe, Sidney, 70, 224
Women's Health Initiative, 209–215
Wood, Alastair, 99
Woodcock, Janet, 245–246
Woosley, Raymond, 224, 246
World Health Organization, 46, 266
Worst Pills, Best Pills, iv
www.clinicaltrials.gov, 256
www.getbetterhealth.com, 262

Y

Yahoo!, 67
Young, Neal S., 173–176, 187
YouTube, vi

Z

Zeiger, Roni, 264
Zerhouni, Elias A., 175
Zoloft, 145, 149, 159

ABOUT THE AUTHOR

ROBERT GOLDBERG, PHD, is Vice President and co-founder of the Center for Medicine in the Public Interest, a nonprofit institute dedicated to promoting the use and understanding of technologies that make healthcare more predictive and personalized. He earned his doctorate in politics from Brandeis in 1984. With Peter Pitts, he co-hosts the controversial blog www.drugwonks.com, and his reporting has appeared in numerous publications, including the *Wall Street Journal* and the *Los Angeles Times*. Formerly a senior fellow at the Manhattan Institute for Public Policy Research, where he directed the Center for Medical Progress and chaired the 21st Century FDA Reform Task Force, Dr. Goldberg lives in New Jersey.